DATE DUE

OC 28 98		
NO 6 00		
DE 05 00		
MT 28 01		
NOV 21 2001		
DE 10 02		
DE 17 05		

DEMCO 38-296

Heart Fitness
for Life

Heart Fitness

~~~~~~

for Life

The Essential Guide to Preventing

and Reversing Heart Disease

MARY P. McGOWAN, M.D.

with

JO McGOWAN CHOPRA

New York   Oxford

OXFORD UNIVERSITY PRESS

1997

iversity Press

New York

~~Athens~~ ~~Auckland~~ ~~Bangkok~~ Bangkok Bogota Bombay
Buenos Aires Calcutta Cape Town Dar es Salaam
Delhi Florence Hong Kong Istanbul Karachi
Kuala Lumpur Madras Madrid Melbourne
Mexico City Nairobi Paris Singapore
Taipei Tokyo Toronto Warsaw

and associated companies in
Berlin Ibadan

Copyright © 1997 by Mary P. McGowan

Published by Oxford University Press, Inc.
198 Madison Avenue, New York, New York 10016

Oxford is a registered trademark of Oxford University Press

All rights reserved. No part of this publication may be reproduced,
stored in a retrieval system, or transmitted, in any form or by any means,
electronic, mechanical, photocopying, recording, or otherwise,
without the prior permission of Oxford University Press.

Library of Congress Cataloging-in-Publication Data
McGowan, Mary P., 1959-
Heart fitness for life : the essential guide
to preventing and reversing heart disease/
by Mary P. McGowan, with Jo McGowan Chopra.
p. cm.   Includes bibliographical references and index.
ISBN 0-19-511624-0
1. Heart—Diseases—Prevention.
2. Heart—Diseases—Treatment.
1. McGowan Chopra, Jo.   II. Title.
RC682.M387   1997   616.1'2—dc21   97-29834

135798642

Printed in the United States of America
on acid-free paper

For Pat and Owen McGowan,
the wonderful parents we share

For Tom Synan and Ravi Chopra,
the wonderful husbands we don't

And for Patrick and Liam Synan
and Anand, Cathleen, and Moy Moy Chopra,
the wonderful children whose hearts and
minds inspire all we do.

WITH THE ASSISTANCE OF

JOHN MILLER, M.D.

MARY CARD, R.D.

JUDY CURRIER

SUSAN CUPOLA

Contents

Acknowledgments

Of course, one has to say this never would have been possible without . . . , but it is perhaps more true in my case than most. Without my patients, there would have been no stories, without my colleagues, there would have been no experts to assemble, and without my family, there would have been no me, so dependent am I on them for their loving support. My first thanks go to my husband Tom, whose belief in me has never wavered, even when my own faltered. For his sense of humor alone, he deserves mention—he is the funniest person I know and kept me laughing even on the days when this book had me near tears.

A close second is my sister and co-author, Jo McGowan Chopra, who is a gifted writer and one of my dearest friends. Jo lives in India where she is the director of a school for children with mental handicaps. We worked on this book long distance for over a year, during which time Jo had neither E-mail, a fax, or even a telephone! The fact that it came through to the publisher all in one piece is a tribute to the U.S. and Indian posts.

My parents were my first teachers and I will always be grateful to them for the love of books they instilled in all seven of their children. I can't remember not knowing how to read. My father's work as a librarian and my mother's as a journalist and editor gave me a deep respect for and delight in the written word, a legacy I am now trying to pass on to my own children. A special thank you to my mother who pitched in with the editing at several critical junctures.

My sister-in-law and good friend, Kathy Felski, looks after my two boys, Patrick and Liam, as lovingly as any mother could ever wish. Her presence in our home makes it possible for Tom and me to go to work every day and without her I could never have written this book.

I am especially grateful to my aunt, Sheila MacGill Callahan, who suggested that I send the manuscript to her agent, Susan Cohen of Writer's House. Susan's input has been valuable and insightful; it is a pleasure to work with her. Joan Bossert, our editor at Oxford University Press, has gone out of her way to critique the manuscript—her suggestions having tightened and sharpened its focus. I especially appreciate her understanding for my desire to reach as many people as possible with the message of preventing and reversing heart disease.

My cardiology professors at the University of Massachusetts Medical Center—Joe Alpert, Joel Gore, Linda Pape, and Bonnie Weiner—had an enormous influence on my choice of a career. Not only as teachers but also as human beings, they are all wonderful and I consider myself lucky to have been their student. Drs. Ira and Judy Ockene, who developed the preventive cardiology program at UMASS, gave me my first glimpse at what such a program should involve, and Judy's smoking cessation program is the same one I still use today with my own patients.

My understandings of the role that inherited cholesterol abnormalities have to play in the development of early cardiac disease and the need to get this information more widely known to the general public are largely due to my friends and teachers, Drs. Peter Kwiterovich and Stephanie Kafonek, at the Johns Hopkins Hospital where I did a two-year fellowship. Both Peter and Stephanie were instrumental in helping me establish my own lipid clinic in New Hampshire, and have remained close friends.

As the director of the Cholesterol Management Center of the New England Heart Institute, I have been involved in the MED-PED FH Project (Make Early Diagnosis—Prevent Early Death in Familial Hypercholesterolemia), through which I have met some of the leading researchers in the field of lipid metabolism. In particular, I would like to mention Dr. Roger Williams and Dr. Evan Stein, both of whom are not only superb scholars but also marvelous human beings, unstinting with their time and tireless advocates for their patients. Roger also found the time to review this manuscript, for which I am very grateful.

One of the offshoots of the MED-PED FH Project has been the development of a national resource center for persons with familial hypercholesterolemia called the Inherited High Cholesterol Foundation, of which I am a board member. Through this association I met Kitty Fixx, the sister of Jim Fixx, the well-known athlete and author who died tragically of a heart attack while still in his forties. Kitty's advice and insight were invaluable as this book was being written.

Several other friends and colleagues have reviewed this book, including Drs. Joe Alpert, Jorge Plutsky, and William Castelli. Dr. Castelli, the former director of the famous Framingham Heart Study and one of my heroes since medical school, took the time to review it almost line by line, resulting in a number of important additions.

Finally, and most important, I would like to thank my patients. Although you will meet only a few of them in the following pages, there are literally hundreds more who have been successful in their battle against heart disease. They are courageous people and determined to win—you can do it too!

Foreword

This is an important book *everyone* needs to read. After all, if you live in the United States or any of the industrialized countries where exercise has been engineered out of your life and a fatty diet engineered in, half of you are headed for a blocked artery. If it's a blocked artery to your heart, you will have a heart attack; if it's a blocked artery to your brain, a stroke; if it's a blocked artery to your legs, an amputation. Many of you already suffer from a vascular problem and are on the fast track to your next heart attack, stroke, or blocked artery in your legs. For you, this book is a must read.

Heart Fitness for Life is written by a doctor with long and extensive experience helping people to prevent these blockages in the first place and even to shrink the blockages that they have. Bypass surgery and angioplasty can alleviate these blockages, but they are only the first steps in the rest of a life that needs to change the cholesterol numbers and other risk factors—hypertension, smoking, and blood sugar elevations—to a point where these deposits stop growing or begin to shrink.

You need to understand everything your doctor suggests about ways to change your lifestyle to avoid getting a blocked artery, or to avoid a repeat blockage if you've already had one. This means learning firsthand about how these blockages occur and what you can do to prevent them. You need to understand your numbers so that you can work with your doctor to get your cholesterol, blood pressure, and weight down to acceptable levels that allow you to live a full and healthy life, free of heart disease. Having a healthy heart starts with a better diet and an exercise program and may eventually require drug therapy. All this is clearly explained by Mary McGowan, a doctor who has helped tremendous numbers of people enjoy a healthier way of life.

Most people take better care of their cars than they do their own bodies. The time has come to take better care of yourself and to learn *all* the techniques, new and old, that will help you live a healthier, longer life. In this new era of medicine, we all need to be better informed about what we should obtain from the medical profession to keep ourselves healthy. Ask what your cholesterol numbers are, your blood pressure numbers, your blood sugar numbers, and read this book to find out what these numbers mean and how you *and* your doctor can best improve them so that your quality of life stays at its highest level.

The vast majority of people who live on this earth do not get the kinds of artery blockages that account for almost half the deaths in the United States each year. Someday, our society will learn to live like those societies who don't suffer such high rates of vascular diseases. But it will take an enormous educational effort to bring people the knowledge they need to prevent these diseases. You don't have to wait for this to happen. Read this book and you can start today to pursue a much healthier way of life.

William P. Castelli, M.D.
Medical Director
Framington Cardiovascular Institute

Heart Fitness
for Life

Introduction

I have always wanted to be a doctor. I actually cannot remember a time when I was not interested in the prevention of cardiac disease. When I was seven (I was an intense little girl), I learned that cigarettes were linked to heart disease and stroke. From that point on I became a self-appointed chieftain in the war against smoking. No one escaped. Guests in my parents' house would often find that their cigarettes had been removed from their overcoat pockets while they ate dinner, and I can still remember stealing my aunt's cigarettes and flushing them down the toilet. "It's for her own good," I insisted, when my parents scolded me.

I hope I've grown up a bit since those days, but I still feel just as strongly about the prevention of heart disease. Don't worry: if you come to my clinic, I won't flush your cigarettes down the toilet. But I will do my best to persuade you to do it yourself.

When I entered medical school, I knew I would learn a great deal about the diagnosis and treatment of particular diseases. This remains one of my favorite parts of the practice of medicine: like solving an intricate puzzle, I find it challenging and rewarding. But as an idealistic young student, I was also hoping to learn about preventive medicine—How could I help patients to avoid disease in the first place?

This question, unfortunately, was not part of the curriculum. In the United States, there has been so much emphasis placed on the treatment and cure of established disease that the vital connection between lifestyle and physical and emotional well-being has often gone unrealized, even by professionals in the field.

Like most of my fellow students, I got totally caught up in the treating and curing aspects of medicine, especially during the early part of my residency when I admitted many patients to the intensive care and coronary care units of the hospital with which I was associated. These people were very sick, often close to death, and being their doctor meant racing frantically in all directions to perform complicated procedures, which used to give me nightmares and anxiety attacks.

There was so much to learn and so many patients to admit that I began to forget why I had become a physician in the first place. Patients whose conditions were less than critical seemed to present no challenge and no opportunity to learn. Such patients often had lots of complaints and many stress-related ailments. I discovered that if I allowed it, the simplest questions would elicit a stream of what I then considered irrelevant information regarding emotions, fears, and worries. Although I don't recall ever consciously thinking it through, I believe I was instinctively protecting my own very fragile psyche when I avoided getting too involved with my patients.

I know now that I was wrong, and I am thankful to the patients and attending physicians at the University of Massachusetts Medical Center and later at Johns Hopkins Hospital in Baltimore, Maryland, for helping me to see the importance of treating the whole person.

My first glimpse of what a doctor's role could be came early in my internship (which is the first year of residency) when I spent a month in the outpatient (primary care) clinic, where we were taught how to develop a clinical practice. During this time I was assigned new patients and was expected to follow them throughout my three-year residency. My first reaction was boredom. "Where's the challenge in this?" I remember asking my supervisor, Dr. Sarah Stone. "These people are all relatively healthy."

She just looked at me for a moment and I will never forget her answer. "Mary," she said, "don't you see? Primary care is the biggest challenge of all. We have to help these people stay healthy."

I thought about this a great deal, and the more I thought, the more sense it made. I also learned that people will do a great deal to become healthy if you just ask them to. The trick is in remembering to ask.

I learned this in the same month in the primary care clinic when I participated in a research study run by Dr. Judy Ockene. The study was based on a very simple idea: people would stop smoking if their doctors asked them to, simultaneously presenting them with a plan for quitting. I was a bit skeptical, but I did attend the smoking cessation training sessions. Even after I completed the program, however, I still had doubts about my ability to change a person's habit—my aunt, after all, was still smoking years after my sabotage.

The study continued with my being assigned smoking patients. With each assignment I would be given an envelope containing a randomly selected smoking cessation technique that I was to use with this patient. This could range from a brief suggestion to an in-depth discussion, offering nicorette gum (the nicotine patch wasn't available at that time), and finally asking the patient to sign a contract promising to quit on a particular day.

My first envelope told me to go the whole nine yards with a patient who had been smoking since the age of 12. Ken was a 45-year-old truck-driver who didn't seem to me to be very likely to want to quit. "Keep an open mind," I thought. "It just might work."

I delivered my whole lecture, hoping that Ken wasn't feeling as bored as he looked. At the end, I asked him whether he thought he might be able to quit. "Well" he said, "I've never thought about it before." He wouldn't sign my contract, but he did promise to go home and think about it.

I was very disappointed and quite sure he would never actually do it. Nonetheless, several weeks later, I called him to check as the study required me to do. To my amazement, he said he had thrown his ciga-rettes out on the way home from my office and hadn't smoked since. When I asked him what made him decide, he said it was simple: I had asked him to and I was his doctor.

I almost dropped the phone. I couldn't believe that what I said had made such a difference. But the more I thought about it, the more I realized what important opportunities I had as a doctor. This first success became the inspiration for my practice of medicine. In the primary care clinic I learned one essential truth: I could ask my patients to do almost anything—quit smoking, cut back on alcohol, reduce fats in their diet, or begin exercising—provided I did two things. First, I had to help them develop a plan to implement the change; second, and more important, I had to make them understand I was asking them to change because I cared about them.

For my next rotation, I returned to the coronary care unit. This time, however, I wasn't so afraid of all the procedures: although I recognized their importance, I knew now that it was equally important to arm pa-tients with the confidence and information that would prevent a second heart attack.

I learned a great deal just watching my professors in their approach to cardiac patients. Dr. Joseph Alpert, in particular, became a role model for me. I noticed that even with patients whose lifestyles were atrocious, he was always positive, never critical or judgmental. He had a way of motivating people to stop smoking, to lose weight, to exercise regularly. His standards were high, but his confidence in his patients was even higher.

"Empowerment" is a trendy word these days, and not one that I generally care to use, but it is difficult to find a better way to describe what I saw happening with Dr. Alpert's patients. His faith in them be-came their own faith in themselves: they began to believe that they could transform their lives, and slowly and surely they did just that. Their diets changed, the cigarettes got tossed, the weight came off. The best part was that for most of his patients, the changes were permanent.

Dr. Alpert didn't limit himself to patients, however. He was also a genius at motivating tired residents. During my second year of residency, he convinced me to run with him in the 3.5 mile American Heart Association Doctors' Road Race in Boston. I was astonished when I actually won first place in the women's division.

But I don't include this story to brag. I do it to illustrate the point that we are all capable of more than we think we are. Sometimes all that is missing is the challenger, the person who goads, cajoles, encourages, prods—the person who believes in us. I am writing this book to challenge you. You can dramatically reduce your risk of developing heart disease. Even if you already have heart disease, you can make lifestyle changes that will reduce your risk of having another cardiac event, and may even reverse some of the disease itself.

Although it may seem difficult to believe, the program outlined in this book is not about deprivation. Giving up smoking, switching to a low-fat diet, taking up exercise, and reducing stress—all these are large changes which certainly take getting used to. And in the beginning, let's be honest, they may seem onerous. But again and again, as you will see from the personal stories in this book, people who do make the changes say they have never felt better in their lives. Their bodies, rather than being things they drag around and feel uncomfortable in, have become a source of pleasure and pride. As Susan, one of my patients, whom you will meet shortly, says, "Whatever I do now, I want it to be physical. I'm so much more energetic—I really enjoy my body now."

One way to understand a disease is to study the people who develop it—to see how it affects their lives and what they are doing about it. For this reason, I thought it would be helpful to include some cases of people I have worked with. I have learned a great deal from each one of them, and I am grateful to them for allowing me to share their stories.

In the chapters that follow I discuss the risk factors leading to the development of cardiac disease and outline a practical program of lifestyle changes for its prevention and reversal. You will find a complete diet plan with menus and recipes, an exercise program, an approach to quitting smoking, and advice on how to handle stress.

But in some cases, in spite of our best efforts, diet, exercise, and weight loss cannot completely normalize levels of cholesterol, a white waxy substance made by the liver and found in many high-fat foods. Such deposits can block the heart and other arteries. This is especially true for the hundreds of thousands of Americans with genetic cholesterol abnormalities. While diet and exercise can help, for a person with familial hypercholesterolemia medications are not only essential, they are lifesaving. The same can be said for the millions of Americans who already have heart disease. Most people with heart disease require cholesterol reductions beyond those that can reasonably be achieved with diet and exercise. For these people, studies have proven that cholesterol-lowering medications can dramatically reduce the risk of heart attack, stroke, bypass surgery, angioplasty, and death.

When I first suggest cholesterol-lowering medications, many of my patients feel like failures. But taking a cholesterol-lowering medication doesn't mean you are weak or unable to stick to a diet and exercise program. It simply means that for whatever reason, these lifestyle changes are insufficient.

In order to achieve maximum benefit, your cholesterol-lowering medications must be taken properly and faithfully. Chapter 8 reviews all currently available medications and describes those likely to become available in the next few years. Don't deprive yourself of the chance to achieve your cholesterol goal: doing so could save your life.

At times lifestyle changes (weight loss, exercise, increased potassium intake, salt and alcohol restriction) may also be insufficient to fully normalize blood pressure. In such a case, blood-pressure-lowering medications are essential. Chapter 7 explains the importance of good blood pressure control and discusses many of the currently available blood pressure medications.

Finally, any woman who lives long enough goes through menopause. At the time of menopause estrogen levels fall and cardiac risk increases dramatically. It is well known that estrogen replacement therapy can reduce the risk of cardiac disease by about 50 percent. So why isn't every postmenopausal American woman on estrogen? By the end of Chapter 5, in which the risks and benefits of estrogen replacement therapy are thoroughly discussed, I think you will be in a much better position to decide if estrogen is right for you.

Although for simplicity's sake this entire book is written in the first person, I must acknowledge the immense assistance of several colleagues. Registered Dietitian Mary Card will show you how to design a low-fat, low-cholesterol diet, based on our program in the Cholesterol Management Center at the New England Heart Institute, in Manchester, New Hampshire. In general, we ask that people consume only 20 percent of their calories in the form of fat. Mary will tell you how to figure the number of fat grams you can have each day—her meal plans are all based on this allowance.

We know that people will only stick with a diet if the food is both delicious and easy to prepare. My old college classmate, Susan Cupola, is a gourmet chef and co-owner with her husband Mark of the very popular Victor Grilling Company Restaurant in Victor, New York. She promised to provide recipes that were quick and great tasting, and I think you will be impressed with her results. We have purposely avoided the use of exotic ingredients, including only items easily available in local supermarkets, and no recipe takes more than an hour to prepare (some take less than half an hour).

We have also been cost-conscious in our menu suggestions. Since legumes and beans, always inexpensive, are an important part of a low-fat diet, you will probably find that your food bill drops. And finally, if you follow our plan carefully, you can't help but lose weight. (Some of the recipes have been provided by people whose stories you will read in this book. One of my patients, Wayne, and his wife Sarah, have been especially generous in sharing their favorites.)

Exercise is a critical part of any cardiovascular fitness program. Its physical benefits are both many and obvious: lower blood pressure, weight loss, improved cholesterol and blood sugar levels, and increased muscle tone. The psychological benefits, however, are perhaps less well known: there is a positive delight that comes with a well-toned body and one needn't be an Olympic athlete to experience it. Many people find that even a simple walking program, if it is consistent, gives them a sense of well-being and more energy than they have ever had before. Others report that regular exercise wards off depression, and many will happily admit to being addicted to it. Exercise should become as much a ritual in your day as brushing your teeth—you shouldn't feel right going to bed without your quota.

In the exercise section, Judy Currier, an exercise physiologist and former member of the junior U.S. Olympic ski team, will help you design a personalized exercise program that will work for you. I generally ask people to commit to exercising at least four times a week for 30 minutes per session. More is certainly better, but your greatest benefit comes when you go from doing nothing at all to doing something. As you review Judy's suggestions, however, remember that no one with or at high risk for developing heart disease should undertake a new exercise program without first consulting his or her doctor.

Giving up smoking is extraordinarily difficult. While I offer guidance and hints on ways to liberate yourself from this habit, ultimately the commitment to quit must come from you. I include information on the various nicotine patches, as recent studies indicate that those who use them achieve better results than those who don't.

With the assistance of John Miller, a great friend and medical school classmate, I address the question of stress and the important role it plays in the development of heart disease. Over the years we have had many long discussions on the role of stress in health and disease. John, now a practicing psychiatrist, has studied mindfulness meditation with the internationally known Dr. Jon Kabat-Zinn (author of *Full Catastrophe Living* and *Wherever You Go There You Are*). John has helped many of his patients develop ways of dealing with the stress that is ever present in our lives today. In the chapter on stress reduction we review the mechanisms by which stress can and does cause physical and emotional symptoms, and provide you with a stress-reduction program that has the potential to dramatically improve the way you react to the tensions in your life.

The actual writing of this book has been done with the help of my sister, Jo McGowan Chopra. Jo is a professional writer who, at the start of this project, had a serious butter addiction. After meeting all the patients in this book and working with Mary, Judy, and Susan she has improved her eating habits and begun a daily exercise routine. She is willing to admit these changes have made her "feel great." She says she tolerates my missionary attitude toward cholesterol with good spirit, and I have to agree with her, she does.

I do hope that this book will provide you with the necessary tools for cardiovascular health and fitness. No book, however, can be a substitute for a consultation with a physician. If you do not already have a personal physician but have concerns about your risk for cardiac disease, you should contact your local hospital for help in finding the right doctor.

1

^^

Am I at Risk

for Developing

Heart Disease?

In the chapters that follow you will meet nine extraordinary people, all of whom have changed their lives dramatically to reduce their risk of future cardiac disease. Each person has a cholesterol abnormality, and most have at least one other cardiac risk factor as well. In this chapter, we look at what we mean by cardiac risk. Learning where you may be at risk is the first step. Each chapter that follows addresses steps you can take to get your risk factors under control.

To begin with, cardiac disease is the number one cause of death in adult Americans. Each year in the United States

- 478,000 people die of coronary artery disease.
- 1.5 million suffer a heart attack.
- 407,000 have bypass surgery.
- 300,000 undergo angioplasty.

What makes these grim statistics particularly difficult to accept is the fact that much of this suffering is preventable. We now know how to reduce the number of people suffering and dying from heart disease. But there must be widespread knowledge of its risk factors to allow people to implement changes in their lives. Once people know exactly *where* their risks lie, they can take positive steps to reduce them.

What are the risk factors for coronary artery disease?

1. Being a male over the age of 45
2. Being a female over the age of 55, or a female having undergone premature menopause (generally as a result of surgery)
3. Family history of cardiac disease
4. Diabetes
5. Cigarette smoking
6. High blood pressure
7. Obesity (especially the potbelly type)
8. Sedentary lifestyle
9. Elevated cholesterol levels (whether related to poor diet or to a genetic abnormality)
10. Elevated levels of lipoprotein (a)
11. Elevated homocysteine levels
12. Stress

Men Over 45

While men cannot change their age, most men who develop heart disease in midlife can still do a great deal to improve their cardiac health. Reducing cholesterol levels, controlling diabetes and high blood pressure, giving up smoking, and taking up exercise are all steps that can be taken. It is very important for men to recognize their vulnerabilities and to take positive action to avoid the development of heart disease.

Women Over 55

It is not until women go through menopause that they begin to catch up with men for cardiac risk. This does not mean that cardiac disease is a predominantly male problem. Contrary to popular belief, more than half of all deaths from cardiac disease occur in women. The average age at which an American woman begins menopause is 51. Although it cannot be prevented, the increase in cardiac risk that follows menopause can be modified by estrogen replacement therapy (ERT). Women who take estrogen after menopause are much less likely to have a heart attack than those who don't. Studies have shown that women on estrogen reduce their risk for heart disease by 35 to 50 percent. If they already have heart disease and begin ERT, they can reduce their risk by as much as 80 percent.

In 1993, the National Cholesterol Education Program (NCEP) acknowledged the importance estrogen plays in improving cholesterol levels and lowering cardiac risk when it recommended estrogen replacement therapy for postmenopausal women for whom diet and exercise failed to normalize cholesterol levels fully.

For more information on how estrogen works to protect against heart disease, see Chapter 5.

Family History

A family history of heart disease is, in one sense, something you can do little about. You certainly cannot change the fact that members of your immediate family have had cardiac problems. However, if this is your situation, it is crucial for you to look closely at the risk factors you can change. If your mother, for example, had high blood pressure and developed heart disease, your own chance for developing it is increased, but there are many ways for you to reduce this possibility. Nondrug therapies for lowering blood pressure work for many people; for those who must take medication, there is a wide range of safe drugs from which to choose.

A family history of cardiac disease often is the result of an abnormal cholesterol profile. In our clinic we recommend cholesterol testing in anyone over age two with a family history of cardiac disease. The earlier a person is tested, the longer he or she has to make changes aimed at cholesterol reduction.

Family history is no longer a death sentence. You can change your destiny. And several chapters and cases in this book will show you how.

Diabetes

Diabetes is defined as repeated fasting blood sugar levels greater than 140 milligrams per deciliter (mg/dl). "Fasting" refers to the fact that the blood sugar is tested after a patient has fasted from food and drink (except water) for 12 hours before the test; and "milligrams per deciliter" or mg/dl are the units used to measure many substances in the blood. In the case of diabetes, anyone with a fasting blood sugar level above 100 mg/dl is at risk for developing symptomatic diabetes within the next five years or so. The symptoms include increased urination and thirst in addition to fatigue and weakness.

Most diabetics do not die from elevated blood sugar levels, but from cardiac complications of their condition. Diabetics who develop the problem as adults are usually overweight and have family members who have diabetes. Diabetics also frequently have cholesterol abnormalities and are at high risk for the development of cardiac disease. Diabetes is an even greater cardiac risk factor for women than for men, but both sexes can dramatically improve their cholesterol profiles and their blood sugar levels with the following lifestyle modifications:

- Exercise
- Avoidance of concentrated sweets
- Weight loss or maintenance of ideal body weight
- Avoidance of alcohol

Diabetics who lose weight, modify their diet, and exercise regularly are often able to stop taking medications aimed at controlling their blood sugar. Just because an individual has a tendency to develop diabetes does not mean that he or she is doomed to do so.

Cigarette Smoking

Cigarette smoking is not only a modifiable risk factor—it is one that can be totally eradicated. Giving cigarettes up is one of the greatest gifts you can give to yourself and the people who love you.

Each time you light up, your body is put at risk. Smoking increases the heart rate, decreases the heart's ability to carry and deliver oxygen, reduces the blood level of HDL-C (the good cholesterol), and leads to activation of platelets, the blood-clotting cells. Clots have a tendency to form in heart arteries, especially if a cholesterol deposit is already present in the artery.

One common objection smokers make when advised to quit for the sake of their hearts is that giving up cigarettes will make them gain weight. In effect, they argue, that's just trading one cardiac risk factor for another—why not stick with the devil you know? The fact is, however, that to equal the cardiac risk of smoking, one would need to gain 100 pounds—not very likely, no matter how difficult the quitting process is.

Two bits of good news: first, the cardiac risk of a person who smokes declines immediately upon quitting and, even better, at the end of one year is the same as that of a nonsmoker. And second, Americans are smoking less. In 1965, fully half of the men in the United States smoked. By 1992 only 27 percent were still at it. In 1965, 34 percent of U.S. women smoked. By 1992, that figure was down to 25 percent. Only among adolescent females are the numbers still rising. A nation of nonsmokers is the ultimate goal, but in the meantime, anti-smoking campaigns must be especially directed toward young women.

High Blood Pressure

Blood pressure (BP) which is measured in millimeters (mm) of mercury (Hg) is the force with which blood pushes against the walls of the arteries. When the heart beats, it pumps blood into the blood vessels and the pressure peaks. This is the systolic blood pressure (top number). As the heart relaxes (between beats), blood pressure falls to its lowest level. This is known as the diastolic blood pressure (bottom number). When the blood pressure is consistently above 140/80, it becomes more difficult for your heart to pump effectively. And over time, high blood pressure increases the risk of developing cardiac disease.

In a classic study of untreated middle-aged hypertensive males, it was found that exercising on a stationary bike for 45 minutes three times a week for six weeks led to an 11-point mercury drop in systolic and a 9-point mercury drop in diastolic blood pressure.

When the same experiment was repeated with participants exercising seven instead of three times per week, the fall in blood pressure was even more dramatic: a 16-point drop in the systolic and an 11-point drop in the diastolic.

Weight loss is likewise very important. Often the loss of even five or ten pounds will lead to a substantial reduction in blood pressure. Salt restriction in the 50 percent of Americans who are salt-sensitive can also produce impressive reductions.

Finally, alcohol can strongly affect one's blood pressure, with as little as two drinks per day leading to significant elevations. In fact, it is estimated that 5 to 10 percent of hypertension in American males is directly caused by alcohol consumption. Blood pressure medications often fail to work effectively in individuals who consume more than two drinks per day.

Some people, however, do require medications to control BP, regardless of whatever other changes they make. They should be aware that some blood pressure medications have an adverse effect on blood sugar and cholesterol levels, whereas others lead to favorable changes in both. If you have high cholesterol or diabetes in addition to high blood pressure, it will be very important to make sure that the drug your doctor chooses to treat your blood pressure will not aggravate or create a new cardiac risk factor.

Take the drugs known as beta-blockers, for example. While they do normalize blood pressure and have been shown to prolong life after a heart attack, they also adversely affect both blood sugar and cholesterol levels. More important to many patients is the fact that beta-blockers affect their sexual responses, decreasing libido and sometimes causing impotence as well.

It is crucial for you to be aware of the various side effects of any drug you are taking. You should never hesitate to ask your doctor why a particular drug has been prescribed.

If elevated blood pressure is your major cardiac risk factor, turn to Chapter 7 for a complete discussion of the lifestyle changes—weight loss, salt restriction, stress reduction, alcohol reduction, and exercise—that may help you achieve a healthy blood pressure reading.

If lifestyle changes alone fail to fully normalize your blood pressure, medications are likely to be necessary. Don't deprive yourself of good blood pressure control because of fear of side effects from these medications. Chapter 8 reviews the risks, benefits, and side effects of the currently available anti-hypertensives (blood-pressure–lowering medications). Once you understand how the medications work and read about their potential side effects you can help your doctor pick the medication that will suit your lifestyle and have few, if any, side effects.

Obesity

Obesity is a major problem in America. In spite of a national passion for slimness and the wide availability of diet foods and drinks, over the past 20 years, Americans have been getting fatter. The National Health and Nutrition Examination Survey (NHANES III) found that in 1991, about 33 percent of adult Americans were overweight—in 1980, only about 25 percent were.

Central obesity (the dreaded potbelly) is the worst form that overweight can take. While all obese people are predisposed toward cardiac risk factors, those with potbellies are especially so. Diabetes, hypertension, and hypercholesterolemia—a predisposition to high cholesterol—are all the more likely to be found in overweight people than in slim ones.

Many studies have shown that one of the major predictors of childhood obesity is the number of hours spent watching TV. Such sedentary habits, begun early enough, can establish a lifelong pattern that becomes increasingly difficult to break. Contrary to popular belief, most obese people do not eat much more than their slimmer acquaintances—they simply eat the wrong foods, and they eat them in front of the television set.

In the United States people often begin gaining weight (on average, a pound a year) once formal education stops. Out of school, organized sports generally cease and easy access to pools and gyms becomes a thing of the past. Getting enough exercise becomes a bit of a chore, one that is all too easy to let slide. My experience, however, has been that diet without exercise is a losing battle. People lose weight, but without regular physical activity, they cannot keep it off.

When I first met Jane, she was 52 years old and had just had a heart attack. Her cardiac risk factors were almost overwhelming—she was postmenopausal, obese (5 feet 2 inches and 170 pounds), diabetic, hypertensive, and had high cholesterol. As I went down the list with her, she was close to tears. "With so many problems," she asked, "how can I possibly correct them all?"

"One step at a time," I told her. Once I had convinced her to start on estrogen replacement therapy (she had had a hysterectomy some years before so she didn't require progesterone therapy), I got her to agree to a low-fat diet. Exercise, however, required all my persuasive powers. "I'm too fat to be seen out walking," she protested. Finally, she agreed to start off in her own backyard. She must have kept at it—within one month she had lost 10 pounds, her blood pressure was normal, and her blood sugar and cholesterol levels had come down significantly.

Once she had seen for herself how much her body could change, I recommended that she join the formal exercise program offered through cardiac rehabilitation. (See Glossary.) I was sure that the group spirit would be a real inspiration for her and knew she would benefit from the educational programs on diet, stress reduction, and other lifestyle changes.

Three months later, I didn't recognize her. She had lost 30 pounds, her hair was done in a becoming new style, her nails were polished, and she was wearing a lovely teal-colored suit. The changes were not just cosmetic, however—her blood pressure, cholesterol values, and blood sugar were all absolutely normal.

When I told her how wonderful she looked, she said that her heart attack was the best thing that could have happened to her because it forced her to confront her obesity. It also led to meeting the new man in her life—a colleague from cardiac rehabilitation with whom she now shared a passion for long walks and gourmet (low-fat, of course!) meals.

Sedentary Lifestyle

A sedentary lifestyle is now so much the norm in America that even moderate physical activity is seen as excessive. How many times have you seen people circling mall parking lots over and over again, looking for a spot as close as possible to the entrance? It is essential to realize that the so-called good life of comfort and ease is in fact a disaster for our health and well-being. A sedentary lifestyle is one of the root causes of cardiac disease—abandoning it in favor of vigorous physical activity is one of the most radical steps we can take. Just how to go about it is discussed in detail in Chapter 3.

High Cholesterol

Elevated cholesterol levels have already been mentioned in discussing most of the other risk factors. While this clearly indicates the interrelatedness of the various factors, high cholesterol levels must be looked at individually as well. A desirable blood report, first of all, would look something like this:

	Desirable level (in milligrams per deciliter)
Total cholesterol	Below 200
LDL	Below 130
HDL	Above 45
Triglycerides	Below 200

Having a total cholesterol of less than 200 mg/dl doesn't always mean a person is out of the woods in terms of cardiac risk. In the famous Framingham Heart Study, 35 percent of cardiac events (heart attack, bypass, angioplasty, cardiac death) occurred in people with total cholesterol levels below 200 mg/dl. Most of these people were also found to have very low (protective) HDL cholesterol levels. It turns out that the best predictor of cardiac risk is the total cholesterol/HDL ratio (obtained by dividing the total cholesterol by the HDL level). People with a ratio greater than 4 need to take action, regardless of their total cholesterol level.

For individuals with diabetes or documented heart and blood vessel disease, it is important for the LDL to be below 100 mg/dl. At this level cholesterol deposits within the arteries are unlikely to progress and may actually get smaller. This is called "regression." We will look at regression further when we discuss the case of Jack.

In a study published in January 1997 in the *New England Journal of Medicine*, bypass patients who lowered their LDL cholesterol to below 100 mg/dl were compared with those who only achieved an LDL cholesterol of around 130 mg/dl. During this four-and-a-half-year study, patients achieving an LDL cholesterol below 100 mg/dl were 29 percent less likely to return to the operating room for repeat bypass surgery.

The National Cholesterol Education Program recommends that people strive to lower their triglyceride level to below 200 mg/dl. I ask my patients to try to lower it even further to below 150 mg/dl. This request is based on several studies published by Drs. Melissa Austin and Ron Krauss.

What exactly are all these things we look at when performing a cholesterol profile? Let's consider triglycerides first since they are the toughest to understand. Triglycerides are used as fuel by the liver for the production of cholesterol. Almost all the fat you eat is in the form of triglycerides: the more fat you eat, the more cholesterol your liver will produce.

Certain diseases—like diabetes, hypothyroidism, kidney and liver disease, alcoholism, and lupus—can cause the liver to overproduce triglycerides. Obesity, usually caused by diets rich in concentrated sweets (candy, cake, soft drinks, cookies, sugar, honey, jam), fats, and alcohol, also leads to high triglycerides. People who do not exercise also tend to have higher triglyceride levels than those who do. And there are also some genetic conditions which can predispose to elevated levels.

To lower your triglycerides, without taking medication, you can take several steps:

- Lose weight
- Cut back on concentrated sweets (this includes simple sugars and even fruit juices)
- Reduce your intake of fat and cholesterol
- Exercise more
- Cut back on alcohol. In people with this problem, even a single drink can dramatically elevate the triglyceride level
- Make sure that your doctor checks you for diabetes as well as kidney, liver, and thyroid diseases

High-density lipoprotein cholesterol (HDL) is the protective or good cholesterol. Its role in the body is that of the police: rounding up the bad cholesterol (LDL) and bringing it back to the liver for processing.

Although HDL levels are largely genetically determined, there are positive steps you can take to raise yours. If you have a high triglyceride level, anything you do to lower it will in general raise your HDL, as the two are metabolically related. Other steps include the following:

- Lose weight.
- Stop smoking.
- Increase your exercise.

Occasionally, when a person is actively losing weight, HDL levels actually fall. However, once the weight has stabilized, HDL will increase and often exceed its previous level. By giving up cigarettes, you can expect to see an average increase in HDL of 8 to 10 mg/dl, although this may take up to six months to appear.

Vigorous and sustained (in my experience, at least 2 ½ hours per week) aerobic exercise will also improve HDL levels. Men and women differ with respect to the speed at which they respond to an aerobic exercise program. A man's HDL level tends to increase steadily for about a year and then levels off. On the contrary, a recent study suggests that a woman may exercise regularly for a full five years before reaching her peak HDL level.

Low-density lipoprotein cholesterol (LDL) is the one almost everyone knows about. It is a well-publicized fact that LDL leads to cholesterol plaque on the arterial walls and that an elevated LDL is associated with an increased risk for heart disease. The famous Framingham Heart Study has shown that the lower the LDL, the lower the risk of developing heart disease.

To lower LDL cholesterol I recommend the following:

- A low-fat diet
- Regular exercise (which, when accompanied by weight loss, tends to result in decreased LDL)
- If necessary, weight loss

Particular Groups at Risk: Families with Genetic Diseases

We all need to be careful about the amount of fat we consume. Some people, however, need to be more careful than others. People with genetic disorders affecting their cholesterol levels have far less leeway than the general population where fats are concerned. Two well-defined disorders are familial hypercholesterolemia (FH) and familial combined hyperlipidemia (FCH). Both are inherited conditions and are fairly common, with FH striking 1 in 500 persons and FCH, 1 in 100 in the general population. FH tends to occur more frequently in certain populations— French Canadians, Afrikaaners in South Africa, the Finnish, the Lebanese, and Ashkenazi Jews, all run a much higher risk of this genetic disease. Where I work, in Manchester, New Hampshire, approximately 1 in 100 French Canadians has FH.

FH causes very high cholesterol levels (in adults FH should be suspected when total cholesterol is 340 mg/dl or higher, and in children at a level of 270 mg/dl) and greatly increases the chance of having an early heart attack, even as early as age 20. In general, however, most men with untreated FH have had at least one heart attack by age 55 and most women with this disorder have had the same experience by age 65.

People affected with FH have inherited an abnormal gene for the processing of LDL cholesterol and have a 50 percent chance of passing the abnormality on to their children. One of the most striking physical signs of FH is the presence of visible cholesterol deposits in the tendons of the hands and feet.

Once the FH diagnosis is suspected, all first-degree relatives of the patient should be screened. In general, 50 percent of those relatives will also be found to have very high cholesterol levels.

But the situation isn't hopeless. With diet, exercise, and medications, it is possible to normalize, or at least greatly lower, cholesterol levels in most persons with FH. But as a rule, it is not possible to normalize cholesterol levels with diet and exercise alone. Most people with FH will require at least one drug, and often two or three, to help them lower their dangerously high cholesterol levels.

Sadly, studies have shown that more then half of those with FH do not know they have this disorder or even that they have a high cholesterol level. As you can see, such ignorance could be deadly. I urge everyone reading this book to have a cholesterol test. If your level is in the range I have described, please consider contacting the Make Early Diagnosis—Prevent Early Death (MED-PED) Project. MED-PED is an international effort launched in 1993 by Dr. Roger Williams at the University of Utah with the help of Merck & Co., Inc. Its aim is to identify as many people who have FH as possible. (For more information about MED-PED, see the appendix.)

A second genetic disease, Familial Combined Hyperlipidemia (FCH), is actually the most common genetic cholesterol disorder. It was discovered over 20 years ago by Drs. Joseph Goldstein, Helmut Schrott, William Hazzard, Edward Bierman, and Arno Motulsky, all researchers at the University of Washington. The genetics of this disorder are not as well understood as those for FH, but it is quite clear that if a person has FCH roughly half of his or her first-degree relatives will also be affected. Persons with FCH have a high risk of developing premature heart disease, often suffering their first heart attack before age 55.

The words "Familial Combined Hyperlipidemia" refer to what is found on the lipid profiles of affected individuals. An FCH patient can have a lipid profile that reveals a high LDL cholesterol level, or a high triglyceride level, or both. And a family with FCH can exhibit all the above abnormalities. So it is possible that if you have FCH and your brother does too, you may have only an elevated triglyceride level, whereas your brother may have both elevated LDL cholesterol and triglyceride levels. Persons with FCH are treated with diet, exercise, and, when necessary, medications. As a rule, individuals with FCH are more responsive to diet than are persons with FH. Weight loss is important for anyone with FCH who is above his or her ideal body weight. Exercise and alcohol restriction can also have a marked effect on triglyceride levels. But, in many cases, persons with FCH may require medication. The drug chosen will depend on whether a person has primarily a triglyceride or an LDL problem.

If you have a strong family history of early cardiac disease and have been told that you have a very elevated cholesterol level, it is likely FH or FCH is the cause. Make sure to discuss this with your doctor and also be sure you take steps to normalize your cholesterol level with diet, exercise, weight loss, and, when necessary, medications.

Whether you have FH or FCH, the dietary advice and exercise program described in this book will assist you in greatly improving your overall cholesterol profile.

Drugs for the treatment of stubbornly high cholesterol levels are now available in a range unknown only a few years ago. Depending on your cholesterol problem(s), your doctor will recommend different medications, alone or in combination. When I start patients on any medicine, I find it helpful to give them written information about how the drug will work, the appropriate dosages, and the possible side effects. Because it is written down, it is always available for future reference. See Chapter 8 for more detailed information on cholesterol-lowering medications.

Lipoprotein (a)

An elevated lipoprotein (a) (we call this one "Lp, little a") level lies in a gray area as far as risk factors go. No well-controlled clinical studies have yet been conducted to prove that lowering Lp(a) will in fact reduce cardiac risk. Common sense, however, suggests precisely that.

In the general population, an Lp(a) level of 2 mg/dl is average. Above 20 to 30 mg/dl is considered elevated, and persons with such a level appear to have a significantly higher risk of developing cardiovascular disease. If a person has had a bypass, she or he also appears to be at risk for developing blockages in the bypass grafts.

In addition to blocking the coronary arteries—(Lp(a) has been found in the plaques in diseased arteries), where it acts as a clotting agent. The two in combination (a plaque-caused blockage and a clot on top of that) could completely block a coronary artery and ultimately lead to a heart attack.

Lp(a) levels are entirely genetically predetermined and do not seem to be reduced by diet or exercise. To date, the only medications shown to reduce Lp(a) are niacin (a B vitamin) and estrogen.

I use a specialized laboratory test to detect Lp(a), which costs around $50. Occasionally, people complain about the cost, which many insurance companies refuse to pay, citing a lack of evidence regarding the value of reducing it in the blood. I believe, however, that knowing a patient's Lp(a) level allows me both to more accurately determine overall risk and to decide which medications would be most appropriate.

For example, I would treat a person with a high LDL and a high Lp(a) level with a drug that would address both problems, rather than simply prescribe a medication for the LDL. Even with the lack of hard data regarding the benefits of reducing Lp(a), it can't hurt to try. The drugs I would choose—niacin or, for a postmenopausal woman, estrogen—would still reduce the LDL we are sure must come down. If it is possible to simultaneously reduce Lp(a) levels as well, all the better.

Since not everyone with a high Lp(a) level responds to niacin or estrogen, it is reassuring to know that one recent study has suggested that if LDL is lowered, significantly elevated Lp(a) levels pose less of a cardiac risk. In other words, at high levels, Lp(a) and LDL may interact to dramatically increase cardiac risk, but if LDL is lowered, the risk is considerably reduced even if Lp(a) remains elevated. In my opinion, it is still best to try to reduce both LDL and Lp(a) whenever possible.

High Homocysteine Levels

Homocystinuria is hardly a household word, nor should it be, since classic homocystinuria occurs in only one out of every 200,000 people. This disease is characterized by a severe accumulation of homocysteine (an amino acid) in the blood, tissues, and urine and very early vascular (including cardiac) disease.

People with this disorder are missing an enzyme called cystathionine synthase (CS). While the complete absence of CS occurs only once in every 200,000 people, mild deficiencies, which also significantly increase the risk of early vascular disease, are much more common. To make matters worse, because the metabolism of homocysteine is complex and involves multiple enzymes, there are other common genetic and nutritional deficiencies that can result in elevated blood levels of this amino acid. These include an abnormality in the enzyme methylenetetrahydrofolate reductase (MTHFR) and insufficient intake of folic acid in the diet. The MTHFR enzyme abnormality is frequent, seen in about 10 percent of the general population, and folic acid deficiency is commonly seen in people who fail to eat sufficient quantities of fruits and vegetables.

In the last few years numerous studies have tried to determine how important elevated homocysteine is as a heart disease risk factor. All these studies have come to the same conclusion—even mild elevations of homocysteine can significantly increase the risk of heart disease. The good news is that the treatment for all causes of elevated homocysteine is an easy to take oral supplement of folic acid. In general, taking between 1 and 5 mg of folic acid a day (generally no more than 2 mg per day are required) will totally normalize homocysteine levels. In some situations vitamins B_6 and B_{12} may also be necessary.

For people with normal homocysteine levels, a diet rich in folic acid will help prevent an increase. I suggest trying to take in 400 micrograms of folic acid per day. Foods rich in folic acid (also called folate) are listed in the table below. If these foods are not in your current diet, try to work them in. If this is impossible, take a daily multivitamin that contains 400 micrograms of folate or folic acid.

Foods rich in folic acid

Food	Folate (micrograms)
Product 19 (1 cup)	400
Total cereal (¾ cup)	400
Lentils (½ cup cooked)	313
Chickpeas (½ cup cooked)	145
Spinach (½ cup cooked)	131
Spinach, raw (1 cup)	109
Orange juice (frozen concentrate 1 cup)	109
Romaine lettuce (1 cup)	76
Beets (½ cup cooked)	45

Before we leave homocysteine, many patients ask me exactly how it damages the artery and leads to heart and other vascular diseases. The answer is, no one knows for sure (though many people are working on finding the answer). But it appears that homocysteine can directly damage the cells that line the arteries themselves.

In addition, it seems that homocysteine elevations in the blood may lead to an increase in smooth muscle cells, and this in turn would tend to make plaques or deposits in the arteries larger. Finally, some lines of evidence suggest that homocysteine may actually promote clotting within blood vessels.

In our clinic we have just recently begun checking homocysteine levels on our patients. So recently, in fact, that you won't find homocysteine levels in the patient stories that follow. Rest assured they will all be tested at their next clinic visit!

Because this is a very new field, no one knows exactly what a safe level of homocysteine is. After consulting with Dr. William Castelli, the former director of the Framingham Heart Study, we have settled on 10 uμol/L (micromoles per liter) or less as normal. Anyone with levels above 10 uμol/L, we put on 1 to 2 mg of folate per day. The cost for a year of folate replacement is about five dollars.

Stress

Experts in the medical community remain somewhat vague about stress as a risk factor in heart disease, in spite of a general public acceptance of its enormous role in creating this problem. Gradually however, even physicians are coming around to the understanding that has been part of folk wisdom for so long: too much worry and anxiety, too much pent-up aggression and hostility can lead to heart attacks.

Numerous studies have shown that in the face of a stressful situation life-threatening cardiac arrhythmias can occur. Cholesterol levels can increase dramatically when persons are under stress—for example, accountants around April 15 or students during final exams. This same reaction has been documented in military recruits as they enter battle.

What can we do to prevent this from happening to us? Since it is virtually impossible (and probably undesirable) to completely avoid stress and stressful situations, we must focus instead on changing the way we react to stress.

There are many simple things we can do to relieve stress. One of the most important is regular exercise, especially walking. In the middle of a stressful situation, conscious breathing—simply paying attention to your breath—can help you glide right through whatever is causing the tension. Although I say these techniques are simple, I am quick to add that they require commitment and practice if they are to make a difference.

Conscious breathing is really a form of meditation, which we will discuss in more detail in Chapter 6, along with other forms of meditation and stress reduction.

I think you will find that as you become less stressed, you will become more accepting and patient with yourself. Developing the capacity to love yourself *as you are today* will help you believe that you can make the lifestyle changes outlined in this book. It has been my experience that individuals who believe they can change their lives are precisely the people who do it!

The Cases of Susan and Lorraine

~~~~~~

High Cholesterol and Early

Heart Disease—It May

Be Your Genes

Raymond had been planning his boss' retirement party for weeks. He had supervised every detail himself and worried over the inevitable last-minute hitches. Midway through the evening, he began to relax slightly: everything was going well.

At the end of the banquet he stood up to deliver the short tribute he had prepared for his boss. This was the moment he had been dreading—he had never given a public speech before. He smiled as he spoke the last word, thinking that now he could enjoy the rest of the evening.

As he stepped down from the podium amid enthusiastic applause, he had almost reached his chair when he collapsed. Raymond was dead, the victim of a heart attack. He was 45.

At the time of his death 28 years ago, little was understood about familial hypercholesterolemia, but with the subsequent findings in his family members, it is virtually certain that this was what he suffered from. FH is an inherited (genetic) disorder which causes abnormally high cholesterol levels, greatly increasing the chance of having a heart attack early in life, even as early as age 20. In general, however, most men with untreated FH have experienced at least one heart attack by age 55, and most women with this disorder will have an attack by 65.

Individuals with FH have inherited an abnormal gene leading to an inability to process cholesterol properly. A person with FH has a 50 percent chance of passing the abnormal gene to each of his or her children. Unfortunately, it is a common disease, striking 1 in 500 persons in the general population. But certain groups—for example, French Canadians, Afrikaaners in South Africa, Finns, Lebanese, and Ashkenazi Jews—run a much higher risk of this disease than do those of other nationalities.

Raymond had three daughters, each of whom had a 50 percent chance of inheriting the abnormal gene responsible for developing receptors for bad cholesterol. His first two children were lucky—his youngest, Susan, was not.

Susan was 12 years old when her father died, but it wasn't until she was 25 that blood work done after a routine physical exam revealed an elevated cholesterol level. Fifteen years ago, neither she nor her doctor attached much importance to the information. She continued to smoke and to eat a fairly high-fat diet, never dreaming that what had happened to her father could also happen to her.

At age 35, things began to change for Susan. She was slowly becoming aware of the ways in which she and her father were similar. She smoked heavily, as he had. She had a high-stress job which she took very seriously, as he had his. And most alarming, her cholesterol level kept rising. She assumed that the same must have been true for her father.

Susan found a doctor who understood the seriousness of her cholesterol level and, under his advice, she made what she considered drastic changes in her diet, quit smoking, and began a regular walking program. Although her weight fell somewhat, her cholesterol level remained stubbornly high. Susan felt frustrated and hopeless: so much effort and so little to show for it!

Then her doctor asked her to try cholestyramine (Questran), one of the first drugs found to significantly lower cholesterol levels. When this did not bring her level down sufficiently, her doctor switched her to lovastatin (Mevacor), a very powerful cholesterol-lowering drug. Unfortunately, as is often the case with FH, Mevacor alone also failed to achieve the desired result. At about this time, Susan, frustrated with her lack of improvement, discontinued all her medications and her cholesterol levels were as follows:

	Susan's Level	Desirable Level
Total cholesterol	412 mg/dl	Less than 200 mg/dl
Triglycerides	114 mg/dl	Less than 150 mg/dl

	Susan's Level	Desirable Level
HDL cholesterol	38 mg/dl	Greater than 45 mg/dl
LDL cholesterol	351 mg/dl	Less than 130 mg/dl*
Lp(a)	126 mg/dl	Less than 20 mg/dl

Susan's physician told her that he thought it likely she would require a very aggressive approach to lifestyle modification and at least two cholesterol-lowering medications. With this in mind, he then referred her to my lipid disorders clinic.

My diagnosis of FH was a shock to her. She had never heard the term before and the thought of having a genetic disease was, in her words, "very frightening." At the same time, however, she had a curious sense of liberation. As she got used to the idea that she actually carried an abnormal gene that prevented her body from processing cholesterol properly, she began to realize that her unsatisfactory levels were not her fault. Previously, Susan had always felt vaguely guilty about her cholesterol count, believing that if she were only more rigid about her diet or more vigorous in her exercise program her levels would be normal.

But I explained to her that, while diet and exercise were extremely important in the treatment of FH, they were not the entire answer. Persons with FH almost universally require cholesterol-lowering medications in addition to a strict diet and exercise program.

As Susan and I discussed her treatment plan, she saw more and more clearly how close she had come to despair. She had begun, at the age of 39, to believe that the disease process which had ended her father's life at 45 would also claim hers. Now, for the first time, she allowed herself to believe she could rewrite her own story.

Susan's physical exam confirmed my diagnosis of FH even before her blood report came back from the laboratory. Her hands were a dead giveaway. She had what are known as tendon xanthomas, visible cholesterol deposits under the skin within the tendons. These deposits are found in no other inherited cholesterol disorder but FH. They may be found in any tendon but tend to be most pronounced in those of the hands and in the Achilles tendons.

With the FH diagnosis established, it was also clear that Susan needed at least two cholesterol-lowering medications. On her first visit, after reviewing some preliminary diet and exercise information, I started her on

---

* Because Susan has not had a cardiac event (heart attack, bypass surgery, or angioplasty), her goal LDL cholesterol is 130 mg/dl. Once a person has had a cardiac event, the goal is 100 mg/dl.

simvastatin (Zocor), which, while closely related to the lovastatin (Mevacor) she had been on, gives a more dramatic initial result. I believe rapid improvement in the first few weeks of treatment is an important psychological weapon in combating FH. For Susan, it was both exciting and motivating to see the prompt decrease in her cholesterol values. At her second visit she had lost five pounds and had been taking her medication faithfully. Her cholesterol values had improved dramatically:

	Susan's level	Desirable Level
Total cholesterol	219 mg/dl	Less than 200 mg/dl
Triglycerides	71 mg/dl	Less than 150 mg/dl
HDL cholesterol	37 mg/dl	Greater than 45 mg/dl
LDL cholesterol	167 mg/dl	Less than 130 mg/dl
Lp(a)	126 mg/dl	Less than 20 mg/dl

She was therefore better prepared mentally to accept the more challenging treatment plan I now had in mind. Susan's cholesterol profile, as you can see, revealed high levels of both low-density lipoprotein (LDL) cholesterol (the bad cholesterol), and lipoprotein Lp(a).

Lp(a) was discovered in 1963 by Dr. Kare Berg, but only in the past four to five years have physicians realized its significance as a risk factor for the development of coronary artery disease (CAD). Lp(a) is a cholesterol-like particle, which when present in high levels—greater than 20 to 30 milligrams per deciliter, or mg/dl—appears to predispose to early heart attacks.

In general, about 50 percent of persons who have inherited the gene for FH have also inherited an elevated Lp(a) level. To put Susan's Lp(a) level of 126 mg/dl in perspective, the average level in the general population is 2 mg/dl. Like LDL, Lp(a) appears to form cholesterol deposits in the coronary arteries, but, unlike LDL, it also seems to increase the likelihood of blood clot formation. Cholesterol deposits and blood clots are a deadly combination, leading in many cases to a heart attack.

I felt it was essential to try to lower both Susan's LDL and Lp(a) levels. Zocor, which can lower LDL by as much as 45 percent depending on the dose, has, unfortunately, no effect on Lp(a). At present, the only medications for lowering Lp(a) are estrogen and niacin. Estrogen, however, is given only to postmenopausal women and Susan, 39, had a number of years to go. Niacin, therefore, was the only possibility.

It should be stated here that niacin, although a B vitamin and available without a prescription, is, when taken in the high doses required to lower Lp(a), a very potent drug. It should never be self-prescribed by people wishing to lower their cholesterol. Not everyone with high cholesterol should take niacin and not everyone who needs it can tolerate it. It is a drug which can have severe side effects and must be monitored carefully by a physician.

Along with the niacin, we also discussed the importance of diet and exercise. Although it is true that virtually all patients with FH must be on cholesterol-lowering drugs for the rest of their lives, a good diet can reduce the need for very high doses of medications, which may increase the risk of serious side effects.

And, while exercise is known to dramatically improve both triglyceride and high density lipoprotein (HDL) cholesterol levels, it does not reduce LDL levels significantly unless accompanied by weight loss. But regular exercise is still very important in FH patients because it promotes weight loss and improves the overall strength of the heart muscle.

Susan's response to the challenges FH created in her life was nothing short of amazing. I visited her in her home to get a better sense of how she had been able to reorder her world and was not only impressed but inspired.

There is a vividness about Susan to which one is instinctively drawn. Her approach to her situation was wholehearted and energetic: How do I do this thing, she asked herself, and still have fun? Looking around her house, it was clear that Susan is a highly effective, well-organized person, so it was no surprise to see these talents put to work toward her goal of cardiac health.

Her first task was an honest appraisal of her diet. "I thought I was eating well," she said, "but when I went over a typical day's meals with Mary Card [our staff nutritionist], I was amazed to see how much fat I actually consumed." With Mary's assistance, however, Susan was able to devise a diet she could live with—one that cut fat drastically but still satisfied her healthy appetite.

"Working with Mary Card also changed my attitude," she said. "Before, I always seemed to be around people who ate lots of sauces and gravies, and I felt I had to please them by producing those sorts of things. Now when I have guests, they just have to eat what I eat. And really, I'm doing them a favor!"

Her family (Susan is single but visits her mother and sisters frequently) has accepted her diet pretty well and she finds she is even able to cope with the demands of holiday baking and gorging. "Mom will sometimes say, 'Is that all you're going to eat, Sue?' But I just say, 'Oh, yeah, Mom, I'm fine,' and she doesn't make a big deal of it. She's adjusted."

Once on her new diet, Susan lost weight steadily, dropping 20 pounds in her first year. She also began to exercise more seriously, walking about four miles four to five times a week, and she found an exercise partner to ensure her getting up every morning. "When you know someone is standing on the corner waiting for you at 5:30 A.M., it's difficult to ignore the alarm!" she points out.

Her weight loss and improved muscle tone have given her a whole new outlook on life. "I feel so much more energetic—and I really enjoy physical stuff now. Whatever I do these days, I want it to be physical."

All this hard work has paid off. Susan's current cholesterol levels on just 10 mg of Zocor and 1500 mg of niacin are as follows:

	Susan's Level	Desirable Level
Total cholesterol	195 mg/dl	Less than 200 mg/dl
Triglycerides	62 mg/dl	Less than 150 mg/dl
HDL cholesterol	56 mg/dl	Greater than 45 mg/dl
LDL cholesterol	128 mg/dl	Less than 130 mg/dl
Lp(a)	95 mg/dl	Less than 20 mg/dl

Although Susan's Lp(a) is not in the desirable range, all her other levels are so good that together we decided not to run the risk of causing side effects by increasing her dose of niacin. At present, Susan's elevated Lp(a) is her only significant cardiac risk factor.

As explained earlier, however, recent data suggest that when LDL levels drop, a high Lp(a) gives less cause for concern. Since Susan's LDL was in the desirable range, I believe we can afford to relax somewhat regarding her high Lp(a).

Finally, Susan took up yoga. "I read a lot," she explained, "and many articles I've read say that stress can contribute to heart disease. I have a high-pressure job and used to be a very tense person. But since taking yoga, I don't get upset anymore. When things go wrong at work, I just take it in stride.

"I have found that yoga is the perfect way to relax. I take a class three times a week and really look forward to it—it works like meditation and it's such a nice way to end the day."

Susan's story is, in a sense, the ideal. If everyone with familial hypercholesterolemia could be diagnosed before heart disease developed, the risk associated with the condition would be dramatically reduced because, as Susan's experience so graphically illustrates, FH is not a death sentence. Given the proper medication, diet, and lifestyle changes, a person with FH stands a good chance of dramatically improving his or her life expectancy. The problem is not in having FH, but rather in having *undiagnosed* FH. People with undiagnosed FH are walking time bombs. Like Raymond, they could suffer a massive heart attack at any moment and die on the spot.

Lorraine almost became one of those statistics, despite several warnings. In her case, the problem was that the warnings were isolated and confusing: no one ever explained what it all added up to.

In 1965, at the age of 34, Lorraine was told that her cholesterol level was 475 mg/dl. At that time, cholesterol was not the hot subject it has become in recent years. Neither she nor her doctor gave it much importance—she was advised to cut back on butter and eggs, and that's where the matter ended.

Several years later, during a routine physical exam, she was told she had cholesterol deposits in her Achilles tendons. This finding, combined with her dramatically elevated cholesterol, and strong family history of heart disease, indicated without a doubt that Lorraine had FH.

She was not, however, informed of her condition, nor does she recall being told that she was at risk for the development of premature heart disease. This risk was compounded by the fact that she had been a heavy smoker for many years. In spite of the fact that treatment of FH in the late sixties was quite difficult (there were no easy-to-take medications available), if Lorraine had quit smoking and made major changes in her diet, in addition to taking one or more of the medicines then available—niacin, cholestyramine (Questran), or colestipol (Colestid)—she would have substantially lowered her risk. As it was, she did little beyond making slight additional changes in her diet.

In 1980, while having blood work done for an unrelated problem, she remembered her earlier high cholesterol level and asked that it be measured again. A few hours later, her doctor, an orthopedist, called her at work, stunned by the lab reports she had just received. "Are you sure you are alive?" Lorraine remembers her asking. "You have the highest cholesterol level I've ever seen." At 650 mg/dl her doctor said, "You need more than an orthopedist. I want you to be seen by an internist."

The next doctor she saw put her on Questran, but the treatment was not very successful. Lorraine still did not understand the importance of lowering her cholesterol. Her own lack of motivation combined with the unpleasant nature of the medication (Questran is a powder that must be mixed in liquid—and drinking it is remarkably like swallowing a glass of sand) resulted in many "forgotten" doses.

In 1985, Lorraine was referred to Dr. Robert Benson, a cardiologist, for more aggressive treatment. It was under his care that she finally began to see a heart attack as a very real threat to her life. Her new doctor was not only able to persuade her that lowering her cholesterol was absolutely essential, but also that she had to quit smoking and radically change her diet.

Giving up cigarettes was the easy part. Despite a 42-year addiction to smoking, she made the decision to quit in a split second and has never regretted it.

Dietary changes, however, were more difficult. Although Lorraine cut out eggs and most red meat and switched to skim milk, in retrospect she admits she was not as strict with herself as she needed to be. At 5 feet 2 inches, she weighed 160 pounds.

Dr. Benson's extreme concern with Lorraine's continued high cholesterol level led him to try a very new therapy—so new, in fact, that the medication he gave her was not yet on the market. Mevacor, now freely available, revolutionized the treatment of hyperlipidemia (high cholesterol). When prescribed for Lorraine in 1985, it was still in the testing phase, but Dr. Benson was able to obtain it on compassionate grounds and, for the first time, his patient's cholesterol level began to drop.

The drop, however, was nowhere near what it needed to be. Starting at 650 mg/dl, Lorraine's cholesterol level came down to 400 mg/dl— remember, the normal level is 200 mg/dl—and stayed there for the next six years. In 1991, she began to slow down. The slightest exertion caused breathlessness ("What worried me most was that I couldn't sing!" she said), and she found herself unable to perform even the simplest household tasks. She believed (or made herself believe) that this was caused by her chronic back problems and she gradually did less and less, allowing her husband, Omer, to take over the running of the house.

In 1992, however, Omer himself suffered a heart attack and died soon after. While he was ill, Lorraine forced herself to get back on her feet to take care of him ("I was so busy worrying about him, I didn't have time to worry about myself," she remembers), but after his death, she was no longer able to go on kidding herself about her own health.

In December, she finally admitted to her family that she was experiencing not only shortness of breath but also chest pressure. Her son, with whom she was living at the time, insisted that she see a local cardiologist, since she now lived far away from her previous physician. In January 1993 she met Dr. Ed Palank, a physician associated with The New England Heart Institute.

Dr. Palank, quite convinced that her symptoms indicated heart disease, had her go through a stress test. Lorraine, who had succeeded in convincing herself that her heart was not the problem, was truly shocked when the test revealed a serious disorder—so serious, in fact, that Dr. Palank ordered an immediate cardiac catheterization for her. This is a procedure that allows the visualization of the inside of the heart's arteries. (See Glossary.)

A few days later, after much thought and a bit of prodding from her children, Lorraine entered the hospital to undergo the procedure. At this point, she still refused to believe that she had any real heart problem. This is a very common occurrence among people with severe heart disease: even when the symptoms are unmistakable, patients will persist in denying their existence.

The results of the catheterization were so clear, however, that even Lorraine had to admit the truth. She was found to have a 75 percent blockage of the left main artery, the heart's most important artery. A blockage here is a clear indication for bypass surgery, because if it is left untreated sudden death can result.

Nevertheless, Lorraine's first reaction to Dr. Palank's report was outrage. "I kept saying, 'There's nothing wrong with my heart! I've never had a heart attack.' " She had given up smoking, stopped eating red meat and butter, and had been taking medication for years. How could she need bypass surgery?

But the gravity of her situation did not allow time for arguments. Surgery was scheduled for the following day and her family gathered to help support her through the ordeal.

Four days after her operation, the cardiac surgeons asked me to see Lorraine. When I asked her how she was feeling, she said she hadn't been able to breathe this well in years. In fact, when she woke up after the surgery she thought she was getting "too much air"! She said she wanted to do everything possible to keep this feeling and I knew her "teachable moment" had arrived.

I examined her carefully, drawing her attention to the cholesterol deposits in her Achilles tendons, and explaining how these, in combination with her high cholesterol level and family history of heart disease, meant that she most definitely had familial hypercholesterolemia.

I warned her that controlling her cholesterol would probably require two, and possibly three, cholesterol-lowering medications. We also discussed the tremendous importance of diet and exercise and her own cooperation in overcoming her genetic condition.

Finally, we talked about the possibility that both her children and grandchildren could have inherited the same abnormal gene. As it turned out, her son, one of her two daughters, and at least one of her grandchildren were known to have very elevated cholesterol levels.

Given Lorraine's diagnosis, it was highly likely that they had FH as well.

I met her son Ron later that night and tried to impress upon him the gravity of his own condition, which was, in fact, more serious than his sister's, in spite of their having similar cholesterol levels.

Until the time of menopause, women with FH have the protection of estrogen, which works in a number of ways to prevent heart disease (see Chapter 5 for a full discussion of estrogen). But Ron, a 38-year-old man, was statistically likely to experience a heart attack in the next 12 years unless he made major lifestyle changes and agreed to take medications.

During the course of my relationship with Lorraine, I came to see Ron as a very loving son with an exceptional concern for his mother's health. Where his own well-being was concerned, however, he appeared to be more casual. Although he listened intently to what I had to say about cholesterol, he admitted he had yet to be convinced of the urgent need to reduce his own, in spite of its being markedly elevated.

He did agree to my consulting with his primary care doctor and has recently begun to take Mevacor, which has lowered his cholesterol but, as in his mother's case, not to an acceptable level. For many people, Mevacor is all that is needed to normalize their cholesterol values, but people with FH do not respond so dramatically to drug therapy and typically require at least two medications for cholesterol control.

Ron must also be convinced of the need for an aggressive diet and exercise program. My hope is that he will be inspired by the progress that his mother and sister (who is also under my care) have made and refuse to become a victim of FH.

Those of his children who have inherited the abnormal gene are helpless to change their situation until their father decides to change his. The motivating factors could not be closer to home: his own life and those of his children.

Lorraine, however, left the hospital with a new diet and exercise program. Her cholesterol profile on the day of admission looked like this:

	Lorraine's Level	Desirable Level
Total cholesterol	473 mg/dl	Less than 200 mg/dl
Triglycerides	291 mg/dl	Less than 150 mg/dl
HDL cholesterol	42 mg/dl	Greater than 45 mg/dl
LDL cholesterol	373 mg/dl	Less than 100 mg/dl

While she was in the hospital, I asked her to begin pravastatin (Pravachol) at a dose of 20 mg per day. Pravachol is a drug similar to Mevacor. Both have a dramatic effect on cholesterol levels, particularly LDL levels.

Lorraine's elevated triglyceride level surprised me because persons with FH very rarely have this problem; but in her case, I felt it was related to her being overweight.

Three months after her hospital stay, she came to my office for a checkup. It is important for a person on cholesterol-lowering drugs to have his or her liver checked regularly to be sure that it is functioning normally. If there is a problem and it is caught early enough, it can be corrected completely by discontinuing the medication. Lorraine's liver function was fine and her cholesterol profile looked like this:

	Lorraine's Level	Desirable Level
Total cholesterol	388 mg/dl	Less than 200 mg/dl
Triglycerides	196 mg/dl	Less than 150 mg/dl
HDL cholesterol	34 mg/dl	Greater than 45 mg/dl
LDL cholesterol	315 mg/dl	Less than 100 mg/dl
Lipoprotein (a)	96 mg/dl	Less than 20 mg/dl

Although this represented a great improvement, Lorraine still needed further reduction in her LDL, the "bad" cholesterol. Her medication, increased exercise, weight loss, and a low-fat, low-calorie diet had had the desired effect on both her total cholesterol and triglyceride levels, but she also had a rather alarming drop in her level of HDL, the protective cholesterol. How did this happen?

Doctors are not sure why, but when people begin a very low-fat diet and especially when the fat they do consume is polyunsaturated (corn oil or sunflower oil, for instance), their HDL level can fall quite dramatically. This HDL drop is not so extreme when monounsaturated fats such as canola or olive oil are used. HDL drops can also occur during active weight loss, but typically, after a new weight plateau is achieved and maintained for a few months, the HDL level will rise to exceed the original level. Since Lorraine had been following a low-fat diet and had already lost 5 pounds, I was not unduly concerned but encouraged her to change to canola or olive oil in her diet.

This doesn't mean that a person can consume any amount of these oils, because they will cause weight gain, just like any other fat. It is safe to limit yourself to about 30 grams of fat per day.

At her checkup, Lorraine's lipoprotein (a)—Lp(a)—was also measured. As we saw in Susan's case, an increased Lp(a) seems to be associated with FH and also with an increased risk of heart disease.

Of the two medications available to reduce Lp(a) (niacin and estrogen), both of which also reduce LDL (Lorraine's biggest problem), my choice for her was postmenopausal estrogen. I felt that it would offer her a great deal of cardiovascular protection, since it has been shown to reduce the risk of a future cardiac event by as much as 84 percent in women who already have heart problems. I explained this to Lorraine, but she was unconvinced, telling me that she was worried about the possible side effects from estrogen, such as an increased risk of uterine cancer. She was right in that there is an increased risk of uterine cancer if one takes estrogen and does not take progesterone with it, but with progesterone on board the increased risk of uterine cancer is removed.

I told Lorraine that I'd like to have her take both estrogen and progesterone, but her expression told me my idea had been vetoed. I was a graceful loser. After all, it was her body, and she had to feel comfortable with what she was putting in it.

I was disappointed, but she did agree to taking the niacin, which improves all aspects of the lipid profile: LDL, HDL, triglycerides, and Lp(a). Because niacin can have many side effects, including flushing and itching, I always start a patient on it slowly, to allow gradual adjustment of the body to the changes it will induce. In addition to the niacin, her dose of Pravachol was increased to 40 mg per day.

With the niacin, Lorraine was on two cholesterol-lowering drugs. Both Pravachol and niacin may cause liver toxicity, and the combination of the two is more dangerous than use of either one alone. For this reason, liver function tests must be monitored closely and a patient on this combination must be sure to notify his or her physician promptly of symptoms such as abdominal discomfort, nausea, vomiting, or leg swelling—all indicators of liver toxicity.

On the day she began niacin, Lorraine also met with Mary Card, the dietitian in our clinic. Mary developed a diet for Lorraine that restricted fat to 20 percent of her total calorie intake and agreed that she should use primarily olive or canola oil as her sources of fat calories. In addition, Mary asked Lorraine to restrict her intake of concentrated sweets such as cookies, candy, ice cream, and soda, since they tend to cause triglyceride elevations.

Twelve weeks later, her lipid profile showed significant improvement:

	Lorraine's Level	Desirable Level
Total cholesterol	324 mg/dl	Less than 200 mg/dl
Triglycerides	102 mg/dl	Less than 150 mg/dl
HDL cholesterol	58 mg/dl	Greater than 45 mg/dl
LDL cholesterol	247 mg/dl	Less than 100 mg/dl
Lp(a)	66 mg/dl	Less than 20 mg/dl

While things were good, they were not good enough. Given the enormous efforts Lorraine had already made, it was very difficult for me to tell her that she needed to work even harder, but she still had a long way to go. Her by now 10-pound weight loss was an excellent beginning, but it was only a beginning, and though she was already on two strong medications, it was clear she would require a third.

This time I added colestipol (Colestid), a drug very similar to the Questran she had taken in the past. Like Pravachol and niacin, it lowers LDL cholesterol but without causing liver function abnormalities. Colestid and Questran are in fact the safest cholesterol-lowering drugs available, and can even be taken by children and pregnant women.

On the same visit, Lorraine reviewed her diet with Mary and found there were still changes she could make. And I asked her to increase her walking and bike riding program to 45 minutes four to five times a week.

Another 12 weeks later Lorraine had lost eight more pounds and her lipid profile looked like this:

	Lorraine's Level	Desirable Level
Total cholesterol	220 mg/dl	Less than 200 mg/dl
Triglycerides	57 mg/dl	Less than 150 mg/dl
HDL cholesterol	69 mg/dl	Greater than 45 mg/dl
LDL cholesterol	149 mg/dl	Less than 100 mg/dl

She was thrilled, gave me a big hug, and told me she was going to go dancing that night!

"Oh, really?" I asked. "With whom?" With a twinkle in her eye, she told me about Roger, an old high school friend with whom she had lost contact for over 16 years. When he saw her again, he told her she hadn't changed a bit.

"Maybe I look the same to you," she said she told him, "but my cholesterol is a whole lot lower today than it was 16 years ago." Since then, Lorraine and Roger have been nearly constant companions and he has been one of her biggest supporters in her fight against fat.

I have told this star patient that I would love to see her LDL fall a bit further, but given her excellent HDL level, I do not expect to change her medications. At this point, her total cholesterol to HDL ratio is outstanding at 3.2 (with her goal being less than 4). I am encouraging her to lose 5 to 10 more pounds, and I have no doubt that she will do it. Lorraine is a fighter and a winner, and I am challenging her children and grandchildren to fight the cholesterol battle as hard as she has. What she has learned can apply to anyone in her medical situation, and the earlier a person takes control of his or her life the better.[1]

If you think that you might have FH, there is an international program to which you can turn for help. It is called the Make Early Diagnosis—Prevent Early Death Project (MED-PED) and is directed by Dr. Roger Williams at the University of Utah. If you would like more information about it, please feel free to contact me or one of the other five physicians in the United States collaborating on this project. For a list of all MED-PED collaborators in the United States, see the appendix at the end of this book.

2

~~~~~~

A Heart-Healthy Diet:

Planning the Diet

You Can Live With

Where would we be without food? Quite apart from its nutritional value, food plays an important role in most people's lives, filling social, emotional, and cultural needs. We let it speak for us when words are difficult; we use it to express love, sympathy, and friendship. When we feel lonely or restless or bored, food is often the consolation we turn to.

Childhood associations with certain tastes may trigger a whole flood of memories, both good and bad. And rejection of food we have offered to someone we love can wound us more deeply than seems possible. Even being consciously aware of an unhealthy relationship to food is no guarantee of becoming more sensible. The connection between food and bliss is primeval, going back to infancy when feelings of comfort, safety, and joy were inseparable from having a filled tummy. It's no wonder, then, that our relationship to food is often complicated and difficult to unravel.

Changing your diet to prevent or reverse cardiac disease, then, is not just a simple matter of cutting out butter and eggs and counting fat grams. Most Americans get close to 40 percent of their calories from fat— about twice what we recommend to our patients.

If you are like most people in this country, you have probably been eating too much fat and too much sugar for many years. The habits built up over those years—how you spend your coffee breaks, how you celebrate Christmas, Chanukah, and birthdays, what you eat at restaurants

40

and weddings, what you snack on while traveling, what you take along to the beach—all must be reexamined in the light of your commitment to cardiac health. The suggestions offered in Chapter 4 on quitting smoking may also be helpful here—after all, you are "withdrawing" from the high-fat lifestyle.

When patients first begin attending our lipid clinic, the diet plans we offer often seem difficult and daunting. Many people want to give up before even trying. They say they are too busy to cook, they don't have time for such shopping, their families will never adjust—you name it. After beginning our program, however, most people are amazed at how easy it actually is. I speak from many years of experience: try the plan outlined here for a few weeks, and you will be pleasantly surprised by the visible difference in your body and by the way you feel. If you follow a good diet, combined with a sensible exercise program, I guarantee that you will have more energy, you will lose your excess weight, and, most important, as you will see in Jack's story, you may experience shrinkage of the cholesterol deposits in your heart's arteries.

In spite of (or maybe because of) all the nutrition information available these days, there are still many misconceptions about fats and cholesterol. This is partly because of constantly changing reports on nutritional research. Because the press tries to keep the public informed, researchers who formerly battled within the confines of scientific journals now find their debates covered on the national news, often long before they are ready to make conclusive statements.

Several things, however, are known for certain. We know that Americans eat too much fat and that obesity is a major health concern, increasing the risk of cardiac disease, diabetes, back pain, and cancer. We also know that saturated fat, more than any other dietary constituent, is responsible for raising Americans' cholesterol levels.

Dietary saturated fat impairs the liver's ability to remove cholesterol from the blood, resulting in elevated cholesterol levels and cholesterol deposits within the coronary and other arteries. In the United States, children as young as 10 have been found to have cholesterol deposits on their artery walls. With aging, such deposits enlarge, increasing the risk of a heart attack.

Excess cholesterol in the diet may also predispose you to an elevated cholesterol level and can certainly contribute to blockages in artery walls. However, concentrating solely on eliminating cholesterol from the diet may, ironically, lead one to a diet even higher in saturated fats. For example, when Wayne, whose case you will read about in Chapter 3, was told that his cholesterol level was too high, he became a vegetarian and set about giving up cholesterol, switching to margarine and swearing off meat and eggs. What he didn't realize was that the nuts, peanut butter, and salad dressings he was consuming were doing as much, if not more, damage to his heart as had the red meat and eggs he was so carefully avoiding.

The mistake many people make is in assuming that only high cholesterol foods contribute to high cholesterol in the blood. The fact is that all foods rich in saturated fat, whether or not they contain cholesterol, can cause problems.

Most of the people we see in our lipid clinic are overweight. I find that when they focus on fat in their diets rather than on cholesterol alone, they can reduce their calorie intake and lose weight more successfully.

Fat is very calorie dense. A single gram of fat contains nine calories, whereas one gram of protein or carbohydrate provides only four. By replacing fats with protein and carbohydrates, you will automatically consume fewer calories.

This is not to say, however, that you can eat unlimited amounts of these foods. In order to lose weight, you must also consider quantity. I often see people who switch to low-fat cookies, potato chips, and crackers, but consume them in such quantity that they gain no benefits. A snack of four or five low-fat cookies, for example, can add 250 "empty" calories to your daily total, meaning that they give you no nutritional benefits. Can you really afford this? A better snack would be a bowl of cereal and skim milk or a cup of 100-calorie yogurt and a piece of fresh fruit.

Most people are aware of butter, cream, margarine, salad dressing, red meats, and mayonnaise as rich sources of fat. But fat is also found in muffins, chocolate, potato and tortilla chips, cookies, peanut butter, all vegetable oils, crackers, cheese, and ice cream. Restaurant food is famous for hidden fats: a burger and a small order of fries can contain 35 to 40 grams of fat—more than a day's allowance for most adults.

For most women, salad dressings are another big contributor to fat in the diet. One tablespoon of regular Italian dressing contains 6 grams of fat and very few people use only one tablespoon. If you eat lots of salad, consider switching to a fat-free or low-fat variety of dressing. If you want to make your own, try one of the recipes given at the end of this book. If you order salad in restaurants, always ask for the dressing to be served on the side. Dip your fork in the dressing and then spear your salad greens rather than pouring three to four tablespoons of dressing directly onto your salad.

The chemistry of fats can be confusing and their names are hard to pronounce, let alone remember. Most people have at least heard of poly-unsaturated and monounsaturated fats, and may also be aware of the debate among scientists over which is preferable. In the past, polyun-saturated oils like safflower and sunflower oils were commonly recom-mended as good for the heart. We now know, however, that when substituted for saturated fats, the polyunsaturated ones tend to lower HDL (the good cholesterol) and may increase the risk of developing co-lon cancer.

Monounsaturated fat is found in olive oil, canola oil, peanut oil, pea-nuts, peanut butter, olives, and avocados. When this type of fat is sub-stituted for saturated fat, HDL levels may increase and total cholesterol levels will drop.

Some health professionals are intrigued by the concept of the Medi-terranean diet, which calls for 40 percent of calories from fat, with olive oil the major fat source. And it is true that the Mediterranean area has a low incidence of heart disease, even though the average person who lives there consumes far more fat than the average American.

But appealing though it may be, the Mediterranean diet cannot be viewed in isolation from Mediterranean culture. Activity levels, climate, genetic predisposition, food preferences, alcohol intake, and even char-acter traits all play important roles in the connection of diet to health. I do not think it makes sense to try transferring cultural values from one country to another. The American lifestyle differs radically from the Mediterranean, and with obesity a national crisis, we will hardly benefit by switching to an even higher fat diet than we already have.

Trans fat, for years an area of study for researchers only, has just recently received public attention. Trans fat is created when liquid oils undergo hydrogenation—a process by which hydrogen is added to fat. Significant sources include fast foods (especially the fried variety), par-tially hydrogenated oils (you will see this term on food labels), com-mercially prepared baked goods, and stick margarine. The longer shelf life of trans fat makes it popular with food manufacturers, but many studies indicate that it causes a reduction in HDL (the good cholesterol) and an increase in LDL (the bad cholesterol).

When recent media reports suggested that for this reason margarine (which contains trans fat) was no better than butter, I was swamped with calls from confused patients who wanted to know if they could go back to butter if it was really a matter of six of one, half a dozen of the other. Of course I told them not to return to butter, since it was as full as ever of artery-clogging saturated fat. Instead, I suggested that they limit their intake of trans fat as well by using diet margarine (in which the first ingredient should be water), avoiding fast foods, and limiting consumption of commercially prepared baked goods like crackers, muffins, cookies, and pastry.

Recommendations for Reducing Fat in Your Diet

Most people can reduce their cholesterol level and lose weight by focusing on their fat intake. Most adult females will lose weight by restricting their fat intake to 27 grams per day and their calories to 1200. Adult males will lose on 33 grams of fat and 1500 calories.

To figure out your own daily fat allowance, follow these steps:
1. Determine your ideal weight based on the formula on page 45.
2. Multiply that weight by 10.
3. Multiply the number from step 2 by 0.2 (20%).
4. Divide that number by nine. This will give you your fat allowance in grams. Remember that each gram of fat has nine calories.

For example,

1. The ideal weight of a woman who is 5 feet, 4 inches, is 120 pounds.
2. $120 \times 10 = 1200$
3. $1200 \times 0.2 = 240$ fat calories
4. $240/9 = 27$ grams of fat per day

Sometimes I see people try to cut fat completely out of their diet. While it is actually impossible to eat a diet devoid of fat because grain products and starches contain trace amounts, it is possible to eat so little fat that one fails to obtain enough linoleic acid, an essential fatty acid. Such acids are found in fat-containing foods and cannot be obtained elsewhere. I generally advise people to be sure to consume at least 15 grams of fat per day.

Here are the fat allowances for different calorie levels:

Calories	20 percent Fat (grams)	15 percent Fat (grams)
1200	27	20
1500	33	25
1800	40	30
2000	44	33

But What About Triglycerides?

In our lipid clinic we take triglyceride elevations very seriously because many studies have shown that high triglycerides increase risk for the development of heart disease in both men and women. In the past, it was believed that triglycerides themselves were not so bad; it was really the company they kept.

For example, high triglycerides were often noted in persons with diabetes, elevated levels of blood-clotting factors, high blood pressure, and obesity. Scientists believed it was these conditions, not the high triglycerides, that increased the risk of heart disease. Some studies have even identified triglyceride-rich particles within coronary blockages. This being so, it is important to get their levels down, preferably below 150 mg/dl.

Since almost all the fat one eats is in the form of triglycerides, people with high triglycerides must restrict fat. In addition, since excess calories can be used by the liver as fuel to make more triglycerides, sugar and alcohol, both sources of empty calories, must also be restricted. Indeed, a single alcoholic beverage can dramatically raise triglyceride levels.

It is quite common for a person with an elevated triglyceride level to be overweight. Caloric restriction leading to weight loss is an essential component of any triglyceride-lowering program. In addition, initiation of an exercise program can reduce triglyceride levels by as much as 40 percent.

But having elevated triglycerides complicates a cholesterol-lowering program, because it is no longer just fat grams you need to consider but the restriction of fat, sugar, calories, and alcohol, and you must try to add vigorous exercise to your schedule on top of everything else. It is hard work but it can be done. If this is your situation, your program will consist of the fat restrictions already outlined, in addition to the following recommendations. They are the same recommendations I gave Wayne. His is a real success story (see his case on p. 108).

Management of High Triglycerides

1. For weight reduction, try to reach your ideal body weight, using this formula:

	Men	Women
First 5 feet of height	105 lb	100 lb
For every inch over 5 feet add	6 lb	5 lb

For example, a man who is 5 feet, 10 inches tall should weigh 165 pounds. A 5 foot, 4 inch woman should weigh 120.

This chart seems like an impossible dream to many of my patients. Laughing, they tell me they haven't weighed so little since high school. There's nothing wrong with your high school weight, I tell them. The young have no monopoly on fitness, nor is there a law that says middle-aged and older people cannot weigh what they did in their prime.

Researchers at Harvard Medical School recently published a study that concludes that women who gain even small amounts of weight after age 18 significantly increase their risk of developing heart disease. Since in my opinion the same is probably true of men, I ask all my patients to get back to their high school weight—unless of course they were overweight at that time!

Other patients, particularly older ones, insist that the "gaunt" look doesn't appeal to them. They tell me they will look sick and unattractive with their bones sticking out, and that anyway their spouses like them round and soft.

For people who lived through the Great Depression or who come from countries where hunger is still a life and death issue, this concern is real. In many parts of the world (including America not so long ago), the poor and unhealthy are thin, while the prosperous and "healthy" are fat.

I try to help my patients to reexamine this idea. Many of our prejudices and deeply held beliefs are acquired uncritically, usually as children, and we are not even aware of how out of touch with reality they are.

In any case, I am not asking anyone to make the skeleton the ideal to strive for, nor do I expect my patients to take up fashion modeling on the side. The lean look may take some getting used to, but the increase it brings in energy and stamina will make it worthwhile. And the compliments you get from the younger generation won't hurt either!

Where triglycerides are concerned, any weight loss at all will help. Sometimes people can normalize even very elevated levels with only a five-or ten-pound weight loss.

2. For exercise, I recommend at least one-half hour five days a week, with more being better. (See Chapter 3 to design your own program.)

3. Restrict foods high in refined sugar. In particular, restrict the following foods:
   - Fruited yogurt
   - Fruit juice, and limit fresh fruit to 4 pieces per day
   - Pies, cakes, cookies, pastries, doughnuts, regular jello
   - Sherbet, frozen yogurt, popsicles, ice cream

> ### Abbreviations:
>
> | | | |
> |---|---|---|
> | cup = C | milligram = mg | teaspoon = tsp |
> | gram = gm | ounce = oz | tablespoon = Tbsp |

- Sugar (white, brown, confectioners), honey, maple syrup, corn syrup, chocolate syrup, jelly, jam, marmalade, hard candy, chocolate bars
- Regular soda
- Pudding, custard, mousse

Sometimes these simple sugar restrictions can have almost magical effects: I have seen triglycerides fall from over 2600 mg/dl to below 300 just with the elimination of orange juice. I have seen similar reductions with the elimination of regular soda, and in one unusual case, the culprit was maple syrup!

4. Restrict fat as already outlined (see p. 44).

5. Restrict alcohol. In general, I recommend that people cut their alcohol intake in half. If this does not achieve the desired result, I suggest further restriction.

6. If diabetic, improve blood sugar control.

People with elevated triglyceride levels are often very discouraged when they see my list of what to avoid. It is true that lowering triglycerides takes some discipline, but the good news is that many people can achieve terrific reductions (on the order of several 1000 mg/dl at times) without medications.

If you have a triglyceride problem, you may be wondering what snacks are acceptable. I have prepared a special snack list for people trying to normalize their triglyceride levels.

Recommended Snack Foods for Lowering Triglyceride Levels

STARCHES AND BREADS

1 ½ graham crackers, 6 saltine crackers, ½ English muffin
2 popcorn cakes or rice cakes (any flavor)
1 oz fat-free potato chips (20 chips: Louise's, Childers)
1 oz baked tortilla chips (13 chips: Guiltless Gourmet, Baked Tostitos)
5 reduced-fat Ritz crackers
5 melba toast rounds
1 C dry unsweetened cereal

⅓ bag Orville Redenbacher Smart-Pop Popcorn
24 oyster crackers
1 oz pretzels
1 slice cinnamon raisin bread or ½ bagel
½ medium Syrian bread pocket (pita bread)
1 Kellogg's Special K waffle

MILK GROUP
8 oz nonfat sugar-free yogurt (100 calories, Dannon Lite, Columbo Lite
    100)
½ C sugar-free pudding made with skim milk or 1% low-fat milk
½ C Kemps sugar-free frozen yogurt
5 ounces TCBY sugar-free, nonfat frozen yogurt
Good Humor sugar-free creamsicle or fudgsicle
8 oz skim or 1% low-fat milk

FRUIT GROUP
1 fresh fruit
½ C canned fruit in juice or water
½ C fruit salad

VEGETABLE GROUP
Use all vegetables as snacks, with the exception of corn, peas, potatoes,
    lima beans, winter squash, and sweet potatoes.

BEVERAGES
Diet Soda
Sugar-free ice tea
Crystal Lite
Water
Club soda or seltzer water
Black coffee and tea

MEAT AND PROTEIN GROUP
1 oz chicken, turkey
Low-fat cheese (less than 5 grams of fat per ounce)
1 oz 96% fat-free luncheon meat

What About Sugar?

Every day the average American consumes 600 calories in the form of
sugar. This means that most of us are eating over 125 pounds of sugar
per year! Sugar goes by many different names, including dextrose, glu-

cose, maltose, fructose, honey, molasses, maple and corn syrups, corn, cane, brown and confectioners sugar.

Beyond adding to the flavor of food, sugar helps retain moisture, prevents spoilage, and improves the texture and appearance of the food we eat. Manufacturers of fat-free products take advantage of these properties and systematically replace fat with sugar. The resulting foods may be fat free, but loaded with calories and sugar. If you consume fat-free cakes and cookies regularly, you may find that your weight doesn't go down and your triglyceride levels go up.

The physiological consequences of a high-sugar diet can be quite serious. Excess sugar in the bloodstream causes your pancreas to release large amounts of insulin, the sugar-regulating hormone. Insulin, in turn, increases the release of the lipoprotein lipase, an enzyme which promotes the transfer of fat from the bloodstream into fat cells. Once in the cell, fat is more difficult to get rid of.

What's more, insulin is also directly involved with cholesterol production. The higher the level of circulating insulin, the more cholesterol a person's liver produces.

Finally, some studies have shown that insulin level is also critical in determining where a person stores excess body fat. High levels of insulin promote abdominal weight gain, often called "central obesity," the very type of fat that increases the risk of developing cardiac disease.

As a rule, I recommend that people with triglyceride abnormalities try to limit sugar intake to 10 percent of their total calories.

For a 1200-calorie diet, 120 sugar calories = 30 grams of sugar per day.

For a 1500-calorie diet, 150 sugar calories = 38 grams of sugar per day. For people without a triglyceride problem, I suggest trying to limit sugar intake to no more than 15 percent of calories.

For a 1200-calorie diet, 180 sugar calories = 45 grams of sugar per day.

For a 1500-calorie diet, 225 sugar calories = 57 grams of sugar per day.

The following chart gives you the sugar content of some common foods. Sugar is also listed on the new food labels: look for the amount of sugar per serving, and make sure to check whether the size of your serving is equivalent to the serving size listed on the label.

As you can see from this list, it is easy to take in a great deal of sugar without even realizing it. If you need to lose weight or to lower your triglyceride level, it is essential for you to examine food labels closely for *both* sugar and fat.

Sugar Content of Some Common Foods

Food	Serving Size	Calories	Sugar (grams)
Baked beans	½ C	150	8
Barbecue sauce	2 Tbsp	35	7
Catsup	1 Tbsp	15	4
1% low-fat chocolate milk	8 oz	180	30
Coca-Cola Classic	12 oz	140	39
Hot cocoa	8 oz	110	17
Regular iced tea	8 oz	90	22
Lemonade (frozen concentrate)	3 Tbsp	110	27
Ocean Spray Cran-Raspberry drink	8 oz	140	36
Dole Fruit Bars	1 bar	45	10
Popsicle	1 bar	45	11
Sherbet	½ C	120	26
Pudding with skim milk	½ C	140	20
Fruited yogurt	8 oz	240	30
Cereals			
Bran flakes	¾ C	110	5
Cheerios	1 C	110	1
Corn flakes	1 C	110	2
Fruit Loops	1 C	110	14
Kix	1⅓ C	120	3
Life	1 C	120	6
Quaker strawberry and cream oatmeal	1 packet	130	10
Special K	1 C	110	3
Total	1 C	110	5
Dunkin Donuts low-fat muffin	1 muffin	220 to 240	31 to 41
Keebler Vanilla Wafers	8 cookies	130	11
Keebler Elfin Delights Chocolate Sandwich	2 cookies	110	8
Little Debbie Fruit Bar	1 bar	130	20
Snackwell Cereal Bar	1 bar	120	18
Snackwell Devil's Food Cake Cookies	2 cookies	100	18
Quaker Caramel Corncakes	2 cakes	100	8
Freihofer's fat-free cookies	2 cookies	110	11
Honey	1 Tbsp	60	16
Molasses	1 Tbsp	50	12
Jelly	1 Tbsp	50	9
Lite pancake syrup	2 Tbsp	50	10

Facts About Fiber

Fiber, or roughage, has recently received a great deal of attention from both food manufacturers and scientists. In the past, it was primarily seen as a cure for constipation. Now it is clear that a high-fiber diet does more than that. Researchers have determined that a diet rich in fiber can reduce the risk of developing heart disease, colon cancer, and possibly breast cancer. New studies extolling its benefits seem to be published almost every day.

But in spite of all the publicity, most Americans are still not getting enough roughage. Many health organizations recommend the daily consumption of between 20 to 35 grams of fiber, and the 5-A-Day campaign for fruits and vegetables is designed to increase our daily intake.

Fiber is found only in plant foods. Fruits, vegetables, whole-grain breads, cereals, beans, lentils, and legumes are all examples of high-fiber foods. Fresh or frozen fruits and vegetables are much better sources of fiber than juices.

There are two types of fiber: water soluble and water insoluble. It is the water-soluble fiber, found in fruits, oatmeal, beans, and legumes, that helps reduce cholesterol levels. Diabetics who increase their consumption of water-soluble fiber often find that their blood sugar levels are much better controlled. Fiber helps delay gastric emptying, preventing a rapid increase in blood sugar levels immediately following a meal.

Water-insoluble fiber is found in most grain products, wheat bran, and most vegetables. It lessens the risk of constipation and diverticulosis, and has also been associated with a reduction in colon cancer risk.

As you eat more fiber, it is important to drink more water because the fiber acts like a sponge and requires additional fluid as it passes through your digestive tract.

Psyllium, commonly found in products promoting regularity, like Metamucil or Citrucel, is another important source of soluble fiber. Psyllium lowers your cholesterol level in the same way as other water-soluble fibers, and it also helps relieve constipation. If you want to add psyllium to your diet, I suggest starting with two tablespoons per day. Ideally, you should mix it in water, but if you have trouble with this try using the flavored brands of Metamucil and Citrucel. Mixing them in orange juice, as often recommended, adds considerably to your daily calorie and sugar intake.

Adding Fiber to Your Diet

- Choose whole-grain breads with whole-wheat flour listed as the first ingredient. Look for at least 2 grams of fiber per slice of bread. Choose whole-grain crackers and snack foods.
- Use brown rice in place of white rice. If you don't like brown rice, try mixing it half and half with white.
- Have at least three fresh fruit servings per day (for example, one whole pear, apple, banana, orange, or one cup of strawberries or blueberries). Each of these has 3 to 4 grams of fiber.
- Have at least three vegetable servings (½ C cooked or 1 C raw) per day (the more the better).
- Create a nutritious salad using assorted greens rather than plain old iceberg lettuce. Venture out, use romaine, red leaf, green leaf, spinach, or cabbage. In addition to cucumbers and tomatoes, add grated carrots, chopped broccoli, cauliflower, red and green peppers, kidney beans, chickpeas, or thawed-out frozen peas to your salads.
- Whole-wheat flour can be used in recipes for up to 50 percent of the total flour requirement (this works well in muffin, pancake, or quick bread recipes).
- Make homemade bean soups or purchase healthier versions of canned minestrone, split pea, lentil, or black bean soup (good brands include Healthy Choice, Pritikin, and Progresso Healthy Classics).

Use this chart to tally your daily fiber intake

BEANS	Fiber (grams) per serving
Beans (½ C cooked)	5 to 8
Campbell's Black Bean Soup (1 C)	5
Chickpeas (½ C canned)	7
Green Giant Harvest Burger	5
Green Giant Three Bean Salad (½ C canned)	3
Health Valley Real Italian Minestrone Soup (1 C)	11
Lentils (1 C cooked)	7
Morning Star Meatless Grillers (1 patty)	3
Pritikin Split Pea Soup (1 C)	10
Progresso Healthy Classics Lentil Soup (1 C)	6
Progresso Split Pea Soup (1 C)	5

BREADS	Fiber (grams) per slice
Arnold Bran'ola Hearty Wheat	3
Arnold oatmeal	2

BREADS	Fiber (grams) per slice
Arnold pumpernickel	1
Pepperidge Farm 9-grain	2
Pita whole wheat	1.5
Tortilla, whole wheat	1.5
Aunt Jemima Low-Fat Waffles (2 waffles)	1
Wonder light wheat or 9-grain	3
Wonder 100% whole wheat	2

CEREALS	Fiber (grams) per serving
General Mills Fiber One (½ C)	13
Grape-Nuts (½ C)	5
Kellogg's All-Bran with Extra Fiber (½ C)	15
Kellogg's Bran Buds (⅓ C)	11
Kellogg's Complete Bran (⅔ C)	5
Kellogg's Fruitful Bran (1 ¼ C)	6
Kretschmer Wheat Germ (1 ½ Tbsp)	2
Nabisco 100% Bran (⅓ C)	8
Nabisco Shredded Wheat (1 C)	5
Post Raisin Bran (1 C)	8
Quaker 100% Natural Low-Fat Granola (½ C)	4
Quaker Quick Oats (1 C cooked)	4
Ralston Multibran Chex (⅔ C)	3.5
Total (¾ C)	3
Wheaties (1 C)	3

CRACKERS AND SNACK FOODS	Fiber (grams) per serving
Archway Oatmeal Cookies (1 cookie)	1
Baked Tostito Guiltless Gourmet No-Oil Tortilla Chips (15 chips)	3
Health Valley Fruit Bars (1 bar)	4
Health Valley Granola Bar (1 bar)	3
Nabisco Wheat Thins (16 crackers)	2
Nature Valley Low-Fat Chewy Granola Bar (1 bar)	1
Pretzels (all varieties)	0
Quaker Rice Cakes (1 cake)	0
Wasa Fiber Plus Crispbread (3 pieces)	9
Whole Wheat Matzos (1 cracker)	4

GRAINS AND PASTA	Fiber (grams) per serving
Barley (1 C cooked)	6
Bulgur (¾ C cooked)	6

GRAINS AND PASTA	Fiber (grams) per serving
Brown rice (⅔ C cooked)	3
Pasta (1 C cooked)	1 to 2
White rice (⅔ C cooked)	1

FRUITS	Fiber (grams) per serving
Apple (1)	4
Apricots, dried (⅓ C)	4
Banana (1)	3
Blueberries (1 C)	4
Cherries (1 C)	3
Figs, dried (2)	4
Grapes (1 C)	1.5
Grapefruit (½)	2
Nectarine (1)	2
Orange (1)	3
Orange juice (4 oz)	0.5
Peach (1)	2
Plums (1)	1
Prunes, dried (5)	3
Strawberries (1 C)	3

VEGETABLES	Fiber (grams) per serving
Asparagus (½ C cooked)	2
Broccoli (½ C cooked)	2
Cabbage (½ C cooked)	2
Carrots (½ C raw)	2
Cauliflower (½ C cooked)	2
Corn (½ C cooked)	2
Celery (½ C raw)	1
Green beans (½ C cooked)	2
Green peas (½ C cooked)	4
Green pepper (½ C raw)	1
Lettuce, iceberg (1 ½ C)	1
Lettuce, romaine (1 ½ C)	2
Mushrooms (½ C raw)	0.5
Potato, baked with skin (1)	4
Sweet potato, baked with skin (1)	4

Snacking

Snacking, which is probably the world's most popular pastime, is one of those open-ended activities that get a lot of us into trouble. Snacks are tempting, easy, and, especially in America, omnipresent. Unlike a proper meal, snacking is something we just drift into without thinking about. Twenty minutes later, that bag of chips from which we were only going to have one or two is unaccountably empty.

If snacks are your downfall, get into the habit of planning ahead. If the only snack foods you have in your house are cookies and ice cream, you will not do as well as the person who has stocked up on low-fat and low-calorie snacks.

I suggest the following:

- Have vegetables (cleaned and chopped) in the refrigerator.
- Make sure you have a variety of fresh fruit on hand.
- Prepare a fruit salad and use it as a snack for several days.
- Choose low-fat cookies and crackers.
- Make muffins or have bagels on hand, which are better choices than doughnuts or Danish.

Remember that all foods contain calories. Even low-fat snacks should be limited.

For specific snack choices, refer to the list that follows.

- FRESH FRUIT (any kind)

- FRUIT SALAD: Prepare this yourself to be sure that no sugary syrup has been added

- RAW VEGETABLES, including carrots, red and green peppers, tomatoes, celery, broccoli, cauliflower, mushrooms

- COOKIES: Your snack should be approximately 100 calories and 2 grams of fat. Choose from the following:

Archway: Molasses, date oatmeal, apple oatmeal, oatmeal rounds, gingersnaps
Entenmann's: Fat-free cookies and cakes
Granola bars: Kellogg's Low-Fat, Health Valley Fat Free
Hostess Light Cupcakes
Keeblers' Cinnamon crisps
Nabisco's Honey Maid grahams, fig newtons, fruit newtons, ginger-

snaps, animal crackers, pantry molasses, Nilla wafers, Teddy Grahams, Social Tea biscuits, devil's food cakes, arrowroot biscuits

Pepperidge Farms: Wholesome Choice carrot walnut, Wholesome Choice
raspberry tart

Snackwell: All varieties

Sunshine: Animal crackers, golden fruit raisin biscuit, lemon coolers, gingersnaps, honey grahams

- CRACKERS: Your snack should contain 60 to 70 calories and no more than
2 grams of fat. Choose from the following:

Crispbreads: All varieties
Crown Pilot
Finn crisps
Garden crisps
Guiltless Gourmet Baked Tortilla Chips
Harvest crisps
Kavli crackers
Matzo (except egg)
Melba toast
Microwave popcorn
    Jolly Time Lite
    Pop Secret by Request
    Orville Redenbacher Smart Pop
    Weight Watchers
    Oyster crackers
    Popcorn, air popped
    Pretzels
    Rice cakes
    Saltines
    Sea rounds
    Soda crackers
    Triscuits
    Uneeda biscuits
    Wasa crisp breads

- DAIRY PRODUCTS: When choosing a snack from the dairy category make
sure to use either 1 percent (low-fat) or nonfat foods.

Fat-free ice milk or frozen yogurt
Low-fat cheese: 3 grams of fat or less per ounce
Nonfat yogurt: Dannon Lite, Colombo Lite 100, or Weight
    Watchers have no sugar so are fine for diabetics

Sherbet
Sorbet

Individuals who must restrict sugar as well as fat can now find great tasting fat-and sugar-free frozen yogurts. TCBY makes several varieties.

- BEVERAGES
Herbal tea
Hot cocoa made with skim milk
Diet soda or diet beverages
Sparkling water or soda water
Ice water (try to drink 8 glasses a day)

- BREADS: Your snack should contain between 70 and 100 calories. Choose from the following suggestions:

½ bagel
½ English muffin
One slice of whole wheat, pumpernickel, raisin, rye, Italian, or French bread
½ Syrian pocket (pita bread)

- CEREAL: Any unsweetened cereal with skim or 1 percent low-fat milk.
Although many people forget about cereal after breakfast, it really makes a great low-fat, high-fiber snack. It is an especially good choice for women who are having trouble getting the calcium they need.

- SOUP
Clear broth or bouillon
Chicken noodle, chicken rice, chicken vegetable
Vegetable beef
Minestrone

Reading a Food Label

Starting at the top, you first want to pay attention to the serving size. All the nutrition information on the label is based on this amount of food, while your own typical serving might be two or three times the amount listed. Noting the number of servings per package helps you plan how many packages you need to feed your family and may also help you with portion control.

Total calories per serving is another important component of the food label, especially for people who need to lose weight. You may be quite

FDA Food Label

Nutrition Facts

Serving Size 1 cup (253 g)
Servings Per Container 4

Amount Per Serving

Calories 260   Calories from Fat 72

% Daily Value*

Total Fat 8g	**13**%
Saturated Fat 3g	**17**%
Cholesterol 130mg	**44**%
Sodium 1010mg	**42**%
Total Carbohydrate 22g	**7**%
Dietary Fiber 9g	**36**%
Sugars 4g	
Protein 25g	

Vitamin A	35%	▪	Vitamin C	2%
Calcium	6%	▪	Iron	30%

* Percent Daily Values are based on a 2,000 calorie diet. Your daily values may be higher or lower depending on your calorie needs.

	Calories	2,000	2,500
Total Fat	Less than	65g	80g
Sat Fat	Less than	20g	25g
Cholesterol	Less than	300mg	300mg
Sodium	Less than	2,400mg	2,400mg
Total Carbohydrate		300g	375g
Fiber		25g	30g

Calories per gram:
Fat 9   ▪   Carbohydrate 4   ▪   Protein 4

surprised by the calorie content of some of the fat-free items on the market. It is equally important to examine a label for total fat, saturated fat, sodium, fiber, and sugars.

The percentages listed on the right side of the label are based on the recommendations for the nutrient intake at the bottom of each label. These percentages can be confusing and I prefer not to use them at all. Sixty-five grams of total fat per day (which is the amount you see recommended on this label) is simply too much for most adults, especially those with high cholesterol or known heart disease. The other percentages you see (i.e., sodium, carbohydrate content, and dietary fiber) can be used in order to assess your total daily intake.

Your Shopping List

The list below can be used as a guide in constructing your own basic shopping list.

FRUIT
Apples, bananas, oranges
Grapes, pears, grapefruit
Lemons, limes
Nectarines, peaches, plums
Strawberries, blueberries, kiwi
Canned fruit in water or juice

VEGETABLES
Broccoli, carrots, celery
Lettuce: romaine, iceberg, red
  leaf
Spinach, brussels sprouts
Mushrooms, beets
Peppers: red, yellow, green
Corn, peas, cabbage
Tomatoes, zucchini
Onion, garlic
Squash: summer or winter

MEATS AND SEAFOOD
Turkey breast
Chicken or turkey
Ground turkey or 90 % lean
  hamburger meat
Fish or shellfish

OILS, CONDIMENTS, AND SPICES
Oil: canola or olive
Cooking sprays
Nonfat or low-fat salad dress-
  ings
Mayonnaise: light or fat-free

Low-sodium soy sauce
Salsa
Seasonings and spices
Vinegar, garlic, mustard
Natural peanut butter, jam,
  honey

DRY GOODS
Flour: white, wheat
Rice: brown, white
Pasta or no-yolk noodles
Lentils, split peas
Beans: kidney, chickpeas, pinto,
  navy, black

CANNED GOODS
Tuna in water
Stewed tomatoes, spaghetti
  sauce
Tomato sauce, paste
Canned beans: kidney, chick-
  peas, pinto, navy, black
Low-fat soups and broth

BREAKFAST CEREALS
All bran, oatmeal, oat bran
  shredded wheat, wheat germ

BREAD AND CRACKERS
Bagels, English muffins
Bread: whole wheat, rye, pita,
  pumpernickel, multigrain
Crackers: whole wheat, rye, sal-
  tines

SNACKS
No-fat tortilla chips
Pretzels
Fat-free cookies
Raisins
Popcorn
   microwave, less than 1 gm of
   fat per 3 cups

DRINKS
Juice: orange, apple, or grape-
   fruit
Apple cider
Soda water or diet soda

DESSERTS
Nonfat frozen yogurt
Sorbet, sherbet
Fat-free ice cream
Sugar-free popsicles
Nonfat, sugar-free fudgsicles
Angel cake

DAIRY AND SPREADS
Skim milk and 1% milk
Nonfat yogurts
Low-fat and nonfat cottage
   cheese
Low-fat cheeses: Swiss and
   cheddar
Nonfat cheese: ricotta
Part-skim mozzarella
Margarine: diet tub types
Cream cheese: fat-free

FROZEN FOODS
Egg substitute
Frozen dinners (low-fat)
Frozen vegetables
Fat-free breakfast foods
Fat-free frozen yogurt

Dining Out

Almost everyone enjoys a meal out. For many of us, eating out is a way of life. In fact, recent studies estimate that Americans eat one out of every three meals in a restaurant. There is no question that it is more difficult to adhere to a low-fat meal plan if you are not cooking for yourself, but it can be done. If you follow these guidelines, you will be successful at just about any restaurant.

Guidelines for Ordering in Restaurants

- Carefully read menu descriptions: Low-fat items are described as "steamed," "stir-fried," "barbecued," "grilled," "broiled," or "roasted." Fatty preparation methods include "buttery," "crispy," "fried," "in cream sauce," "in cheese," or "stewed."
- Ask questions: If you are not sure of a menu item, ask your waiter for specifics. Be assertive and request what you want. More and more restaurants are catering to the needs and wants of their patrons. Many restaurants have a special section on their menu for low-fat choices.

- Keep an eye on added fat: Have sauces, gravies, salad dressings, mayonnaise, butter, margarine, and sour cream served on the side or not at all. By eliminating 1 tablespoon of mayonnaise, you will save 100 calories and 14 grams of fat!
- Make special requests: Don't be afraid to ask for something special from the kitchen or for substitute items. For example, use mustard in place of mayonnaise, low-calorie salad dressing rather than regular dressing, baked potato in place of french fries, or low-fat milk instead of whole.
- Control portions: Choose regular, small, or child-size servings. If you find the item that you have ordered is too large, take half of it home with you and enjoy it another day.

Eating ethnic foods is fun and different, but unfamiliar names and preparation methods make it difficult to know what to choose. The following listings include some of the best choices you can make while dining in Italian, Chinese, Mexican, and Indian restaurants.

ITALIAN: Remember that shrimp is okay; although it does contain some cholesterol, it is so low in fat that it is an excellent alternative to red meat.
Plain Italian bread or rolls
Pasta dishes with tomato sauce (without meat or cheese)
Chicken or veal cacciatore
Soups: minestrone, pasta e fagioli, tortellini in broth
Salads: arugula and Belgian endive, house salad, insalata frutte di mare (seafood in a light marinade served on greens)
Chicken primavera, chicken in wine sauce
Shrimp primavera, shrimp in marinara, sole primavera
Linguini with white clam sauce
Italian ice, sorbet

CHINESE: Keep your focus on the vegetables, rice, and noodles.
Steamed Peking ravioli
Teriyaki chicken
Soups: hot and sour, wonton, sizzling rice, delights of three
Chicken chop suey, sizzling chicken with vegetables
Yu-Hsiang chicken
Shrimp with broccoli, Moo shoo shrimp, Szechwan shrimp
Spicy green beans, vegetable stir-fry, broccoli and mushrooms
Steamed white or brown rice
Chicken lo mein, vegetable lo mein
To limit sodium, request your order to be prepared without MSG and do not add soy sauce at the table.

MEXICAN: Keep your order simple and avoid combination platters.
Mexican rice
Salsa
flour or corn tortillas
Gazpacho, Black bean soup, Dinner salad, Mexican salad
Fajitas, enchiladas, burritos, chili with beans
Hold the guacamole, sour cream, refried beans, and limit the cheese.

INDIAN: North Indian food is generally much richer than South Indian. Avoid the flaky and fried breads (puris and parathas) in favor of the plain chapatty and tandoori naans. Raitas—chopped vegetable salads in spiced yogurt—are good, but avoid "boondi ki raita." Ask for your lentils (dal) to be served without the "tarka" (spices fried in oil and added at the last minute). Ask which vegetables are "suki" (without gravy) and order those. "Idli"—a steamed rice–lentil cake—is a delicious nonfat meal served with a lentil soup and chutneys (most chutneys are also fat-free).

A Word on Alcohol

I don't think there is an adult in America who hasn't heard that alcohol will protect against heart disease. There is, in fact, some strong evidence that moderate (one drink per day) alcohol consumption can reduce the risk of heart disease in both men and women. It does not appear to matter what type of alcohol is consumed—red or white wine, beer, and spirits—all appear to reduce the risk of cardiovascular disease.

The beneficial effect of alcohol seems to be its ability to raise HDL cholesterol (the good cholesterol) and its tendency to increase blood levels of tissue plasminogen activator (TPA). TPA is a clot dissolver, high blood levels of which may decrease the risk of a blood clot forming in the coronary arteries. Blood clots are commonly the cause of heart attacks. Alcohol also seems to prevent platelets, the blood's clotting cells, from clumping together.

However, before you rush out and buy your heart a drink, you should understand that alcohol is also a drug with many negative effects. With one in nine Americans suffering from alcoholism, taking it up as a virtuous decision is probably not wise. Even moderate alcohol consumption can significantly raise triglyceride levels. Triglycerides are a strong predictor of cardiac risk in both men and women. If you have a triglyceride elevation, my advice is to limit your alcohol consumption as much as possible.

Heavy alcohol consumption (in general defined as more than three drinks per day) is associated with a host of adverse consequences. At this level, the risk of heart disease, including enlargement of the heart and the development of cardiac arrhythmias, increases. Alcohol abuse also increases the risk of cirrhosis of the liver, pancreatitis, gastritis, high blood pressure, some forms of stroke, and cancer of the mouth, pharynx, larynx, esophagus, and liver.

Fetal alcohol syndrome is the most common cause of mental retardation in the United States and has been directly linked to even small amounts of alcohol consumption during pregnancy. Alcohol is implicated in many auto and boating injuries and fatalities, and is often a factor in domestic violence. Finally, evidence is emerging that alcohol use increases the risk of breast and colon cancers.

Quite apart from its toxic effects, it is important to remember that alcohol has calories. For those counting calories, the following chart should be helpful.

4 oz wine (white)	80 calories
4 oz wine (red)	95 calories
8 oz beer	100 calories
8 oz beer (light)	64 calories
1 oz hard liquor (80 proof)	64 calories
1 oz hard liquor (90 proof)	73 calories
1 oz hard liquor (100 proof)	82 calories

Given our national alcohol abuse crisis, I cannot recommend even moderate alcohol consumption to most of my patients. If you have questions about whether you might benefit from moderate alcohol consumption, I suggest that you review this information carefully and then discuss the issue with your personal physician.

Vitamin Supplements

When I was in medical school, the idea of vitamin supplements was pooh-poohed. I was taught that if you ate a good diet you were wasting your money on vitamins. I can still hear myself saying this to my patients—and can only hope that their memories are not as good. Since my medical school days, a large number of excellent research studies have been published which challenge the notion that there is no place for vitamins.

Indeed, there is currently a great deal of evidence that many Americans, especially those who have or are at high risk for the development of cardiac disease, would benefit from vitamin supplementation. Since everyone absorbs vitamins and minerals from dietary sources slightly differently, no one can tell you exactly which vitamin or exactly what dose to take. What I would like to do is share with you some information that has emerged in the last few years regarding the antioxidant vitamins C and E, and also folic acid. These dietary supplements have been linked to reduction of cardiovascular disease.

Dr. Daniel Steinberg and his colleagues at the University of California have researched the antioxidant vitamins extensively. Through their work, we have learned that one of these vitamins' most important functions is to prevent the oxidation of low-density lipoprotein cholesterol, or LDL cholesterol (the bad cholesterol). For LDL cholesterol to enter easily a growing blockage within the artery wall, it must be oxidized. Artery blockages, including those of the important coronary arteries, are made up of cholesterol and cellular debris. If a blockage is large enough, it can fill the entire artery and cause a heart attack. The process of oxidation occurs normally in our bloodstreams but can be slowed down considerably when antioxidants are present.

Two large studies, one of female nurses and the other of male health professionals, looked at vitamin E intake and the risk of subsequent cardiac events (such as heart attacks). Both studies found that individuals who consumed at least 100 international units (IU) of vitamin E per day for at least two years had a significant reduction in cardiac risk. In the recently published two-year Cambridge Heart Antioxidant Study (CHAOS), people with heart disease who took either 400 IU or 800 IU per day reduced their risk of a second heart attack by 47 percent. Of the two doses of vitamin E used, it appears that 400 IU per day is the better choice.

The benefit of vitamin C seems less than that of vitamin E, being mainly related to its ability to regenerate vitamin E after it has acted as an antioxidant.

When evaluating these studies, it is important to recognize that as yet there is no way to say for sure that it is the vitamins and not something else (that we aren't measuring) that was really protecting these people from heart disease. This is, of course, the nature of science. It may be that the vitamins will not prove to provide the protection that we hope they do. On the other hand, the lead looks promising and it is often by this scientific process of observation, followed by planned clinical studies, that very important discoveries are made.

For example, until large clinical trials were performed, many physicians, including me, were convinced, based on observational studies alone, that beta-carotene was a very powerful and beneficial antioxidant.

Over the past two years, however, three studies have raised concern that, especially in smokers, beta-carotene might cause more harm than good, increasing the risk of lung cancer and heart disease. If these large clinical trials had not been performed, we might have continued to suggest that persons at high risk for heart disease take beta-carotene.

No one is sure why the dietary studies of beta-carotene looked so much more promising than the earlier studies in which beta-carotene was given as a pill. One of the most likely theories is that when you eat foods rich in beta-carotene (carrots, melons, green leafy vegetables, tomatoes, and sweet potatoes) you are also getting a whole host of other beneficial vitamins and nutrients. It may be that these other substances and not beta-carotene are really protecting against heart disease. Still another theory suggests that taking huge doses of beta-carotene in pill form may prevent the absorption of other important vitamins in the beta-carotene family.

There are currently several large-scale clinical trials of antioxidants being conducted in the United States and Europe. In these studies, half the participants will take the antioxidants and half will take a sugar pill (neither the participants nor the doctors running the study will know which pill a person is taking; only a central pharmacy will have that information).

After about five years, it will be disclosed which patients took which pills and this will help determine the true effectiveness of the antioxidants. Until that time, we can only say that the studies published to date do suggest a benefit in terms of cardiovascular risk reduction for people taking antioxidants.

If you decide that you want to take them, there are several important questions to ask. These include the following:

1. Can I get enough of these vitamins in my diet? Vitamin C is available from citrus fruits and tomatoes, whereas vitamin E is found in foods such as egg yolks, milk fat, liver, nuts, vegetable oils, and grains.

   As you can see, a low-fat diet is deficient in vitamin E, making supplementation necessary.

2. If I do take vitamin supplements, should I take them on a full or an empty stomach, and how many doses a day should I take? Since vitamin E is a fat-soluble vitamin, it is absorbed best if taken with food, preferably at a meal that contains at least a small amount of fat. This does not mean you should increase the amount of fat in your diet!

   In general, studies indicate that the antioxidants are best absorbed in two doses. Ideally, this means taking them with lunch and supper. However, since for many people it is difficult to remember a lunch-time pill, it is acceptable to take them with breakfast and dinner, even though most people on a low-fat diet take in very little fat at breakfast.

3. Have the vitamins any side effects? The antioxidant vitamins are relatively free of side effects, but a few have been reported. In very high doses, vitamin C can cause stomach irritation and diarrhea. Vitamin E has been safely used in doses as high as 3200 international units (IU) per day, but certain people, for example those on blood thinners such as Coumadin, should ask their doctor to check the time it takes for their blood to clot after taking vitamin E.

4. What doses of these vitamins should I be taking? No one knows the correct dose for sure. I generally suggest the following:

   - *Vitamin E*: 400 IU. When buying vitamin E look for the word d-alphatocopherol, not dl, since the natural form of vitamin E appears to be better absorbed.
   - *Vitamin C*: 1000 mg.

   Since it is difficult to absorb the entire dose at once, I suggest taking half of it—that is, 200 IU of vitamin E, and 500 mg of vitamin C—with breakfast and the other half with dinner.

Many Americans who are quite well informed on antioxidants have heard much less about the importance of folic acid (also called folate) in their diet. In a recent study reported by Dr. Jacob Selhub in *The New England Journal of Medicine,* people with high levels of homocysteine in their blood were found to be at increased risk for the development of cardiac disease. Blood levels of homocysteine rise when people fail to take enough folic acid on a daily basis, or as mentioned in Chapter 1, as a result of genetic enzyme deficiencies. In an editorial accompanying Dr. Selhub's article, Meir J. Stampfer, M.D. of the Harvard School of Public Health recommended a daily folate supplement (generally, a 1 to 2 mg dose is sufficient).

However, if your doctor has determined that you do not have an enzyme deficiency, you can obtain all the folate you need by consuming a diet rich in lima beans, broccoli, spinach, asparagus, potatoes, whole-wheat bread, and dried beans. Other excellent sources of folic acid are Total cereal or a multivitamin.

To summarize, then, the antioxidant vitamins and folic acid (folate) supplements may help protect against cardiovascular disease, and we should know much more about their potential benefit in five to seven years. Until more data are available, all of us must weigh the risks and benefits of these vitamins for ourselves. It is important to understand that neither the antioxidants nor folate supplements can take the place of such proven cardiovascular safety measures as a low-fat diet, exercise, and the cessation of smoking.

Meal Plans for Heart-Healthy Living

The following seven-day meal plan helps get you started on a program that will lower your cholesterol and your weight. As you become comfortable with the principles outlined and the recipes provided at the end of the book, you will be able to develop your own meal plans.

As mentioned earlier, we find that women lower cholesterol and lose weight on a daily diet that includes 27 grams of fat and 1200 calories, and that men achieve similar results with 33 grams of fat and 1500 calories daily.

While on a calorie or fat-restricted diet, I recommend a daily multivitamin and a 500-mg calcium supplement.

A typical 1200-calorie day might be broken down as follows:

BREAKFAST: 2 breads, 1 fruit, ½ cup skim milk, ½ fat serving
LUNCH: 1 bread, 2 meats, 1 vegetable, 1 fruit, ½ fat serving
SNACK: 1 fruit, 1 C skim milk
DINNER: 2 meats, 2 breads, 2 vegetables, 1 fruit, 1 fat
SNACK: 1 bread, ½ C skim milk

If you are allowed 1500 calories per day, add the following: 2 breads, 1 vegetable, 1 oz meat, 1 fat. These servings may be added as snacks or to your meals.

Use these guidelines as you begin to design your own meal plans.

	Servings per day	
Food Group	1200 calories	1500 calories
Bread and starch	6	8
Fruit	4	4
Vegetables	3	4
Skim milk*	2	2
Protein and meat alternatives	4	5
Fat	2	3

* If you use 1% low-fat milk, eliminate 1 fat serving per day.

While following either the 1200-or 1500-calorie plan, feel free to consume moderate quantities of coffee, tea, diet soda, soda water, and Crystal Lite. We encourage you to consume between 6 to 8 glasses of water per day.

What Is a "Serving"?

Since it is important that we all be in agreement on the size of a serving, we ask that you use the following guidelines.

BREADS AND STARCHES: 1 serving provides 80 calories and 15 grams of carbohydrate. Examples include:
1 cup cold cereal
1 slice bread, or ½ bagel, or ½ English muffin
½ cup pasta, or ½ cup rice, or ½ cup mashed potatoes
6 crackers, or 1 oz pretzels, or 2 popcorn cakes
½ cup corn, or ½ cup peas, or 1 small baked potato
1 cup soup
⅓ cup cooked beans or lentils
⅓ bag of Orville Redenbacher Smartpop Popcorn

PROTEIN: 1 serving provides 55 calories, 7 grams of protein, and 3 grams of fat. Examples include:
1 ounce cooked lean red meat
1 ounce cooked skinless chicken
1 ounce fish
2 ounces shellfish (crab, lobster, shrimp, scallops, clams)
¼ cup tuna in water
¼ cup nonfat or lowfat cottage cheese
½ cup egg substitute
2 egg whites
1 ounce low-fat cheese (less than 3 grams of fat per ounce)
1 ounce (less than 96% fat-free) luncheon meat
⅓ cup cooked beans or lentils

MILK: 1 serving provides 100 calories and 8 grams of protein. Examples include:
1 cup skim milk
1 cup ½% low-fat milk
1 cup 1% low-fat milk
⅓ cup dry nonfat milk powder
1 cup plain nonfat yogurt
1 cup 100-calorie fruited yogurt with Nutrasweet or aspartame

FRUIT: 1 serving provides 60 calories and 15 grams of carbohydrate. Examples include:

½ cup fruit juice

½ cup canned fruit (packed in water or juice)

1 cup watermelon, honeydew, or cantaloupe cubes

1 cup berries

VEGETABLES: 1 serving provides 25 calories and 3 grams of protein. Examples include:

½ cup juice (tomato, carrot, V-8)

½ cup cooked vegetables

1 cup raw vegetables

FAT: 1 serving provides 45 calories and 5 grams of fat. Examples include:

1 Tbsp diet margarine

1 Tbsp lite mayonnaise or 1 Tbsp lite salad dressing (mayonnaise type)

1 tsp vegetable oil (canola, olive, peanut, corn)

2 Tbsp reduced-calorie salad dressing

1 Tbsp pumpkin or sunflower seeds

2 Tbsp nuts (peanuts, walnuts)

FREE FOODS: The following foods contain less than 20 calories per serving. You can use them as often as you like.

BEVERAGES

Broth or bouillon (fat free)

Sugar-free soda or beverages

Seltzer water or soda water

Coffee or tea

FRUITS

Cranberries or rhubarb (unsweetened)

VEGETABLES

Cabbage, celery, cucumbers, mushrooms, radishes, salad greens, zucchini

CONDIMENTS

Horseradish, mustard, taco sauce, vinegar, Worcestershire sauce, all herbs and seasonings

SUGAR-FREE SWEETS

Sugar substitute and sugar-free gelatin, jams, jellies, gum, hard candies or mints, pancake syrup

Day 1

BREAKFAST   1 C cold cereal
              1 slice whole-wheat toast
              ½ banana
              4 oz skim milk
              ½ Tbsp lite margarine

LUNCH   ½ whole-wheat pita pocket
              2 oz sliced chicken
              lettuce and tomato
              1 apple
              ½ tsp reduced-fat mayonnaise

SNACK   1 orange
              1 C of 100-calorie yogurt

DINNER   3 oz shrimp cocktail
              Cocktail sauce
              ½ C rice pilaf (see recipe p. 276)
              ½ C broccoli
              1 Tbsp lite margarine
              1 C whole strawberries

SNACK   1 popcorn cake (any flavor)
              4 oz skim milk

Individuals following a 1500-calorie diet may add:
              ½ C rice pilaf
              1 popcorn cake
              4 oz tomato juice
              1 oz chicken
              1 Tbsp of diet margarine

Day 1	1200-calorie plan	1500-calorie plan
Calories	1239	1498
Protein (grams)	80	95
Fat (grams)	17	24
Saturated fat (grams)	3	4
Cholesterol (milligrams)	281*	300*
Sodium (milligrams)	1961	2381
Fiber (grams)	21	21

* Cholesterol is from the shrimp.

Day 2

BREAKFAST	1 English muffin 1 orange ½ C 100-calorie yogurt 2 tsp strawberry jelly
LUNCH	4 Wheat n' Bran Triscuits ½ C 1% low-fat cottage cheese Tossed green salad 2 Tbsp reduced-calorie French dressing 1 pear
SNACK	1 small banana 1 C skim milk
DINNER	2 oz spicy grilled chicken (see recipe p. 266) 1 small baked potato 1 slice whole-wheat bread 1 C steamed asparagus ½ C unsweetened applesauce
SNACK	1 ½ graham crackers 4 oz skim milk

Individuals following a 1500-calorie program may add:

> 1 C vegetable soup
> 6 saltines
> ½ C beets
> 1 oz chicken
> 1 tsp canola oil

Day 2	1200-calorie plan	1500-calorie plan
Calories	1262	1501
Protein (grams)	72	76
Fat (grams)	12	18
Saturated fat (grams)	3	4
Cholesterol (milligrams)	62	67
Sodium (milligrams)	2012	2313
Fiber (grams)	24	27

Day 3

BREAKFAST	½ C bran cereal
	½ cinnamon raisin bagel
	½ C orange juice
	1 Tbsp lite cream cheese
LUNCH	1 C gazpacho soup* (see recipe p. 242)
	1 oz low-fat cheese
	1 oz sliced turkey
	Spinach salad with mushrooms
	2 Tbsp reduced-calorie Caesar dressing
	1 nectarine
SNACK	1 fresh apple
	4 oz skim milk
DINNER	One serving meatless chili (see recipe p. 255)
	⅓ C brown rice
	1 C steamed carrots
	½ C fruit salad
SNACK	4 reduced-fat vanilla wafers
	4 oz 100-calorie yogurt

Individuals following a 1500-calorie program may add:

    2 slices whole-wheat bread
    1 whole tomato sliced
    2 oz chicken
    1 tsp canola oil

Day 3	1200-calorie plan	1500-calorie plan
Calories	1212 calories	1489 calories
Protein (grams)	64	88
Fat (grams)	15	23
Saturated fat (grams)	4	5
Cholesterol (milligrams)	47	94
Sodium (milligrams)	3286	3681
Fiber (grams)	30	36

* Use low-sodium tomato juice in the gazpacho soup if concerned about sodium content of today's meal plan.

Day 4

BREAKFAST	1 slice cinnamon raisin toast
	1 apple (sliced and chopped)
	4 oz plain nonfat yogurt
	1 tsp vanilla
	1 Tbsp brown sugar
LUNCH	1 ½ C vegetable soup with tortellini (see recipe p. 239)
	6 saltines
	Carrot sticks
	1 orange
	4 oz skim milk
SNACK	1 C cantaloupe cubes
DINNER	1 serving fettuccine Alfredo (see recipe p. 261)
	Tossed salad
	2 Tbsp fat-free dressing
SNACK	1 C blueberries
	1 C 100-calorie yogurt
	1 ½ graham crackers

Individuals following a 1500-calorie meal plan may add:

1 slice raisin bread
1 C steamed zucchini
2 Tbsp grated Parmesan cheese
1 tsp olive oil

Day 4	1200-calorie plan	1500-calorie plan
Calories	1278	1472
Protein (grams)	55	63
Fat (grams)	16	26
Saturated fat (grams)	5	9
Cholesterol (milligrams)	34	44
Sodium (milligrams)	2248	2578
Fiber (grams)	17	20

Day 5

BREAKFAST   1 whole bagel (2 oz)
                  ½ grapefruit
                  2 Tbsp reduced-fat cream cheese
                  4 oz skim milk

LUNCH   2 slices low-calorie bread
                  2 oz turkey
                  Romaine lettuce, sliced tomato
                  1 Tbsp reduced-fat mayonnaise
                  1 small banana

SNACK   1 C strawberries
                  1 C 100-calorie yogurt

DINNER   3 oz baked haddock (see recipe p. 274)
                  1 baked sweet potato
                  1 Tbsp lite margarine
                  1 C green beans
                  1 orange

SNACK   ⅔ C complete bran cereal
                  4 oz skim milk

Individuals following a 1500-calorie meal plan may add:
                  1 C chicken noodle soup
                  6 saltine crackes
                  4 oz V-8 juice
                  2 Tbsp peanuts

Day 5	1200-calorie plan	1500-calorie plan
Calories	1214	1541
Protein (grams)	80	98
Fat (grams)	17	30
Saturated fat (grams)	3	5
Cholesterol (milligrams)	129	154
Sodium (milligrams)	1420	2113
Fiber (grams)	23	26

Day 6

BREAKFAST   1 pumpkin muffin (see recipe p. 246)
½ banana
4 oz skim milk
½ C 100-calorie yogurt

LUNCH   ½ whole-wheat pita pocket
2 oz tunafish with celery and onion
1 Tbsp reduced-calorie mayonnaise
Green leaf lettuce
Green and red pepper strips
1 apple
1 C skim milk

SNACK   1 pear

DINNER   2 oz grilled balsamic chicken (see recipe p. 267)
1 baked potato
1 dinner roll
1 Tbsp lite margarine
1 C broccoli
Tossed salad with fat-free dressing

SNACK   6 saltine crackers

Individuals following the 1500-calorie meal plan may add:
½ whole-wheat pita pocket
1 ½ graham crackers
1 whole carrot
1 oz tuna

Day 6	1200-calorie plan	1500-calorie plan
Calories	1220	1525
Protein (grams)	68	82
Fat (grams)	16	24
Saturated fat (grams)	4	5
Cholesterol (milligrams)	58	58
Sodium (milligrams)	1389	1959
Fiber (grams)	24	27

Day 7

BREAKFAST	⅓ C Grapenuts cereal
	1 C strawberries
	8 oz skim milk
LUNCH	1 C chunky minestrone soup (see recipe p. 240)
	1 slice whole-wheat bread
	1 oz turkey
	Lettuce, tomato
	Mustard
	8 oz skim milk
SNACK	Orange
DINNER	3 oz teriyaki swordfish (see recipe p. 272)
	½ C brown rice
	1 C steamed zucchini and summer squash
	1 C peaches
SNACK	1 oz pretzels
	1 apple

Individuals following the 1500-calorie meal plan may add:

⅓ C Grapenuts cereal
1 slice whole-wheat toast
½ C tomato juice
1 oz teriyaki swordfish
1 Tbsp lite margarine

Day 7	1200-calorie plan	1500-calorie plan
Calories	1199	1548
Protein (grams)	49	66
Fat (grams)	11	20
Saturated fat (grams)	2	3
Cholesterol (milligrams)	64	80
Sodium (milligrams)	3668*	4086*
Fiber (grams)	24	30

*Sodium is high due to teriyaki marinade. It is difficult to determine how much is absorbed by the swordfish.

The Case of Jack

~~~~~~

Using Diet to

Increase Your Odds

What more could anyone want? Jack was in love with a beautiful woman and very happy with his job as a plastics engineer. His weekends were free to spend with Kathy, and there was plenty of time for his other passions: tennis, hiking, and camping. Physically and emotionally, he was at the top of his form.

Yet still, something was missing. Sometimes in the evening as he drove home from work, the thought would cross his mind that perhaps he had settled for too little in life and he wondered what had become of the dreams he'd once had of doing something positive for society. Finally one night, he asked himself a question. "Do I really want to be remembered as the guy who invented a great plastic bag?"

The answer was No. After four years in the field of plastics, Jack gave up engineering and entered medical school. Almost immediately, his stress level began to rise. Having been away from the academic world for a long period, he was not sure that he could cope with the enormous demands of medicine and he found himself constantly anxious. Long hours and little sleep took their toll. He was already thin and full of nervous energy, and the pounds just kept coming off.

But by the end of his second year, Jack was confident. His hard work had paid off in terms of excellent grades and he began to believe he might make it as a doctor. Nothing, however, in the first two years of medical school prepares one for the last two. Jack's experience till then had been entirely classroom based. He had a good memory, he did his homework, took his exams, and passed with flying colors.

Then suddenly, without warning, he was in his third year and expected to act like a real doctor. His time was no longer his own and he was frequently expected to function on little more than an hour's sleep. He found out what it meant to have to tell someone he had AIDS or that the child who seemed so healthy in fact had leukemia.

By nature a perfectionist, Jack rapidly became almost obsessive during his third and fourth years. He remembers that time as a blur of work and too few snatched hours of precious sleep. At the hospital his eating habits deteriorated; living on high-fat snacks, he almost never found time to sit down for a proper meal—it was a pizza here, a burger there. In spite of his eating habits, Jack graduated from medical school at a slim 150 pounds. But the scales became less forgiving as he continued with his medical training.

By now, he and Kathy were married and he had decided on a career in interventional radiology: a very technical specialty involving evaluation of arteries for cholesterol blockages and clearing them by means of balloon angioplasties. It was a logical choice for an engineer.

The young couple moved from Pennsylvania to Massachusetts for Jack's final years of training. In spite of his overall satisfaction with what he was doing, Jack found the next few years extremely demanding. His time was not his own and he felt stretched. In addition to a heavy load at the hospital, he was now the father of two small children.

Exercise moved to the bottom of his list, and healthy eating was among the least of his worries. By the time Jack had finished his training, he weighed 175 pounds. No one meeting him at that time could have imagined he had once had a passion for outdoor activities.

In 1990, Jack, Kathy, and their two children moved to Manchester, New Hampshire, where Jack joined the staff of a medical center. His reputation as a superb radiologist grew rapidly and he was frequently invited to lecture at medical conferences. In addition, he made himself so accessible to all members of the hospital staff, that he generally did not get home until 7 or 8 P.M.

The demands of work and family obligations kept his stress level high, but far from objecting to the situation, Jack found it invigorating and believed it brought out the best in him.

His weight, however, continued to increase and by the time he was made a partner in his radiology group, he was up to 192 pounds. On a routine checkup, he learned that his cholesterol was at 260 milligrams per deciliter (over 60 milligrams higher than it should have been). Neither Jack nor his primary care physician was particularly worried about this finding. At age 38, a nonsmoker, with normal blood pressure, no family history of cardiac disease and not a diabetic, Jack was quite sure he was safe. In fact, he felt invincible. He continued to snack on donuts and candy bars at work, while at home it was not uncommon for him to consume a full bag of potato chips before dinner.

A scene in the hospital cafeteria at this time now comes back to haunt him. He was about to begin his lunch of a hamburger and french fries when a colleague asked him whether he ever worried about his high-fat diet. "You know," Jack answered, "I think this whole cholesterol thing is overrated." Jack laughs now. "I guess I ate my words."

In late February of 1992, Jack and Kathy decided impulsively to take a vacation aboard a cruise ship. Work had become nightmarishly demanding and even Jack, with his taste for stress and tension, admitted that he needed a break. The week immediately prior to departure was so busy he felt it wasn't worthwhile to go home at night since he would no sooner get there than it was time to go back to the hospital. When the week finally ended, he felt a palpable sense of relief. At last, he was going to relax.

The first day of the cruise was exactly as Jack and Kathy had hoped it would be. The children were happy and excited, and the parents were enjoying the experience of being together as a family. The food on the ship was delicious and rich, and they overindulged happily, reasoning that this was a once-in-a-lifetime vacation. By the second day, however, Jack began to feel a little odd.

On the third day, still queasy, he had a light breakfast and noticed a distinct improvement. By lunch he felt almost normal. He and his family were just about to start eating when three-year-old Joseph, recently toilet trained, announced that he had to go to the bathroom. Unfortunately, all the bathrooms in the dining area were being cleaned. Given the average three-year-old's inability to wait in such a situation, Jack's only option was to scoop Joe up in his arms and sprint the two flights of stairs to their cabin. Once there, he felt winded and as if there were a tight knot in his stomach. He and Joe returned to the dinner table, but while Jack managed to finish his meal, his discomfort increased.

Back in the cabin, he asked Kathy to get some motion sickness medicines. While she went to the ship's pharmacy to request it, he became nauseated and began sweating profusely. After swallowing the medicine Kathy brought, he went into the bathroom to take a cold shower, but once inside, he found he was too weak to stand up.

After giving the medicine a chance to work and feeling worse rather then better, Jack decided he'd better see the ship's doctor. Just as he made the decision, he began to have discomfort in his arms, shoulders, and jaw. The possibility of a heart attack flashed through his mind, but he quickly dismissed it—he knew he was just too young. It had to be motion sickness.

The doctor on duty thought otherwise. One look at his patient's ashen color persuaded him that it was Jack's heart and not his stomach that needed attention. An electrocardiogram (ECG) confirmed his fears. Jack was indeed having a heart attack. As a radiologist, Jack didn't read many electrocardiograms, but there was no mistaking what he was seeing on the screen across the room. Even without that as confirming evidence, it would have been difficult for him to continue ignoring how he felt. He was now experiencing severe chest pressure and continued jaw, arm, and shoulder pain. Morphine, commonly given to control heart attack pain, caused him to vomit repeatedly, making matters worse. Finally, he got some relief with a combination of nitroglycerin and heparin. Nitroglycerin helps dilate the heart's arteries, allowing better blood flow to areas not getting enough oxygen. Heparin, while not able to break up blood clots in the coronary arteries, can prevent an existing clot from becoming larger and new clots from forming.

In general, a heart attack occurs when a cholesterol deposit or plaque within a coronary artery cracks, exposing the inside of the plaque to the blood, which instantly activates the body's clotting mechanisms, causing a large clot to form on top of the plaque. This can lead to a complete or nearly complete blockage of the coronary artery.

Had Jack been in a hospital, he would have been given one of the so-called clot-busting medications which act to break up an existing clot and can, if given early enough, prevent the damage that a heart attack can cause.

With heparin and nitroglycerin, the ship's doctor had exhausted his resources for treating Jack. He needed to reach a hospital as quickly as possible and receive a clot-busting medication. Speed was essential because these medications only work well on fresh clots, and should be given during the first six hours after chest pains begin. The decision was made to turn the ship around and head for the Bahamas (the trip seemed endless), and from there, get Jack on a medi-jet back to the United States.

The next few hours could have been lifted from a made-for-TV-movie: the handsome young radiologist, gray-white in color, lying in the ship's infirmary, the frantic wife making desperate calls on the ship's radio to arrange for medical transport to Miami, the dramatic lowering of the entire family from the cruise ship to a smaller boat, the journey through the dark ocean waters to the Freeport, Bahamas dock, where an ambulance crew was waiting to administer the clot-dissolving medication—with only minutes to spare before the six-hour deadline—the medi-jet flight to Florida, and the final wild ambulance ride through the streets of Miami, with Kathy and the children following in a taxi. The taxi driver, urged on by Kathy, managed to beat the ambulance to the hospital, giving her what seemed like hours to pace the corridors of the emergency room, certain that Jack had been brought to a different hospital, and wondering why they had ever gone on the cruise in the first place.

When the ambulance finally arrived, Jack was taken immediately into an examining room where a team of doctors began to evaluate him. Kathy, almost speechless with relief at seeing him still alive, was then able to turn her attention to her exhausted children, who were overwhelmed by all that was happening.

Jack was soon moved to the hospital's cardiac intensive care unit (CICU), and Kathy did her best to settle the children in the waiting room for the night. Although it was Jack who had suffered the physical pain, Kathy was perhaps in the more difficult situation, grappling alone with visions of a nightmarish future. What should she say to her children? Was it encouraging false hopes to tell them that Daddy would be fine? And what to say to Jack himself? Heavily medicated for pain and feeling worlds better, he was now refusing to admit that he'd had a heart attack.

The next day Jack's aunt arrived to escort the children back to New England to stay with Kathy's sister. Once they left, Kathy was better able to focus on Jack, but he continued to deny that anything serious had occurred. Kathy kept wondering what was going on in Jack's mind: "Didn't he see that cardiogram himself? Didn't he say he could read it from across the room? Has he really forgotten what happened on the ship?" At that point she was very grateful to Jack's doctor who explained to her that denial is a commonly experienced first phase in the emotional adjustment to heart disease and that Jack's reaction was perfectly normal.

On Monday, Jack was scheduled for a cardiac catheterization—a procedure that allows visualizing the inside of the heart's arteries. (See Glossary.) Early that morning the CICU nurse stopped his heparin (the medication which prevents formation of new blood clots), a routine practice that prevents significant bleeding during the catheterization procedure. Almost within minutes, Jack began experiencing the same nausea he had had on the cruise ship. At first, he tried to dismiss it as a psychosomatic reaction to the heparin being turned off, but when it increased, he called the nurse.

The electrocardiogram she immediately ran showed the same grim picture Jack had seen on the cruise ship. Within minutes he was whisked to the catheterization laboratory for an angiogram, a procedure in which dye is injected into the coronary arteries to determine if they are being blocked by cholesterol. The doctors told him that if a large blockage was found they would want to perform an angioplasty. Now Jack was on his home turf. As an interventional radiologist, he spent his days evaluating arteries in the arms, legs, and neck for blockages, and he was very skilled at performing angioplasties of these blood vessels. Even though his practice did not include the heart arteries, he knew what a blockage looked like, and he could see for himself that his right coronary artery (RCA) was completely blocked and his circumflex artery about 85 percent blocked. These graphic findings finally persuaded him that the impossible had in fact occurred: he had had a heart attack.

Because Jack's electrocardiogram indicated that the RCA was causing his symptoms, his doctors decided to try an angioplasty only on the right artery and to leave the circumflex artery alone. Angioplasties have about a 70 percent success rate and Jack was one of the lucky ones. With the blockage in his artery reduced from 100 to 20 percent, he was ready to begin cardiac rehabilitation.

In the midst of all the drama and chaos in the hospital, Kathy had had little time to think about herself. But just before Jack's discharge, it occurred to her that she had missed her menstrual period. Jack's cardiologist, amused at the unusual request, ran a pregnancy test for her, and she and Jack were delighted when it came back positive. It seemed to them a beautiful promise of the future, and they resolved that when the new baby arrived, it would be into the arms of a healthy father.

They decided not to rush back to New Hampshire. Both felt instinctively that they needed time alone as a couple to adjust to the experience they had just gone through. They took long walks together, talking endlessly about what had happened and what they wanted for the future.

As a result, they began to change their eating habits and develop a daily exercise program. Kathy, however, was clear about one thing: as supportive as she wanted to be for Jack, she had no desire to take responsibility for his health. She told him she had no plans to nag or even cajole him into eating properly or exercising regularly. That had to be his own decision. Jack's immediate response was that he was going to conquer his heart disease. He refused to allow it to conquer him.

By the time the couple returned home, they felt strong, ready to meet their families and friends, and to endure the onslaught of advice that began coming their way almost immediately.

"It was difficult meeting people afterward," Jack recalled. "There were a lot of platitudes." Everyone seemed to have some sage bit of advice to offer, but the most popular line was, "Take it easy, Jack. Just remember to smell the roses." He heard that cliché so often that he began carrying a little card in his pocket. When he sensed that the moment was at hand, he would pull out the card and hold it up. It read "I am smelling the roses."

Keeping a sense of humor helped a lot, but more important was the support Jack got from his family. Kathy took a heart-healthy eating class at the hospital and became a very creative low-fat cook. Even the children, once they understood the importance of new eating habits, were eager to change their diets and quickly learned which foods were high in fat and which were not. By the age of seven, Ashley could read labels and determine for herself whether a particular food was acceptable or not. She couldn't understand why other people were not as sensible as her family—in restaurants, she has been known to ask, quite audibly, why the people at the next table weren't eating "heart-healthy" foods.

But as anxious as Kathy and Jack were that their children develop good eating habits, they were determined not to make them feel different from their friends. So rather than send carrots and celery in their school lunches, snacks that they happily eat at home, Kathy packs them treats like fresh strawberries, blueberries, grapes, and little packages of raisins. They go to McDonald's occasionally, but even the children don't want to do it very often.

For Jack, the new routine of diet, exercise, and cardiac rehabilitation classes proved much easier to adjust to than he had expected. On the emotional level, however, things were more difficult. The fleeting thoughts of death that had come to him in Florida came much more frequently in New Hampshire, and nightmares about Kathy struggling to raise three children on her own began to haunt his sleep. Finally, he confided in his cardiologist, Dr. Bill Bradley, and learned to his surprise that many people had such feelings following a heart attack. Somehow, just knowing that he wasn't abnormal was a great comfort to Jack.

Dr. Bradley also thought Jack might benefit from talking to a psychiatrist. Although somewhat taken aback by this idea at first, Jack decided to give it a try. The stress-reduction techniques Jack learned and the insight he gained during his sessions with the psychiatrist did make a big difference. Gradually, the nightmares stopped, and Jack's confidence in his ability to survive grew steadily.

I met him about six months after his heart attack. I had just come to The New England Heart Institute in Manchester to begin a clinic for the treatment of cholesterol disorders. Jack gave me a tour of the radiology department, in the course of which he asked which medical group I was going to join. When I said I would be in cardiology, he mentioned that he had had a heart attack six months earlier.

I had to admit it took me by surprise. Jack was fit, trim, and looked in excellent condition. Must have a bad family history, I thought, just as he volunteered the information that he had totally changed his life with a new diet, an exercise program, and a 30-pound weight loss. Since he was being so open, I asked about his cholesterol level.

He said it had been quite high, but that with the help of dietitian Mary Card, he was following a diet with no more than 20 percent of its total calories derived from fat. In contrast, most so-called low-fat diets obtain a full 30 percent of their calories from fat. Such diets are not usually very successful, typically achieving only about a 5 percent reduction in low-density lipoprotein cholesterol (the bad cholesterol). Mary Card had explained to Jack that a diet consisting of only 20 percent fat is often successful in lowering a patient's total cholesterol by a matching 20 percent. Such a substantial drop may allow a person to avoid drug therapy entirely, or at least be on very low levels of medications. Jack, however, was already on a cholesterol-lowering medication.

I suggested a more thorough cholesterol evaluation and Jack agreed. In order to evaluate his cholesterol profile independent of drugs, I asked him to stop his cholesterol-lowering medication for one month. Sometimes such a halt reveals that a patient is on the wrong medication or even that medication is no longer necessary.

After a month without medications, Jack's profile looked like this:

	Jack's Level	Desirable Level
Total cholesterol	233 mg/dl	Less than 200 mg/dl
Triglycerides	115 mg/dl	Less than 150 mg/dl
HDL cholesterol	43 mg/dl	Greater than 45 mg/dl
LDL cholesterol	167 mg/dl	Less than 100 mg/dl

Although these values represented about a 20 percent improvement from his preheart attack level, they were still too high for Jack. Once a person has documented heart disease, the National Cholesterol Education Program (NCEP) guidelines recommend an LDL (bad cholesterol) level of no more than 100 mg/dl. At that level, existing heart disease may regress—in other words, some of the cholesterol deposits in the coronary arteries may get smaller.

The desirable level for triglycerides listed for Jack is actually somewhat lower than the upper limit of 200 mg/dl allowed by the National

Cholesterol Education Program. I use an upper limit of 150 mg/dl because many studies have shown that, once triglycerides rise above 150 mg/dl, cardiac risk increases. In part this happens because, when triglycerides rise above 150 mg/dl, persons tend to have a particularly dangerous kind of LDL cholesterol (bad cholesterol) called small, dense LDL-C.

Jack had not been aware of the possibility that he could reduce the cholesterol deposits in his arteries and was delighted to hear of it, since it addressed an issue that had worried him ever since his heart attack.

Before leaving Florida he had undergone an exercise stress test. It had revealed that the area of his heart served by the circumflex artery (which had the 85 percent blockage) was not getting enough blood flow during exercise and that he was therefore at risk for another attack. Jack's concern was whether his efforts to prevent future cardiac problems would be useless because of his past medical history.

With the possibility of regression in mind, Jack was eager to try out the new therapy I was suggesting. I told him that he would probably benefit from niacin and began him on a low dose of 250 mg three times a day. Although this dose has virtually no effect on cholesterol levels, it allows the body to accustom itself to the medication. Over time, Jack was gradually able to increase his niacin dose to 2500 mg per day, and his resulting cholesterol profile showed a dramatic improvement.

	Jack's Level	Desirable Level
Total cholesterol	146 mg/dl	Less than 200 mg/dl
Triglycerides	18 mg/dl	Less than 150 mg/dl
HDL cholesterol	63 mg/dl	Greater than 45 mg/dl
LDL cholesterol	79 mg/dl	Less than 100 mg/dl

Both of us were very excited by these numbers. I told Jack that it would not be surprising if the cholesterol deposit in his circumflex artery began to diminish. This is not an overnight process, but it has been documented as early as one year after beginning a very aggressive cholesterol-lowering program. I told Jack that the only way to be absolutely certain that regression had occurred would be to perform a repeat catheterization of the artery involved, but because of the inherent risks of the procedure, I didn't think it was appropriate to perform it just to satisfy our curiosity.

Jack, Dr. Bradley, and I decided that the best approach would be to monitor him according to his symptoms and to have him undergo an occasional stress test to look for improvement. Improvement on the stress test would give us some idea as to whether or not his circumflex blockage had decreased in size.

Jack continued in excellent health for over a year until suddenly one weekend he began experiencing the same sort of nausea and vague chest discomfort he had had on the cruise ship. Concerned, he went to see Dr. Bradley, who immediately performed a cardiogram. When that was normal he put Jack on the treadmill for an exercise stress test, which was also normal. Although these results were reassuring, Dr. Bradley, worried about the same cholesterol deposit that was troubling Jack, reccommended a repeat catheterization. Jack agreed to this and the procedure was performed the following morning.

The results were cause for rejoicing. The deposit in Jack's circumflex artery was now only 65 percent—a significant reduction. In other words Jack's cardiac disease had regressed. His nausea proved to have been caused by an intestinal bug, and within a few days, he was back on his feet and feeling fine.

With such positive evidence of his cardiac well-being, he and Kathy decided to celebrate. For years they had been longing to go to Italy for a holiday, but after Jack's heart attack, uncertainty about the availability of medical facilities abroad had made them hesitate. Now there was nothing to stop them.

Their trip was a blissful dream and they returned rested, refreshed, and ready to continue with a life that now looked better than ever: their marriage was strong, their three children (John was born nine months after his father's heart attack) healthy and happy. The two older children had been tested for cholesterol abnormalities and thanks to their excellent diet, their results were perfect; John's level will be checked when he is two. Jack's work was satisfying and challenging, and his heart almost as good as new.

3

‿‿‿‿‿‿‿‿‿‿‿‿‿‿‿‿‿‿‿‿‿‿‿‿‿‿‿‿‿‿

Making Exercise a

Lifetime Commitment

The exercise enthusiast has never had it so good. Most cities now have extensive and well-designed bicycle paths, many parks provide workout areas (often called vita courses), shoes for every possible sort of activity are widely available, and sports shops stock equipment in a range that only a few years ago was unimaginable.

So why are so many Americans still on the sidelines? A single scan of the supermarket magazine racks confirms our national obsession with slimness and quick weight loss. But an equally quick glance at the contents of most shopping carts explains why we remain fat.

Like the magic pill many Americans continue to long for in the quest for a thin body, the desire is equally great for a magic piece of equipment that will give all the benefits and power of exercise without having to go to the trouble of actually breaking a sweat.

Unfortunately, in the pursuit of fitness, there is no magic anything. The fact is starting and sustaining an exercise program is difficult. Rememember learning to ride a bike? Remember how you teetered and tottered precariously across two squares of the sidewalk before losing your balance and toppling over? But remember how you kept at it, getting on again and again until suddenly everything clicked into place and you were sailing down the street, on your own at last.

Exercise is like that. However, unlike children, many of us are unwilling to fall, get up, and try again. But if you can make it through the

87

first few weeks of an exercise program, picturing yourself as a six-year-old, rediscovering your childish stubbornness, gritting your teeth, and staying with it, you will experience the same delicious sense of pleasure you felt when for the first time you coasted off on your own.

Your body can become fit beginning today. We in America have become accustomed to letting machines do our work, believing them to be more efficient, faster, and stronger than we are. But do you know any machine that can adapt itself endlessly and become leaner and stronger even when 60 or 70 years old?

Your body is you. If you follow the diet outlined in Chapter 2 and the exercise program outlined here, your life will change. Your body will become a source of pleasure and pride and a reflection of the you inside, rather than a thing you drag around like some distant and unloved relative.

The benefits of regular exercise go far beyond just weight control. People who exercise have leaner muscles and stronger bones than those who do not. Their hearts are more efficient at pumping blood and their muscles better at extracting oxygen from that blood. Active people have lower blood pressure, better sleep patterns, less stress, and in general a longer life span than their sedentary friends.

Many people are willing to change their diets because they see this as the key to weight loss, but when it comes to exercise, they just don't have the time. Nice try, I tell them. In fact, when patients tell me they can't find time to exercise, I tell them, politely, of course, that they are mistaken. They have the same 24 hours a day that everyone else has. The difference is that they haven't yet learned to regard exercise as an essential part of their lives—as essential, in fact, as eating or sleeping. Once they really understand this, they make time for it. No matter how important the job or how busy the day, everyone can find time for exercise if he or she is determined to do so.

People who diet without exercise are really only making things more difficult for themselves. They go through the misery of deprivation and hunger pangs without the satisfaction of long-term weight loss. Americans spend a staggering $30 billion a year on diets while the statistics on obesity continue to rise: between 1980 and 1991, the number of overweight Americans climbed 8 percent. At present, 33.4 percent of American adults are overweight.

The logic is fairly simple. When calories are drastically restricted (especially when the individual fails to exercise) the body utilizes both fat and muscles for energy. Fat loss is desirable, but muscle loss is not. It is our muscle which is responsible for burning calories. Maintaining your weight after a diet without exercise is difficult because fewer calories are required when you have diminished your muscle mass. Almost inevitably, the lost weight creeps back, this time in the form of fat. The person ends up in worse shape than when he or she began.

If, on the other hand, moderate caloric restriction is combined with exercise, the result will be weight loss and muscle gain. Since muscle is more efficient than fat, more calories will be burned whether the person is active or at rest. People undertaking such a program should realize that in the beginning, progress will appear slower then when on a crash diet, because they are replacing fat with muscle and muscle weighs more than fat.

This can be quite discouraging: enormous discipline and effort translate into only a five-or six-pound difference on the bathroom scale. It is important to look for other evidence: How do you feel? Do your clothes fit better? Has your blood pressure improved? Are your cholesterol and blood sugar levels lower? Are you sleeping better at night? Do you have more energy during the day? Weight loss is only one indicator—you don't want to become a slave to your scale.

With this understanding of the importance and the benefits of regular exercise, let's get down to the practical details—how to design a program that will become an integral part of your life, something you not only look forward to but cannot imagine doing without.

Your program should consist primarily of aerobic exercise. Aerobic means "with oxygen." When you exercise at a steady pace without becoming exhausted or out of breath, chances are you are performing an aerobic exercise. During aerobic exercise, your muscles use oxygen to burn both glucose (sugar) and body fat. Anaerobic exercise (weight lifting, for example), by contrast, is performed in short bursts, does not require oxygen, and burns only glucose, not fat. Since burning fat is your goal, you will want to choose an aerobic exercise. This does not mean that you might not benefit from the toning that anaerobic exercises such as weight lifting provide. If you do choose to include anaerobic activities in your fitness program, I recommend that they be in addition to your aerobic program and not in place of it.

In order to achieve aerobic fitness, it is not necessary to join an aerobics class (although the camaraderie of a class can be invaluable in helping novices stick with it): walking, jogging, cycling, and swimming are all good aerobic exercises.

These activities, however, can all become anaerobic if you push yourself too hard. You have probably switched into anaerobic metabolism if you find yourself totally out of breath while exercising vigorously. Another tipoff is painful, burning muscles, which are a direct result of the buildup of lactic acid which is a typical result of anaerobic exercise. If you experience these symptoms, just slow down. As your fitness improves, it will become more difficult to shift into anaerobic metabolism. Pat yourself on the back then: not only have you reached an important milestone in your program, but your body will automatically become more efficient at burning fat.

The F.I.T. Principle

When designing your exercise program, we recommend that you use the F.I.T. principle: Frequency, Intensity, and Time.

Frequency

Since I have met very few individuals who overtrain when first starting an exercise program, I find it is safe to ask the beginner to exercise as often as possible. In order to achieve a conditioning effect, however, you will need to exercise at least three times per week.

Walking has a very low injury rate, particularly compared with jogging. It is certainly reasonable to start off walking five times per week. If you decide to initiate jogging or another high-impact sport, you must allow sufficient time between sessions to avoid muscle fatigue and injury. Cross training is a great way to exercise daily while decreasing the risk of injury. In cross training, one alternates sessions of high (jogging, aerobic dancing) and low (walking, bicycling, or swimming) impact sessions.

Intensity

To make the most of your exercise, it is important to work at the proper intensity. This is achieved when your body is working hard enough to start changing fat into muscle, but not so hard that it switches into anaerobic metabolism. Gauging intensity takes practice, but there are several tools to help you judge.

Your heart rate (the number of times your heart beats per minute) is an indirect measurement of how hard your body is working. Determining a "target heart rate range" for safe, effective aerobic exercise is a common method of measuring exercise intensity.

First, figure your maximum heart rate, using this simple formula:

220 − Your age = Maximum heart rate per minute (MHR)
Example: 45-year-old male or female
220 − 45 = 175 beats per minute

Luckily, it isn't necessary to exercise at your maximum heart rate to become fit! About 50 to 85 percent of your MHR is your "target heart rate range." As you can see, this is a wide range. People who are less fit or who have medical conditions will typically begin at the lower range, while active, healthier individuals may strive for higher heart rates.

> Example: 45-year-old male or female
> Target heart rate: 175 × 0.50 = 88 beats per minute
> 175 × 0.85 = 149 beats per minute
> Range: 88 to 149 beats per minute

Once you have determined your target heart rate, you need to know how to take your own pulse. It is easiest to find and count using the carotid (neck) pulse. To locate the exact spot, place two fingers of one hand on the voicebox (center of your neck), then move one inch to the right or the left (you have two carotid arteries). You should be able to feel your pulse. Never apply pressure to both carotid arteries at the same time, since this decreases blood flow to the brain and can cause dizziness. A radial or wrist pulse (located on the thumb side of the wrist) can also be used.

A 10-second pulse count, which is then multiplied by six, for your one-minute heart rate is the best way to monitor intensity without seriously interrupting exercise. Always begin your count with zero. Checking your pulse before, during, and after exercise will ensure ideal intensity and give valuable insight into your progress. As your body adapts to the new regime, your heart rate will be lower for a given amount of work. You can use the following chart for an estimate of your target heart rate and 10-second pulse.

Another method of determining exercise intensity is the Borg Scale of Rated Perceived Exertion (RPE). On a scale of 6 to 20, the level between 12 and 14, "Somewhat hard," is your training zone.

Because it is a relative measure, using the RPE scale takes some practice.

By far the easiest method of determining whether you are working hard enough is to use the "Talk Test." If you can't talk without gasping or stopping your routine altogether, you are working too hard. On the other hand, if you find you can deliver a short lecture (say, on the value of exercise), you could probably work a little harder.

Time

This is determined by the amount of time needed at your target heart rate to improve your fitness. We recommend that you spend 30 minutes in aerobic exercise on most days. The minimum I recommend for cardiovascular

Target Heart Rates

Age	Max HR	50 to 85% (target HR)	10-second pulse
20	200	100 to 170	17 to 28
25	195	98 to 166	17 to 28
30	190	95 to 162	16 to 27
35	185	92 to 157	16 to 27
40	180	90 to 153	15 to 26
45	175	88 to 149	15 to 26
50	170	85 to 145	14 to 25
55	165	82 to 140	14 to 25
60	160	80 to 136	13 to 24
65	155	78 to 131	13 to 24
70	150	75 to 128	12 to 23
75	145	72 to 123	12 to 23

fitness is 30 minutes, three times a week. Some studies do indicate that benefit can be derived with as little as 20 minutes, three times a week. In general, however, most people need more because they also need to lose weight or to improve their lipid profile. This amount of time does not include warming up and cooling down (more on this later).

There is mounting evidence that several short sessions in one day are as beneficial as one long one. So people who are short on time, or who don't yet have the stamina for a 30-minute session, may find two 15-minute sessions easier to manage. The only drawback here is you will spend more time warming up and cooling down, as this really is essential both before and after each exercise session. If you have time, then, for a quick bicycle ride in the morning and a walk at noon, do it. Don't worry that you don't have the full half-hour.

Do Calories Count?

Tracking calories expended during an exercise session is another helpful means of monitoring your progress. The American Heart Association Scientific Statement on Exercise recommends that "individuals should be encouraged to engage in activities requiring up to 2000 calories per week for maximum health benefits. Walking 20 miles each week is one way to accomplish this goal." I do not recommend that you start out walking this distance; instead, I suggest that you build up gradually. Remember

Borg Scale of Rated Perceived Exertion (RPE)

6	
7	Very, very light
8	
9	Very light
10	
11	Fairly light
12	
13	Somewhat hard
14	
15	Hard
16	
17	Very hard
18	
19	Very, very hard
20	

Source: Borg GA, Psychophysical basis of perceived exertion. Medicine and Science in Sports and Exercise 1982; 14: 377–381. With the generous permission of Williams & Wilkins.

you will still derive cardiovascular benefit if you exercise as little as 20 minutes, three times a week (an expenditure of about 300 calories). See the following table for information on the caloric expenditure of various activities.

Getting Started

The first essential is to choose an exercise you like and that you think you may grow to love. Walking is emphasized in this book because it is an aerobic activity that has a very low injury rate. The beauty of walking is that it requires no special skills or equipment, it can be done year round, alone or with friends, and can easily be incorporated into your daily routine—by getting off the bus two stops early, or walking to the post office rather than driving.

If you decide to purchase a piece of exercise equipment, do your homework. Make sure that the exercise you will be doing on it is aerobic, and that it works large muscle groups rhythmically and continuously. Ask yourself if this is really an exercise you will stick with. It may be possible to borrow or rent a piece of equipment for a month or two before investing in it. There is nothing quite so discouraging as an expensive stationary bicycle gathering dust in the family room.

Caloric Expenditure* of Various Activities

Activity	Calories per Hour
Aerobic Dancing	280 to 700
Backpacking	350 to 770
Badminton, competitive singles	480
Basketball	360 to 660
Bicycling	
10 mph	420
11 mph	480
12 mph	600
13 mph	660
Calisthenics, heavy	600
Gardening, much lifting, stooping, and digging	500
Golf, pull/carry clubs	280 to 490
Golf, power cart	140 to 210
Handball, competitive	660
Hiking	210 to 490
Horseback riding	210 to 560
Mowing, pushing hand mower	450
Rope skipping, vigorous	800
Rowing machine	840
Running	
5 mph	600
6 mph	750
7 mph	870
8 mph	1020
9 mph	1130
10 mph	1285
Shoveling, heavy	660
Skating, ice or roller, rapid	700
Skiing, downhill, vigorous	600
Skiing, cross-country	
2.5 mph	560
4 mph	600
5 mph	700
8 mph	1020
Snowshoeing	490 to 980
Swimming, 25 to 50 yards per min	360 to 750
Tennis (singles)	420 to 480

Activity	Calories per Hour
Tennis (doubles)	300 to 360
Walking	
Level road, 4 mph (fast)	420
Upstairs	600 to 1080
Uphill, 3.5 mph	480 to 900
Wood chopping	560

* Caloric expenditure is based on a 150-lb person. There is a 10 percent increase in caloric expenditure for each 15 lb over this weight, and a 10 percent decrease for each 15 lb under.

Sources: Adapted from E. L. Wynder, The Book of Health: The American Health Foundation. New York: Franklin Watts, 1981. W. D. McArdle, F. I. Katch, and V. L. Katch, Exercise Physiology. Philadelphia: Lea & Febiger, 1981.

Avoiding Injury

Since you want to continue your walking program for life, it is important to take precautions aimed at avoiding injury. I recommend the following:

1. Always walk with your head erect, back straight, and abdominal muscles tightened slightly. Swing your arms slightly as you stride. Step off the ball of your foot and land on your heel.
2. Invest in a good pair of walking shoes.
3. When possible, opt for walking on soft surfaces such as a jogging track, dirt road, or grass. Walking on the sidewalk is not as desirable, but is certainly better than not walking at all. If you must walk on concrete, it is even more important to invest in a good pair of walking shoes.
4. Warmup and cool-down periods prepare your body to start and end exercising. Make sure you include adequate time for each of these in your walking program. I recommend the following warmup and cool-down programs.

Warmup

A 5-to 10-minute period of gradual aerobic exercise allows your body to safely and comfortably reach its target heart rate. This warmup generally consists of a less intense version of whatever exercise you will be doing. A muscle that is adequately warmed up performs better and is less likely to be injured. The warmup can, but does not have to, include stretching. You will find diagrams of some basic stretches at the end of this chapter.

They will look familiar and can easily be integrated into any warmup routine.

Cool-Down

The purpose of a cool-down period is to gradually bring your heart rate down to the preexercise level. To cool down, slowly (over the course of 5 to 10 minutes) decrease the intensity of exercise. The cool-down phase prevents blood from pooling in your legs, reducing the risk of fainting and dizziness. In general, a heart rate below 100 beats per minute (16 beats per 10-second count) indicates sufficient cooling down.

This is the best period for stretching. Static stretching is performed by lengthening a particular muscle and holding the stretch position for 10 to 30 seconds. Relax and breathe while stretching and focus your attention on the muscle you are working with. If a particular muscle seems tight or painful, direct your breathing to that area and relax. (This is a common yoga technique.) Each major joint and muscle group of the body should be stretched.

Because conditioning effects occur at the target heart rate, the warm-up and cool-down are in addition to the recommended minimum 30 minutes of aerobic exercise. Thus your total workout time will be about 45 minutes. As you reach the maintenance phase of the walking program outlined in this chapter, your total workout may often be as long as an hour and 20 minutes, including warmup and cool-down.

Rate of Progression

We all enjoy making progress. It is especially exciting to see our strength increase while our waistlines shrink. The American College of Sports Medicine defines three stages for an aerobic exercise program.

Initial Conditioning Stage

During the first four to six weeks of your new program, your body will gradually adapt to the demands of aerobic exercise. During this time period, exercise intensity should be at the lower end of your target heart rate range (50 to 70%). Many beginners have difficulty sustaining the exercise intensity necessary to reach their target heart rate.

Don't worry: If you stick to it, you will get there (in some cases, the initial conditioning stage can be extended to two or three months). Be patient with yourself. Beginning an exercise program isn't easy.

The most important thing during this initial phase is consistency. Be conservative: People who progress gradually are less likely to injure themselves than those who try to reach and sustain 85 percent of their maximum heart rate on the very first day. We recommend beginning with an exercise program (generally walking) for a total of 12 to 15 minutes per session. During the initial conditioning stage you will gradually build up to 20 minutes of uninterrupted exercise. (See Initial Conditioning Stage in The Walking Program section which follows.)

Improvement Stage

During this 12- to 24-week stage, the rate of progression is more rapid. Intensity may be increased to 85 percent of your target heart rate range and the duration of an exercise session is increased every two to three weeks. During this phase you will work your way up to a total of 30 minutes of uninterrupted exercise, and by its conclusion you should be exercising at least four to six times per week. (See Improvement Stage in The Walking Program section which follows.)

Maintenance Stage

When the desired level of fitness is reached, maintenance begins. The maintenance phase typically begins six months after you initiate training. You now need to make your lifetime commitment to staying fit. Now that you have succeeded in making exercise a part of your daily routine, you never want to break stride again.

Now is the time to increase your exercise sessions to a maximum of 60 minutes. You should find by now that the whole business has actually become enjoyable. With your new strength and muscle tone, you may want to try different types of exercise, including some which you may have thought beyond you. Do discuss your plans with your primary care physician, however, before embarking on any new program.

At this point many people consider participation in walking events, generally for a good cause, or fun runs. Maybe you are ready to try a day hike up a nearby mountain. The possibilities are endless. (See Maintenance Stage in The Walking Program section which follows.)

The Program

Many people I work with say that they enjoy reading about exercise and its merits, but that when it comes to planning their exercise routine, they aren't exactly sure what to do. In the next few pages, you will find specific instructions on how to proceed through the three phases I have outlined here. This is a generic exercise program that many people will be able to use as is. At the end of this chapter, however, you will find my recommendations for people with "special concerns": high choles-

terol, cardiac disease, diabetes, weight loss goals, arthritis, and pregnancy.

The Walking Program

INITIAL CONDITIONING STAGE

This stage lasts from four to six weeks, depending on your initial fitness
level. If you feel comfortable, you can progress more rapidly than suggested here.

Weeks	Frequency (per week)	Intensity	Time (minutes)
1 and 2	3 to 5 times	50 to 60% THR[a] "Talk Test"[b]	12 to 15
3 and 4	3 to 5 times	50 to 60% THR "Talk Test" Borg Scale: 11 to 13[c]	15 to 20
5 and 6	3 to 5 times	60 to 70 THR "Talk Test" Borg Scale: 11 to 13	15 to 20

[a]THR, or Target Heart Rate Range; see pages 90–92.
[b]The "Talk Test" is described on page 91.   [c]The Borg Scale is described on page 93.

Your goal is a caloric expenditure of 100 to 200 calories per session, and
300 to 800 calories per week. Walking one mile generally expends 100
calories.

IMPROVEMENT STAGE

This stage lasts between 12 to 24 weeks, again depending on how your
body adjusts to the demands of the program.

Weeks	Frequency (per week)	Intensity	Time (minutes)
7 and 8	4 to 5 times	70 to 80% THR "Talk Test" Borg Scale: 13 to 15	20
9 and 10	4 to 5 times	70 to 80% THR "Talk Test" Borg Scale: 13 to 15	20 to 25
11 and 12	4 to 6 times	70 to 80% THR "Talk Test" Borg Scale: 13 to 15	20 to 25
13 to 24	4 to 6 times	70 to 85% THR "Talk Test" Borg Scale: 13 to 15	25 to 30

MAINTENANCE STAGE

After six months of aerobic conditioning, you have achieved a significant improvement in your fitness level—isn't it wonderful? Prolonged exercise sessions are no longer so difficult as they were early in your program. You are well on your way to a lifetime of fitness, weight control, and cardiovascular health.

During the maintenance stage, you should extend the length of your exercise sessions to a maximum of 60 minutes. For example, the following would be a typical F.I.T. (frequency, intensity, time) plan during your maintenance stage:

Exercise	Frequency (per week)	Intensity	Time (minutes)
Walking	5 to 6 times	70 to 85% THR	45 to 60

Other Activities

Throughout this section I have stressed that maximum health benefits occur when you expend 2000 calories per week. One way to do this is by walking 20 miles per week.

Walking has been emphasized because it has a high success and low injury rate. Walking is, however, not the only acceptable aerobic exercise. During the maintenance stage you may continue to use walking as your primary form of exercise, as already outlined, or you may add some variety to your program by cross training.

Cross training allows you to exercise different muscle groups and is an excellent hedge against bad weather. Following is a review of some other aerobic activities that are suitable for cross training. Use the table on page 94 to determine, based on your speed, the length of time you need to exercise to expend about 300 calories. For example, a 150 lb individual who runs at a speed of 5 miles per hour will need to run for 30 minutes to expend 300 calories.

AEROBIC DANCING

This is a group activity which offers aerobic conditioning in a fun environment. High-impact aerobics, which can involve considerable joint stress, should be avoided by individuals with diabetic retinopathy (a disease of the eye) and by those who have joint, back, or other musculoskeletal problems.

Low-impact aerobic classes are easy to find and offer an excellent workout. With practice, you will become more supple and flexible, and your muscular definition will improve. When you choose an aerobics class, make sure that your instructor is professionally qualified.

CROSS-COUNTRY SKIING

Cross-country skiing has the potential to greatly improve cardiovascular fitness. It is the ultimate "fat-burning" aerobic exercise because it uses the large muscles in both your arms and legs. Although it is strenuous, it is low impact and has a very low injury rate (much lower than running, for example). Becoming proficient at cross-country skiing takes some practice, skill, and, of course, snow. Many people take a lesson or two when first beginning a skiing program. For the nonwinter months, indoor cross-country skiing simulators are also an excellent choice.

CYCLING: (STATIONARY, ROAD, OR TRAIL)

Cycling is a low-impact exercise that provides excellent cardiovascular conditioning. While cycling does emphasize your leg muscles, some home equipment incorporates arm conditioning as well.

Outdoor (road, trail, or mountain) bicycling is higher impact than stationary cycling because of the added challenges, such as wind and hills, to say nothing of traffic.

JOGGING

Jogging is a high-impact activity but has a fairly low injury rate when performed only once or twice per week as part of a cross-training routine. It is very important to make sure that you warm up adequately before jogging.

The best way to begin jogging is a walk/jog program. Based on your own level of fitness, alternate periods of walking with periods of jogging. I recommend jogging for two to three minutes, followed by a similar period of walking. Gradually lengthen your jogging and shorten your walking periods. Keep in mind that the walking periods should not be "rest." While walking, you should aim to keep your heart rate within your target range. Ultimately, you may feel comfortable jogging for 30 to 45 minutes at a stretch. As with any new exercise program, I recommend discussing jogging with your primary care physician before you begin. If you already have an orthopedic problem, such as a knee or back injury, I strongly recommend working only on the previously described walking program. Why risk further injury. You want an exercise you can continue for life.

ROWING (STATIONARY)

There are several excellent rowing machines on the market. This aerobic activity is low impact and incorporates arm and leg conditioning for a balanced effect. As you can see from the table on page 94, rowing is a very efficient way to expend calories.

STAIR CLIMBING

Stair-climbing machines are very popular and are an excellent aerobic activity. Stair climbing is a great way to expend calories. In fact, it is possible to burn 2000 calories during just two hours of this exercise a week. The drawback is that it is difficult for many people who have just entered the maintenance phase of an exercise program to sustain the intensity necessary to stair climb for two hours per week (that is, 30 minutes, four times a week).

SKIPPING ROPE

This is a high-intensity, high-impact exercise. I recommend it for only short periods of time, on the order of 15 minutes, followed by a brisk walk. I suggest this aerobic activity only to the well-conditioned person.

Individuals with Special Concerns

People with special concerns can in most cases follow the walking program already outlined. Here I discuss modifications and precautions that should be taken in certain situations. People with cardiovascular disease are encouraged to participate in a hospital-based cardiac rehabilitation program before beginning a program at home. In the case of individuals with arthritis, I suggest a swimming rather than a walking program.

Hyperlipidemia

People with elevated cholesterol levels can benefit significantly from a regular aerobic exercise program. Depending on your particular lipid abnormality, you may be more or less responsive to exercise.

High Triglyceride Levels

People with elevated triglyceride levels may lower their blood level of this fat up to 40 percent quickly and dramatically with regular and vigorous aerobic activity. In order to achieve such a significant reduction, I recommend advancing to the point where you are walking at least five times per week.

Low HDL Cholesterol Levels

People with low levels of HDL (the protective cholesterol) need an aggressive aerobic exercise program in order to improve their cholesterol profile. In one well-known study, Dr. Peter Wood of Stanford University found that in order to improve HDL significantly, participants had to jog at least eight miles per week, and the more than that, the better. This doesn't mean that you absolutely must jog to improve your HDL, but Dr. Wood's results do indicate that serious exercise is essential. I recommend walking at least five days and 20 miles a week when trying to improve your HDL cholesterol level.

High LDL Cholesterol Levels

People with elevated LDL cholesterol levels should know that unless an exercise program is accompanied by weight loss, little reduction in this blood fat occurs. This doesn't mean exercise doesn't have other benefits (I have mentioned many of them earlier in this chapter), but in order to lower LDL levels with exercise, one must exercise frequently enough and long enough to promote weight reduction. I recommend a walking goal of at least five times per week for a minimum of 30 minutes per session (longer sessions, up to 60 minutes in duration, are even more desirable).

Cardiac Disease

There is no substitute for a hospital-based cardiac rehabilitation program. After you have completed phase II of a standard rehabilitation program, you will probably be ready for a home- or community-based exercise program. If you choose a home program, it is likely that you will have no trouble beginning the walking schedule outlined in this chapter, but it is important to discuss your exercise plan with your cardiac rehabilitation staff and your primary care physician.

Diabetes

People with Type II (adult onset) diabetes can benefit greatly from exercise. It, like insulin, helps to lower your blood sugar level. It is, however, very important for diabetics to be under good control and to consult their physician prior to initiating an exercise program. Because of the insulin-like effects of exercise, hypoglycemia, an abnormal decrease of sugar in the blood, is the most commonly encountered problem among exercising diabetics. This can occur during or up to six hours after an exercise session.

In addition to concerns about hypoglycemia, a diabetic must pay close attention to foot hygiene. It is very important to invest in a good pair of walking shoes. Finally, diabetics with advanced retinopathy (a disorder of the retina of the eye) should not participate in activities that are high impact and cause excessive jarring of the body and marked increases in blood pressure.

Walking is the optimal exercise for diabetics. After a discussion with your primary care doctor, you should be able to progress through the walking program outlined in this chapter.

Weight Loss

Reduction of body fat is the primary exercise goal for many people. If this is your situation, I recommend frequent walking sessions of low intensity and long duration to burn fat most efficiently.

If you are obese or very out of condition, it is not imperative to reach your target heart rate. It is more important to strive to increase the duration and frequency of your exercise sessions. After your initial conditioning stage, you may be able to reach your target heart rate range.

As mentioned previously, caloric expenditure is another useful means of measuring exercise. I recommend trying to expend 300 to 500 calories per exercise session or between 2000 to 3000 calories per week. The table on page 94 gives estimates of caloric expenditure for various activities. Keep in mind that these are estimates and should not become your sole focus while exercising.

Arthritis

For people with arthritis, non-weight-bearing activities offer cardiovascular conditioning while avoiding joint stress. Swimming, cycling, and arm exercises are good choices for those with osteoarthritis or rheumatoid arthritis, while strength and range of motion exercises help limit the effects of arthritis on the joints. Your local YMCA, YWCA, or swim club may have such programs, which are usually held in a pool and have been developed specifically for people with arthritis.

With arthritis, pain is a fact of life and is often the limiting factor in terms of frequency and duration of exercise. In such cases, sessions of short duration and increased frequency will help the arthritic person exercise during periods of increased inflammation. The intensity of exercise must be guided by pain tolerance.

However, exercising inflamed joints may worsen your situation. Analgesics can be a double-edged sword, controlling pain so effectively that you feel free to exercise vigorously but end up with increased tissue damage. During periods of severe inflammation, no matter how good your pain relievers are, exercise with greater caution and check with your doctor to be sure that your routine is safe for you.

In general, people with mild arthritis can safely participate in the walking program outlined in this chapter. Those more severely affected should consider other forms of aerobic activity. I recommend swimming or the use of a stationary bike as an initial conditioning program. The following guidelines may help you plan your exercise program.

Weeks	Frequency (per day)	Intensity	Time
Weeks 1 and 2	1 to 2 times	50 to 60% THR*	10 to 12 minutes
Weeks 3 and 4	1 to 2 times	50 to 60% THR "Talk Test"	Increase as tolerated up to 15 minutes
Weeks 5 and 6	1 to 2 times	50 to 60% THR "Talk Test"	Increase as tolerated up to 20 minutes

*THR = Target Heart Rate Range.

Always consult your physician prior to beginning and when considering an increase in your exercise program.

Pregnancy

Women are exercising in record numbers and they often want to continue their routines during pregnancy. In the past, most physicians did not recommend this because of fears that exercise might impair growth and development by decreasing the supply of oxygen and glucose to the fetus. But actually, up until about 15 years ago, little research had been done in this area.

However, many well-designed studies have now shown that moderate exercise during pregnancy benefits the mother without causing harm to her developing baby. Indeed, such exercise has been shown to result in improvements in cardiovascular and muscular conditioning and may shorten labor and promote rapid postpartum recovery.

But pregnancy is not a time to start a new unsupervised exercise program other than low-intensity walking or stationary cycling. It is better to join supervised prenatal exercise programs, which are often offered at hospitals and health clubs and are generally appropriate for a woman who has not previously engaged in formal exercise activities.

In 1994, the American College of Obstetricians and Gynecologists published its second set of recommendations for exercise during and after pregnancy. They are summarized in the following list.

1. During pregnancy women are encouraged to participate in a mild to moderate exercise program. Exercise on a regular basis (at least three times per week) is preferable to intermittent activity.

2. Exercise while lying on your back is not recommended after the first trimester.

3. Women should take great care to modify exercise intensity according to symptoms of fatigue. Use the Borg Scale of Rated Perceived Exertion (p. 93) or the "Talk Test" (p. 91) to monitor exercise intensity. Stop when fatigued; do not exercise to exhaustion. Although weight-bearing exercise may in some cases be continued throughout pregnancy, non-weight-bearing exercises such as swimming and cycling are preferred. If you choose a non-weight-bearing exercise, you are more likely to be able to continue your exercise program for your entire pregnancy than if you choose something like jogging.

4. Since pregnancy results in an altered center of gravity, it is best for pregnant women to avoid exercises that require balance and agility and activities such as downhill skiing, which may result in abdominal trauma.

5. Pregnant women require an additional daily intake of approximately 300 calories. Women who exercise during pregnancy must be careful to take in sufficient calories.

6. Drink plenty of water to avoid dehydration and take care to avoid significant increases in body temperature.

Although beginning an exercise program requires discipline, the rewards are great. Not only will you become proud of your outward appearance, the inner you will become stronger—both physically and emotionally.

Give the exercise program profiled in this chapter a try. You will soon see differences and wonder why it took so long for you to get started.

Basic Stretches

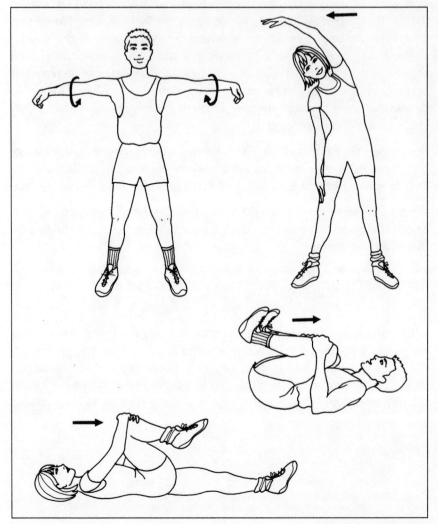

Fran Slattery Design LLC

Basic Stretches

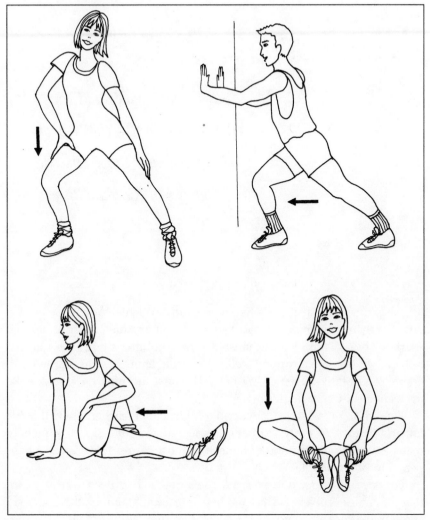

Fran Slattery Design LLC

The Case of Wayne

▼▼

High Triglycerides and Low

HDL Cholesterol—The Impact

of Exercise and Other Lifestyle

Changes on Cardiac Risk

"I guess this is what it feels like to get old," Wayne commented to his wife Sarah one evening. It had been an ordinary day, with no special exertion, but Wayne was exhausted. The troubling thing was that his fatigue had become a routine feeling. Every evening he was washed out, and a good night's sleep didn't help. The next morning he would wake up feeling only marginally better.

Even though Wayne, a 53-year-old high school teacher, knew that his father's history of early cardiac disease put him at risk, he somehow managed to avoid thinking of himself in those terms. Heart attacks happened to other people.

For several years, however, Wayne's doctor had been warning him that his cholesterol levels were too high. He and Sarah took this seriously enough to adopt an almost total vegetarian diet. Unfortunately, because they were not well informed on the subject of fats in food, they substituted eggs, cheese, and nuts for red meat. These replacements turned out to be even higher in fat.

In early 1991, Wayne's fatigue increased. Added to this was an occasional vague chest discomfort. At first, he wrote it off as muscle strain, but when it increased in frequency and became associated with left arm numbness, he became concerned. Things deteriorated to the point that one afternoon in the spring of 1991, Wayne recalls being in so much pain that he was unable to open the door to his classroom. Because he did not want to worry any of his colleagues, he called Sarah at work and asked her to bring him to the Emergency Room (ER).

In the ER his electrocardiogram (ECG) was normal and he was told his symptoms were probably stress related.

It was exactly what he wanted to hear. Understandably anxious not to be having a heart attack (the more so because his own judgment told him that it was a distinct possibility), he grabbed eagerly at the first plausible explanation he was offered for his discomfort. If the ER physician could accept stress as the most likely cause of his chest pain, then why bother asking him about all the other risk factors he knew he had? That would only bring up the one thing he didn't want to consider—cardiac disease, with all that came along with it—and the need to change his self-image and his whole lifestyle. And, even more disturbing, he would have to face his own mortality.

Somehow he made it through another year marked by bouts of gradually increasing chest pressure and arm numbness. After one particularly bad episode, he again consulted his physician and again got the reassuring diagnosis of stress.

By November of 1992, his discomfort had become more intense and seemed to occur with even minimal exertion. At this time, for insurance reasons, he changed physicians. Wayne was by now growing uneasy with the diagnosis of stress and was more willing to consider the possibility of his problems being cardiac related. Even though he knew he was opening a Pandora's box, he decided to insist that his new physician perform a more complete cardiac evaluation.

That doctor didn't need to be convinced. After hearing Wayne's story, he immediately ordered an electrocardiogram combined with exercise (a stress test). He explained to Wayne that sometimes an electrocardiogram, which measures the electric activity of the heart while a person is lying still, can appear normal even in the face of significant heart disease. An electrocardiogram obtained during exercise gives much more information about the health of the heart and its blood vessels.

On December 23, in preparation for his stress test, electrodes were attached to Wayne's chest wall, arms, and legs and he was then instructed to begin walking on a treadmill. Two minutes into the test, he was abruptly told to stop exercising. Not only had he developed his by now familiar chest pain, but his electrocardiogram revealed worrisome changes indicating that his heart muscle was not getting enough oxygen.

Wayne was sent home with strict orders to "do nothing" over the Christmas holidays and to go directly to the emergency room in the event of a prolonged episode of chest pain.

It was the worst holiday the family had ever spent. Wayne lay practically motionless for days, terrified that the slightest movement could bring on a heart attack. Sarah and the children crept around the house as if a wake were in progress. Sarah remembers playing a cassette of Gregorian chant over and over during the weekend as its solemn tones seemed to suit the situation. Now, however, none of them can listen to it; it brings back the painful memory of those days too vividly.

No one spoke of death or dying, but Wayne was all too aware of what they were thinking. For the first time that any of them could remember, the family did not attend Christmas Eve services together because Wayne didn't think he could manage the trip to church in the cold New England night. The next day, he and Sarah sat down to discuss their new reality. After a long talk, they agreed that they were ready to make whatever lifestyle changes were necessary. Although nothing in Wayne's condition changed as a result, the situation seemed a little brighter once that decision had been made.

On December 27, in order to determine the extent of his cardiac disease, Wayne underwent a cardiac catheterization. During this procedure a narrow tube called a catheter was inserted into an artery in Wayne's groin, then threaded up under X-ray guidance to his heart. A contrast agent was then injected through the catheter into his coronary arteries, allowing his cardiologist, Dr. Bob Dewey, to determine how extensive his blockages were. Wayne was found to have a 95 percent blockage of one of the heart's most important blood vessels, called the left anterior descending artery, or LAD.

That evening, Dr. Dewey visited Wayne and Sarah to explain the results of the catheterization. He told them there were two ways to approach the problem: by balloon angioplasty or bypass surgery. Because Wayne's blockage was mainly confined to one coronary artery, an angioplasty was recommended. Dr. Dewey explained that as with the catheterization, an angioplasty would involve threading a catheter through a groin artery up to the heart.

The difference would be that the angioplasty catheter has a plastic balloon at its tip. Once the cardiologist performing the procedure determines with the help of X-ray equipment that the balloon has reached the blockage, it is inflated under pressure, squashing the cholesterol deposit against the inside wall of the artery, thus enlarging the artery's diameter and allowing more blood to flow through it. Dr. Dewey told Wayne that, as with his previous catheterization, he would be awake and able to view the entire procedure on the X-ray screen. Wayne consented and his procedure was scheduled for the following day.

On December 28, the angioplasty was successfully performed, reducing the cholesterol deposit in Wayne's blood vessel from 95 percent to 20 percent. He was discharged from the hospital two days later and he and his family immediately began to make dietary changes. Grateful for their second chance, they were determined to make heart health a priority.

Very soon, however, they were brought sharply down to earth. After a few days recuperation, Wayne started a walking program, but much to his dismay, began experiencing the same old chest pain. A second stress test revealed a recurrence of the changes which had caused the initial concern. Although he had been warned that 30 percent of all angioplasties fail within the first six months, it was still hard to accept the findings of the repeat catheterization: the blockage was back.

In the weeks that followed, Wayne's whole life seemed to focus on his heart and the turbulent changes it was experiencing. On January 19, he underwent a repeat angioplasty, but again his pain was back within days. A repeat exercise test failed to reveal any worrisome changes that suggested a recurrence of the blockage, but although Wayne hoped that the discomfort would improve, it continued as before. The physical turmoil he was experiencing was now being reflected in almost every aspect of his emotional life. Full of self-doubt, he began to question his own interpretation of his symptoms. Was he imagining things? Overreacting to what should be tolerable pain? Other people he knew had been fine within days of their angioplasties. What was wrong with him?

At home he was touchy and out of sorts, while at school he found himself losing his temper with students he'd once found easy to relate to. When several students actually suggested that he consider retiring, Wayne realized that things had gone too far. On February 26, alone at home, he decided to test himself. If his arteries were still clear, he reasoned, there was no reason why he couldn't chop some wood.

Sarah recalls coming home that day to a house that was eerily silent. Wayne was lying on the couch, looking gray and drawn, and without his saying a word she knew that his condition had deteriorated. Two days later, another stress test revealed that his blockage was very likely back. This time, however, the news was almost a relief to him—at least, he hadn't been imagining the whole thing.

The following Monday Wayne returned to the hospital for yet another catheterization. By now he was familiar enough with the laboratory procedure to interpret what he saw on the X-ray monitor. As the contrast agent was injected into his arteries, he could see for himself that the stress test had been accurate: the blockage was back and with a vengeance. He was no longer a candidate for angioplasty. The only option left was bypass surgery.

That afternoon, Dr. Dewey sat with Wayne and Sarah to detail what the surgery would entail. First he explained that all the coronary arteries spring from the aorta. In order to restore blood flow to the areas of the heart served by Wayne's blocked arteries, a piece of vein from his leg would be used, with one end attached to the aorta and the other sewn to his diseased coronary artery just beyond the blockage. In this way all areas of the heart would receive enough blood flow.

Dr. Dewey also told Wayne that his heart would be stopped while the bypass was being performed, and that his breathing and circulation would be handled by machines until the surgery was complete and his own body could take over again.

Although the prospect of such major surgery was terrifying, Wayne realized that he didn't have much choice. He knew he couldn't go on as he was, either in fear of pain or actually experiencing it. He and Sarah spoke briefly in privacy and then told the doctor that they were ready for the operation.

I met Wayne the day before the operation and he, Sarah, and I spent a long time discussing the importance of lifestyle modifications. Their commitment to change was obvious: Wayne had been on a low-fat diet since Christmas and had already lost 10 pounds. The whole family had joined him in this and were also benefiting from the new regime. However, while his cholesterol values had improved substantially, they were still quite worrisome to me. These were his values before his surgery:

	Wayne's Level	Desirable Level
Total cholesterol	230 mg/dl	Less than 200 mg/dl
Triglycerides	347 mg/dl	Less than 150 mg/dl
HDL cholesterol	22 mg/dl	Greater than 45 mg/dl
LDL cholesterol	138 mg/dl	Less than 100 mg/dl

Wayne's total cholesterol level might seem rather low, considering that he was about to undergo open heart surgery. At only 30 mg/dl above the desirable 200, one might conceivably wonder what all the fuss was about. But while it is true that Wayne's total cholesterol level was not, in fact, dramatically elevated, it would be a mistake to assume that his values were nearly normal.

Total cholesterol value is a composite of several different kinds of cholesterol, specifically low-density lipoprotein cholesterol (LDL), popularly known as "bad" cholesterol; high-density lipoprotein cholesterol (HDL), or "good" cholesterol; and very-low-density lipoprotein cholesterol (VLDL). VLDL is composed primarily of triglycerides. In general, if you divide your triglycerides by 5, you arrive at a rough estimate of your VLDL. Total cholesterol, then, is equal to the sum of your HDL + LDL + triglycerides, divided by 5.

Individuals can have a variety of cholesterol abnormalities. People with very depressed HDL are at risk for heart disease (even though their total cholesterol may be within the normal range), whereas people with very high HDL are at a low risk of heart disease even when their total cholesterol is quite high. It is also commonly known that individuals with elevated LDL are at high risk.

What about triglycerides? High levels seem to predict development of cardiac disease in postmenopausal women. In men, the impact of high triglycerides on the risk of developing heart disease has not been so easy to determine. But in a recent evaluation of the results of many published scientific studies, Dr. Melissa Austin found that elevated triglyceride levels increase the risk for developing heart disease in both women and men, with the risk greater in women.

In both men and women, high triglycerides are also a marker for other cholesterol abnormalities, including very low HDL and small dense LDL (a type of LDL that is more dangerous than larger, more buoyant LDL particles). It can happen that a person has a fairly normal total cholesterol level but still has significant cholesterol abnormalities.

For this reason, people should insist that their doctor measure both total cholesterol and HDL levels. If any abnormality is detected, then a full fasting profile (total cholesterol, LDL, HDL, and triglycerides) should be obtained.

Although Wayne's most serious problem was his very depressed HDL, he also had an elevated triglyceride level. His ratio of total cholesterol to HDL (that is, the total cholesterol number divided by the HDL number) was 10.5. This ratio is often used as a predictor of cardiac risk, and a level greater than 4 in a person with cardiac disease is considered undesirable. Wayne and Sarah's first question, then, was both logical and obvious: How could they raise his HDL level?

I explained to them that although some measures can be taken to improve a person's HDL, it is largely genetically determined and therefore not always affected by lifestyle changes. However, when trying to decide how difficult or easy it will be to raise a person's HDL, I do look at the triglyceride level, weight, exercise level, and whether or not the patient smokes.

Because triglycerides and HDL are metabolically related, when triglycerides are high, HDL tends to be low. As shown in a study by Drs.

Michael Miller and Peter Kwiterovich of Johns Hopkins Hospital, Baltimore, individuals with high triglyceride levels who manage to reduce them will tend simultaneously to raise their HDL level, in some cases quite dramatically. (This may not be the case if triglycerides are only marginally elevated.)

People who are very overweight tend to have depressed HDL levels. But as a person is actively losing weight, his or her HDL may actually decline for a time. Once a new weight plateau is achieved and maintained for a few months, however, the HDL will often increase and even exceed the previous baseline.

Individuals who do not exercise regularly often have lower HDL levels than do those who engage in regular aerobic activity. Simply beginning an exercise program can significantly improve a person's HDL level. Dr. Peter Wood of Stanford University found that when sedentary men initiated an exercise program they improved their HDL levels on average by about 4.4 mg/dl, if the exercise burned off at least 800 to 1000 calories per week. The more calories burned, the greater the improvement—up to about 4500 calories. So more is better, and the exercise must be vigorous.

This study was performed only with men. In the past it was believed that women did not respond as well to exercise programs aimed at HDL improvement. But more recent data suggest that women simply have a slower response to exercise than men: in some cases, they do not reach peak HDL levels until five years after initiating regular exercise. Knowing this can help women avoid discouragement and keep them focused on the more immediately obvious benefits of vigorous exercise.

Giving up smoking is one of the most important things a person with low HDL can do to raise its level. On average, smoking men have HDL levels about 5.3 mg/dl lower than nonsmoking men. In smoking women, the difference is even more dramatic: their level is, on average, 9 mg/dl lower than that of nonsmoking women.

I told Wayne, himself a nonsmoker, that these were the general things one could do to improve HDL levels. In his particular situation, I pointed out that his recent weight loss could have caused a slight drop in his HDL which might gradually improve as his weight stabilized. Lowering his triglycerides, a priority in my treatment plan, would also improve his HDL. And finally, since he did not engage in a routine exercise program when I met him, I hoped that beginning one would raise his HDL level. But in spite of there being quite a few positive changes he could make, I told him it was unlikely that he would totally normalize his HDL cholesterol with lifestyle modifications alone.

Reviewing the steps to be taken to improve his triglyceride level, I gave Wayne and Sarah the following instructions written by Mary Card.

Management of High Triglycerides

1. Limit calories to promote weight reduction.

2. Exercise at least one-half hour five days a week.

3. Restrict simple sugars and foods high in refined sugar. Restrict the following foods:
   - Fruited yogurt
   - Fruit juice and fresh fruit (limit to 4 pieces per day)
   - Pies, cakes, cookies, pastries, doughnuts, regular jello
   - Sherbet, frozen yogurt, popsicles, water ice, ice cream
   - Sugar (white, brown, confectioners), honey, maple syrup, corn syrup, chocolate syrup, jelly, jam, marmalade, hard candy, chocolate bars
   - Regular soda
   - Pudding, custard, mousse

4. Restrict fat.

5. Restrict alcohol.

6. If diabetic, improve blood sugar control.

Some of the items on this list are self-explanatory, but a few deserve comment. Most people know, for example, that restriction of fat is critical for improving cholesterol levels. What is not so well known is that *to lower triglycerides*, it is very important *to cut down on sugars*.

Consider the case of Carl, a police officer referred to me with a triglyceride level of over 2600 mg/dl and an HDL of only 17 mg/dl. In spite of a strict low-fat diet for over a year, Carl's triglyceride level hadn't budged.

Questioned about his diet, it turned out that he was drinking quantities of fruit juice and soft drinks, using sugar in his coffee, and eating popsicles whenever he felt like a snack (reasoning that none of these things contained fat). With only a few simple changes in his diet, one month later his triglycerides were down to 298 mg/dl and his HDL up to 24 mg/dl. Clearly, then, the impact of diet on lipid levels is enormous. The body, by the way, cannot distinguish between healthy and unhealthy sugars—a glass of orange juice and a chocolate bar will both raise triglyceride levels.

Alcohol also deserves a comment. Many people have heard (to their delight) that alcohol will, in all cases, improve cholesterol levels and reduce the risk of heart disease. For individuals with triglyceride abnormalities, however, even a single alcoholic beverage can dramatically elevate triglyceride levels.

What do I tell such people who drink? I never begin by telling anyone to give up alcohol entirely, primarily because in my experience, most people just won't. I first ask them to cut their intake in half, or to a maximum of three to four drinks per week. Many people can bring their triglycerides to normal levels simply by cutting back. If cutting down fails to normalize their triglycerides, then I do suggest abstinence.

Wayne decided then and there that once he left the hospital he would drink less (he was drinking 3 to 4 beers a week), restrict concentrated sweets, and develop a regular exercise program.

Before leaving Wayne's room that day, we discussed the impact of stress on cardiac health. Although he believed that he generally handled stress well, he admitted that with his own three children going through the struggles of young adulthood and the challenges of his job as a high school teacher, the past few years had not been easy. When he asked if I thought a stress reduction program would help him, I told him that given the world we live in, almost everyone could benefit from such a program.

I recommended that Wayne get in touch with a former professor of mine, Dr. Jon Kabat-Zinn, who runs a stress reduction clinic at the University of Massachusetts Medical Center in Worcester, Massachusetts, and has written several books on the subject. I suggested either taking Dr. Zinn's eight-week course or reading his book, *Full Catastrophe Living*. I also told Wayne that as a very busy and quite stressed intern, I had taken Dr. Zinn's course myself and found it very helpful. It gave me a new way of looking at challenging situations and taught me relaxation techniques that I truly needed at that time and continue to use to this day.

That night Wayne and Sarah prepared themselves emotionally for his surgery. He sailed through and recovered rapidly: within eight days he was home. Given his angioplasty experiences, however, he half expected to experience chest pain again, once he began to exercise. His first week at home, he quite nervously began walking around the house—but no pain. The following week, he tried walking in the yard—still no pain. By the third week, he was confident and walking outside for a mile. Within a few weeks he was unstoppable, logging up to five miles a day.

Sarah labels this period Wayne's postsurgical euphoria, and her husband agrees that he felt he had been given a new lease on life. Now he was determined to stay healthy.

I saw Wayne in my office eight weeks after his bypass surgery. It is important to wait at least that long after this operation before checking cholesterol levels, since they will temporarily fall immediately following surgery. By the end of eight weeks, Wayne had lost 10 more pounds, was walking five miles a day, and was down to only two beers a week.

His lipid profile was also much improved and now looked like this:

	Wayne's Level	Desirable Level
Total cholesterol	177 mg/dl	Less than 200 mg/dl
Triglycerides	226 mg/dl	Less than 150 mg/dl
HDL cholesterol	27 mg/dl	Greater than 45 mg/dl
LDL cholesterol	125 mg/dl	Less than 100 mg/dl

His ratio of total cholesterol divided by HDL was better at 6.5, but not good enough. However, when I suggested medications to improve his profile further, Wayne was reluctant. He had achieved so much through his own efforts that he really wanted to give diet and exercise more time.

I saw Wayne again several months later. He looked wonderful. He had joined a cardiac support group which met once a month to exchange insights, ideas, and low-fat recipes. He had also begun traveling to Worcester to attend the stress-reduction clinic and had incorporated meditation into his daily routine. He really was like a different person. I was as anxious as he to see the results of his blood work. Once again, the numbers were all better:

	Wayne's Level	Desirable Level
Total cholesterol	158 mg/dl	Less than 200 mg/dl
Triglycerides	203 mg/dl	Less than 150 mg/dl
HDL cholesterol	28 mg/dl	Greater than 45 mg/dl
LDL cholesterol	89 mg/dl	Less than 100 mg/dl

But in spite of a total cholesterol that would thrill most people, his HDL was still very low. I hated to have to tell him there was still work to be done. I pointed out the significant improvement in his LDL and triglyceride values, and that at 5.6 his total cholesterol to HDL ratio was also much better. However, he himself commented that this was still too high, and I had to agree that it was.

Wayne and Sarah were very discouraged, wondering what more they could do. One option I offered them was to use a medicine to raise Wayne's HDL level. This approach, however, is controversial: although it is known that a low HDL puts a person at greater risk for heart disease, it has not been proven that a drug-induced rise in HDL will reduce that risk.

The Veterans Administration is currently conducting a study called the HDL Intervention Trial that should answer this question. In this study, persons with documented heart disease and low HDL levels are being asked to take Gemfibrizol (Lopid), a drug which lowers triglycerides and generally raises HDL. The goal is to determine whether taking Lopid reduces the incidence of cardiac problems such as heart attacks, but the results, unfortunately, will not be available for some years.

Wayne and Sarah, whose main concern was to get through *this* year, commented that they really didn't want to wait for the study to conclude before giving Lopid a try. In the end, we decided to try it for three months and then evaluate the situation.

Three months later, Wayne's profile looked like this:

	Wayne's Level	Desirable Level
Total cholesterol	141 mg/dl	Less than 200 mg/dl
Triglycerides	61 mg/dl	Less than 150 mg/dl
HDL cholesterol	28 mg/dl	Greater than 45 mg/dl
LDL cholesterol	100 mg/dl	Less than 100 mg/dl

His triglycerides were better, and once again his ratio had improved to a new level of 5.0, but still nothing had happened to his HDL. Deciding to focus more on improving his ratio, I switched him from Lopid to a low dose of simvastatin (Zocor) and ultimately, with continued adherence to lifestyle modifications and the Zocor, Wayne achieved the following results:

	Wayne's Level	Desirable Level
Total cholesterol	140 mg/dl	Less than 200 mg/dl
Triglycerides	87 mg/dl	Less than 150 mg/dl
HDL cholesterol	29 mg/dl	Greater than 45 mg/dl
LDL cholesterol	93 mg/dl	Less than 100 mg/dl

Although his ratio, at 4.8, was not the desired 4.0 or lower, it was nonetheless a great deal better than 10.5.

Today, Wayne's risk for heart disease is dramatically lower than it was the year before his problems started. He has learned an entirely new way of living: as he says, "I'm not on a diet—this is my life. And I don't feel deprived, I feel better than ever."

What he has accomplished has not gone unnoticed: he is in part the inspiration for 150 pounds of weight loss at the high school where he teaches. Sarah and one of his children have each lost 25 pounds, and his colleagues and friends think of him as a great resource on dietary questions.

He has compiled over 100 "livable" low-fat and nonfat recipes that allow guilt-free enjoyment of foods like pesto and lasagna (some of his recipes are included in the "Recipes" section at the end of this book). During his free period at school, Wayne meditates, and hopes that his students will notice and perhaps "learn how to avoid their own heart attacks in the future." Exercise is also a regular part of his life—he walks or cycles the six-mile round trip to his school every day.

Although Wayne is not inclined to blame others for his cardiovascular disease, he wishes that the medical community placed more emphasis on preventive medicine. Perhaps if he had been asked to see a dietitian in the years before he developed chest discomfort, things might have turned out differently for him. His advice to people with cholesterol abnormalities is to take a proactive stance—ask to see a dietitian, read all you can, change your lifestyle, and if you are experiencing chest pressure or pain insist on a complete cardiac evaluation.

Wayne has proven resoundingly that even people with a genetic predisposition to cardiovascular disease can turn their lives around. I expect Sarah and him to continue feeling young for many years to come.

4

~~~~~~~~~~~~~~~~~~~~~~~~~~~~~~~~~~~~~~~

Quitting:

A Tough Task with

Great Rewards

You don't need me to tell you about the hazards of cigarette smoking—but I'm going to do it anyway. You've heard it all before, you probably know the statistics by heart and here I am, about to cover the same tired ground again. The reason is simple: you want to quit (80 percent of American smokers say the same), and today may be the day you make the decision to do it. You just never know when the same old facts suddenly become real to a person, or which combination of words will do the trick. As I mentioned in the Introduction to this book, I am a missionary when it comes to convincing people to stop smoking, and I never pass up an opportunity.

Quitting smoking may be the most difficult thing you ever do. Getting hooked was so easy. If you started as a teenager, as most people do, peer pressure and the desire to look cool probably got you through the initial period when you found smoking actually unpleasant. Then, before you knew what was happening, you were addicted.

Cigarettes contain nicotine, a substance which can activate many of the brain's hormones—beta-endorphin, a mood elevator (which explains why many people find smoking a good antidote to depression and anxiety); adrenaline (you aren't just imagining that a cigarette improves your performance and concentration); acetylcholine, norepinephrine, and dopamine. Smokers also have improved metabolism and reduced hunger—

on average, a smoker weighs three to five pounds less than a nonsmoker of the same height and build.

It may sound from all of this as if smoking has a lot going for it, but unfortunately, nothing comes without a price. Ultimately, smoking exacts a toll that fewer and fewer people are willing to pay. The issue is nothing less than control of your own life.

One of my favorite patients, Kathy, told me what a shock it was to realize this. "I was at work—I had gone back to smoking. I decided if I was going to smoke, I would at least try to control the number of cigarettes I put in my mouth every day. I left my pack on the counter in the back room so that if I wanted a cigarette, I would have to make an actual decision, get up, and walk back there to get it. All day I kept thinking about that pack. I was disgusted with myself because I suddenly realized that those cigarettes rule me. I thought even my husband doesn't cling to me the way those cigarettes do!"

Being out of control is a very unpleasant experience. But you don't have to feel it any longer. Quit smoking and get back in charge. You know you can do it! Don't be discouraged by a few temporary setbacks—most people who ultimately became nonsmokers have had to quit a few times before they gave it up permanently. If you have some experience already with quitting, that's all to the good. You know firsthand where the pitfalls are. Of course, if you have never quit before, there is no rule that says that your first try won't succeed.

How do you begin? The program I would like to share with you is based on the one Dr. Judy Ockene taught me very early in my medical training. It has proven very successful for many of my patients, and I think you will find it beneficial for you as well.

How Addicted Am I?

The first step is to test the severity of your addiction to nicotine. The Fagerström Nicotine Dependency Assessment is a simple method for doing this.

Figure out your total score from the table:

- If it is 6 or higher, this indicates a strong nicotine dependency. You may well benefit from participation in a smoking cessation class or use of either the nicotine patch or gum to help you as you become a nonsmoker.
- If your score is 5 or less you have only a low to moderate nicotine dependency.

The next step is to determine your degree of motivation and your

Fagerström Nicotine Dependency Assessment

	0 points	1 point	2 points
1. How soon after you wake do you smoke your first cigarette?	After ½ hour	Within ½ hour	—
2. Do you find it difficult to refrain from smoking in places where it is forbidden, such as the library, theater, doctor's office?	No	Yes	—
3. Which cigarettes would you hate most to give up?*	Any other than the first in A.M.	The first in A.M.	—
4. How many cigarettes do you smoke a day?	1 to 15	16 to 25	26 or more
5. Do you smoke more during the morning than the rest of the day?	No	Yes	—
6. Do you smoke if you are so ill that you are in bed most of the day?	No	Yes	—
7. How often do you inhale the smoke from your cigarette?	Never	Often	Always

*Question number three needs a little explanation. You get one point if some cigarette other than your first cigarette of the day would be the hardest for you to do without. This is because studies have shown that people who smoke the minute they get out of bed are the most strongly addicted. If you *have* to have that first cigarette you get two points, and chances are you will have to work extra hard to become a nonsmoker. If this is your situation, you may benefit from the nicotine patch or gum.

Reprinted from: Fagerström KO. Measuring degree of physical dependence on tobacco smoking with reference to individualization of treatment. Addictive Behaviors. 1978; 3 (3): 235–241. With kind permission from Elsevier Science LTD, The Boulevard, Langford Lane, Kidlington OX51GB, UK.

reasons for quitting. Please take a moment and actually write those reasons down.

Take a look at what you have written, and ask yourself whether these reasons are really enough to make you stop. If you can say yes, you have taken one big step toward becoming a nonsmoker. Whatever your reasons—your own health, the health of your children, social pressures—they have to be good ones. Smoking is a strong addiction: without a clear understanding of why you want to stop, you will find it very difficult to stick with your resolve.

If you have quit before, you can learn a lot about yourself by carefully examining exactly what happened. How soon after you quit did you start smoking again? If you lasted only a few days, you probably succumbed to withdrawal symptoms—your body's craving for nicotine. This can take many forms, among them:

Anxiety	Increased appetite
Irritability	Shakiness
Impatience	Tremor
Restlessness	Sweating
Difficulty sleeping	Lightheadedness
Trouble concentrating	Coughing
Chest tightness	Constipation

The pattern of frequent attempts at quitting that end within a week indicates a heavy addiction to nicotine. This doesn't mean that you won't be able to manage it, but it is important to realize the nature of the problem. Indeed, recognizing the severity of your addiction is part of the battle (but not, unfortunately, half of it). If your addiction is this severe, I would strongly advise considering nicotine replacement (the patch or gum).

Maybe you have been able to quit for up to six months before going back to smoking. But after one month, all physical withdrawal symptoms are over. What is left is a psychological addiction that may last for years. It is essential to understand how this works in your life. Think back to the last time you quit and then restarted. What made you go back to smoking? Was there stress at home or at work? Or perhaps some other activity triggered it?

One of my patients told me that his attempts at quitting were always successful until he had a beer. He could go for months on end without smoking, but the moment he had a beer he would suddenly "need" a cigarette. He decided that the only way to quit once and for all was to stop drinking at the same time. He cut out alcohol for a full year before he felt sure enough of himself. Now he says he can have an occasional beer without craving a cigarette, but he believes that had he not given himself the full year, he never would have become a nonsmoker.

In any case, the fact you were able to quit for several months means that you can do it again. This time, with advance planning to avoid the snares of your last try, it will be for good.

If it was stress that caused you to return to smoking the last time, you can be sure that there will be more of that the next time around. The answer is not to avoid stress, but to change the way you deal with it. Stress-reduction courses are available at many hospitals; Chapter 6 of this book contains many techniques for coping with what is an unavoidable part of everyone's life. Regular exercise is an excellent way of releasing tension. If you initiate a daily exercise routine, you may soon feel so good you don't want to smoke anymore. Even a daily walk is enough. Exercise also helps control the weight gain many people experience when quitting.

Tips for Quitting

What will make it difficult for you to stay away from cigarettes once you have decided to quit? If you have smoked for most of your adult life, there are probably many things you cannot imagine doing without the company of a cigarette. You may also have many smoking friends and perhaps even live with another smoker. Working around all these factors requires careful strategic planning.

- Most offices and public buildings in the United States are now smoke free by law. If this is not the case at your job, ask your boss to consider making the change.
- Ask your friends and family not to smoke in your house or apartment. Throw your ashtrays out.
- Sit only in the nonsmoking section of a restaurant.
- Change your routine. If, for example, you always smoke on the way to work, choose a new route, join a car pool, switch to public transportation.
- If you associate a cigarette with a cup of coffee, switch to tea.
- If you associate a cigarette with the end of a meal, leave the table immediately after you finish eating, brush your teeth, and go for a quick walk.
- If you associate a cigarette with an alcoholic beverage in the evening, give up alcohol until you are comfortable as a nonsmoker. The problem with alcohol is that it weakens your resistance for just about anything—for the purposes of this book, we are mostly concerned with smoking and eating, but I have yet to meet a person for whom drinking provides the incentive to rush out and run a five-mile race.
- If you smoke while watching television, try not to watch any TV for the next few weeks. Instead, pick up a hobby that requires you to work with your hands. Consider knitting, jigsaw puzzles, computer games, model ships, or checkers. Join your children (or grandchildren) in constructing a Lego city.

There are no doubt many situations specific to your life that I have not mentioned. Please consider your own needs and try to come up with tactics for dealing with them that work for you.

Getting Started

And so to work. Before you do anything, I want you to set a quit date. Think hard about it. Make it no sooner than two weeks from now, no later than four. The reason I ask you to wait two weeks is that you need this much time to observe yourself as a smoker. The information you will acquire will help enormously in planning your campaign. Ideally, you will quit in two weeks. Some people, however, prefer a more gradual approach. You may set your quit date a full four weeks from today, but any longer than this is not advised, as your motivation level will tend to wane with time.

Please write your quit date down, and keep it in sight.

Ideally, you will choose a nonworking day to quit. It is important to have as little stress as possible for your first few days as a nonsmoker. You should now spend the next two weeks getting ready for the big day.

For the first seven days, record every cigarette you smoke. Wrap a piece of paper around your pack and make a note of the time of day and the circumstances under which you smoked—for example, "cigarette 16, after supper, in order to relax." Once you have seven sheets of paper, you can easily evaluate your typical smoking habits.

See which cigarettes you are smoking out of habit or boredom—these will be the easiest to do without. Choose the five cigarettes you enjoy or need the most and plan to smoke only these five per day for the next seven days.

At the end of this two-week period, you will be ready to begin your life as a nonsmoker. Let the important people in your life know that you are quitting, and that you will be relying on them for support and encouragement in the next few weeks. If you like team sports, you may consider trying to find a friend to quit with you—many people, however, prefer to go it alone. Try to plan some of your favorite activities (ones you don't associate with smoking) on your first day as a nonsmoker. In the next week or so, you are sure to experience some or all of the withdrawal symptoms listed earlier. Don't lose heart—there is a whole bag of tricks to help you get through what you must keep telling yourself is only a passing phase. Remember always to think of yourself as a nonsmoker.

If you find yourself feeling anxious, irritable, impatient, and restless, this is your body's way of demanding a cigarette. If you wait out each individual urge, you will find that the serious craving lasts only a few minutes. The underlying irritability, however, may last for as long as four weeks. When things get too tense, try the following:

- Take a walk or ride a bike.
- Ask a friend to give you a back rub.
- Close your eyes and inhale deeply through your nose, then slowly exhale through your mouth; repeat this six times.
- Take a warm bath.
- Drink a cup of herbal tea in a rocking chair.
- Brush your hair, snap a clothes pin, play with a rubber band, or pet your dog. These repetitive movements may help you to relax.

You may find that you are very tired during the first few weeks—this is a common reaction. Nicotine is a stimulant to which your body has become accustomed. It often takes two to four weeks to get your old energy back. In the meantime, try the following:

- Take a vacation and, if possible, spend it in a new environment.
- Go to bed an hour earlier than usual.
- Take frequent walks, especially in the cool evening air. Believe it or not, walking may help relieve the fatigue.

Unfortunately, in spite of being more tired than usual, you may still have difficulty sleeping. This is because nicotine can influence your sleep patterns: abruptly deprived of it, your body may take up to a week to work out its own routine. When you finally fall asleep, don't be surprised if your dreams are full of cigarettes.

If sleep is a problem for you:

- Avoid caffeine, especially after noontime.
- Exercise daily.
- Try a cup of herbal tea before bed.
- Take a hot bath, then read for 15 minutes in bed.
- Once in bed, shut your eyes, then try to relax each part of your body in succession (see Chapter 6 on stress reduction for further details).

When you quit smoking, your "smoker's cough" may actually get worse for a few days, often accompanied by a runny nose and dry throat. This phenomenon occurs as the cilia (small fiber-like protrusions) which line your respiratory tract recover from years of abuse. It will pass quickly, but in the meantime:

- Keep your throat moist with sugar-free hard candies.
- Drink plenty of water.
- Suck on ice cubes or ice chips.

One of the most common problems quitters report in the first few weeks is that they cannot concentrate and feel as if they are walking around in a cloud. This is the brain's response to the withdrawal of the powerful stimulant of nicotine. The damage is not permanent; over the next couple of weeks, the fog will lift and your brain will again function normally. While you wait:

- Plan a vacation or, at the very least, avoid major deadlines or projects at work.
- Take regular walks to clear your head.
- Get as much sleep as possible.
- Consider the use of nicotine gum or the nicotine patch.

The withdrawal of nicotine may also affect the movement of your bowels. If constipation becomes a problem, try the following:

- Get plenty of exercise, which is a known stimulant of bowel activity.
- Eat lots of high-fiber foods such as bran cereal, low-fat bran muffins, apples, oranges, and carrots. (See pages 52–54 for further suggestions on high fiber foods.)
- Drink plenty of water.

Not everyone who quits smoking gains weight, but many people do. Cigarette smokers are used to having something in their mouths and in their hands. Many people who quit smoking replace their cigarettes with high-fat candy and snacks. Don't exchange one bad habit for another:

- Drink eight glasses of water a day.
- Suck on sugar-free hard candies or cinnamon sticks.
- Stock up on celery, carrot sticks, and fresh fruit.
- Keep your hands busy, too—take up knitting, or build a model ship.

Even if you don't start snacking on junk food, you may still find that your weight goes up a few pounds. But remember, you would have to gain 100 pounds to equal the negative effect smoking has on your heart. Nicotine does seem to speed up the body's metabolism, but you can prevent weight gain by exercising daily, thereby naturally improving your metabolism.

Throughout these difficult few weeks, go on reminding yourself, over and over again, that these feelings will pass. And remember that almost all withdrawal symptoms disappear within four weeks of quitting. Keep telling yourself that you can win, and in one month you will have done it. It may be the longest month of your life, but once it is over, you will have a much longer life to look forward to.

The psychological addiction to tobacco is harder to gauge—some people still crave a cigarette years after quitting. This is where stress reduction and avoidance of situations that will increase your desire to smoke become critically important. Please see Chapter 6 for the stress-reduction program I recommend.

Now suppose, in spite of all your best efforts, you slip back and have "just one cigarette." Don't despair. Use the experience. Learn from it. Carefully analyze the dynamics of the situation. Why did you smoke? Were you feeling depressed or tense? Had you had a great meal, a cup of coffee, or a drink, and found it just too tempting to pass up a cigarette? There is always something new to discover about what makes you tick—find out why you did what you did and use it to plan a way around the next temptation. Then go on with your life as a nonsmoker.

Nicotine Patch and Gum

Studies have shown that if you are heavily addicted to cigarettes—that is, if you scored 6 or higher on the Fagerström Nicotine Dependency Assessment—nicotine replacement (nicotine gum or patch) may improve your quitting success. This does not mean that you must use these products to quit. After all, people were quitting successfully long before these aids were available. But nicotine replacement may make the transition to smoke-free living a little easier. Some studies have also shown that nicotine replacement can reduce the likelihood of significant weight gain in heavily addicted smokers.

In 1984 the Food and Drug Administration (FDA) approved the use of nicotine-containing gum (2 milligram dose) for use in the United States. Since that time four different nicotine patches and a double-strength nicotine gum have also been approved. Since the summer of 1996, both forms of nicotine replacement have been available without a prescription.

Sometimes, however, people fail to benefit fully from nicotine replacement because they are not using it properly. This is especially true of nicotine-containing gum.

This gum is marketed under the brand name Nicorette by the drug company SmithKline Beecham and is available in 2-milligram and 4-milligram (mg) doses. Both come in boxes of 96 pieces. In general, I suggest using the 4-mg strength. There is definitely a right and a wrong way to use this gum. Here are the instructions I give my patients:

1. Use Nicorette only after totally giving up smoking.
2. Chew gum slowly, and periodically "park" it between your cheek and gums. This is the way the nicotine is absorbed into your system. Park the gum after every 15 to 20 chews or each time you notice a peppery taste in your mouth. After 30 minutes in your mouth, all the nicotine is absorbed.
3. Eating or drinking while chewing the gum tends to impair absorption of the nicotine. Don't eat or drink 15 minutes prior to or while chewing a piece of gum.
4. You may use as many as 30 pieces of gum per day of the 2-mg Nicorette or 20 pieces of the 4-mg variety.
5. After using Nicorette for two to three months, you should begin to taper your use. I recommend a gradual substitution of sugar-free gum for the Nicorette. Within six months, you should be off the gum completely.

Instead of gum, many people opt for a nicotine patch. There are currently four different patches on the market which differ slightly in terms of dosing and length of time worn (see the following table). All patches are changed daily (in the morning), except for Nicotrol which is taken off at bedtime.

Special Populations

In general, if a person is a light smoker (less than 10 cigarettes a day), weighs less than 100 lb, or has had a heart attack (or unstable angina) within the last three months, the individual is started on the first weaning dose rather than the highest dose patch.

Very few people have side effects from the patch, although occasionally a person may develop a skin rash at the site of administration. As with the nicotine gum, you should use the patch only after complete cessation of smoking. Finally, some people find that the nicotine patch keeps them awake at night. This is not a problem with Nicotrol, since the patch is taken off at bedtime. It is certainly possible to take the other patches off at bedtime as well, if this becomes a problem for you.

Finally, I want to leave this subject with some mental pictures for you to muse over: what cigarette smoking actually does to your insides. You may skip this section if you wish, but many people find the graphic images a good source of motivation.

Whenever you smoke a cigarette, you expose your body to thousands of noxious chemicals. Within seconds of lighting up, nicotine enters your

Comparing Nicotine Patches

	Patch Name[a]			
	Habitrol (Ciba-Geigy)	Nicoderm (Marion Merrell Dow)	Nicotrol (Parke-Davis)	Prostep (Lederle)
Initial starting dose				
In most persons	21 mg	21 mg	15 mg	22 mg
Special populations[b]	14 mg	14 mg	15 mg	11 mg
Number of weeks on starting dose	4 to 8	6	4 to 12	4 to 8
First weaning dose	14 mg	14 mg	10 mg	11 mg
Number of weeks on first weaning dose	2 to 4	2	2 to 4	2 to 4
Second weaning dose	7 mg	7 mg	5 mg	none
Number of weeks on second weaning dose	2 to 4	2	2 to 4	none
Recommended total length of program in weeks	6 + 2 + 2 = 10	6 + 2 + 2 = 10	8 to 16	4 + 4 = 8

[a]The drug company is given in parentheses.

[b]Special populations include light smokers and people with cardiac disease. See text for a discussion of these cases.

bloodstream, increasing your heart rate and blood pressure and decreasing the heart's ability to carry and deliver oxygen.

Cigarette smoking also reduces the blood level of HDL (the good cholesterol). On average, a smoking man has an HDL level 5 to 6 mg/dl lower than a nonsmoker, and a smoking woman's HDL level is about 8 to 10 mg/dl lower than that of her nonsmoking friends. The good news is that when you quit, your HDL increases, peaking at about six months.

In addition, smoking activates our platelets—the blood-clotting cells. Clots have a tendency to form in heart arteries, especially if a cholesterol deposit is already present within the artery. If you have an arterial blockage, any cigarette could be the one that will trigger chest pain and cardiac arrhythmias.

The carbon monoxide you are breathing in every time you inhale is a poisonous gas that displaces the oxygen your body needs to function. This explains the shortness of breath that many smokers experience. If you have an underlying heart condition, this lack of oxygen could also lead to a heart attack or a fatal heart arrhythmia.

The tar in your cigarette is a combination of noxious chemicals and gases that deposit inside your bronchial tree which supplies air to your lungs. Tar inflames and destroys your lung tissues. Smokers are more prone to bronchitis than nonsmokers and take twice as long to get over a simple cold.

The thousands of chemicals present in each cigarette you smoke combine to increase your risk of not only lung cancer but also cancers of the esophagus, bladder, head, and neck. Cigarette smokers are also more likely to have peptic ulcers, premature wrinkling of the skin, and gum and tooth problems.

The damage and destruction that result from your smoking habit are not even limited to the lungs and heart. There is virtually no organ in your body which is not affected by cigarettes. When you quit, you will both feel and look better, inside and out, and you'll smell better, too. You have nothing to lose and, literally, everything to gain. Go ahead— you really can do it!

The Case of George

When Smoking and

Genes Don't Mix

To a geneticist, it matters little what relationship a person has to his or her biological parents. Their genetic contribution is made on the day of conception and how they behave after the child is born makes no difference to the youngster's genes. But to the child, genes are a shadowy, meaningless concept compared to the flesh and blood parent.

George never felt related in any way to his father. Abandoned by him at an early age, he and his siblings were brought up entirely by their mother. His father's death from heart disease at the age of 38 had almost no impact on George, nor did he consider it significant to his own life that two of his father's brothers had suffered disabling heart attacks, or that still another had also died young of heart disease. What were they to him? His primary relationship was with his mother, a loving, determined woman who managed to make a life for herself and her children on Baltimore's East Side.

"In my neighborhood, you had to be street smart to survive," George remembers. "And I was." A secret smoker by the age of nine, by the time he was 13 he was addicted. In his mid-teens, he married and had his first child. At 19, his second was born.

In spite of his own history, George was determined to give his children what he had never had: a father they could look up to and rely on. He joined the army and there discovered his special aptitude for mechanical work. For three of his ten years in the military, George was an instructor in biomedical technology, and while in the service, he was in outstanding physical condition. In spite of continuing to smoke heavily, he remembers being able to run five miles without feeling out of breath. Emotionally, however, things were not so good. At age 23 his marriage fell apart and George soon found himself a single father with two young children, ages 4 and 6, to raise.

Three years later, he remarried and settled in New Hampshire. With Sharon he felt that his life was at last coming together. His children adjusted well to their new home and George landed an excellent job as an X-ray field service engineer.

His work was demanding, requiring both travel and a strict adherence to deadlines. Hospitals all over New England depended upon him to keep them on schedule—they couldn't afford to have their equipment down for even an hour. George thrived on the stress and the responsibility: he knew he could fix anything from an infant scale to a CAT scanner, and he loved seeing the looks of relief his arrival occasioned at a hospital where a vital machine was malfunctioning. He took his work very seriously, almost never missing a day due to illness, although he did suffer from irritable bowel syndrome.

But in spite of his insistence that the higher the pressure, the better his performance, in his more honest moments he had to admit that stress sometimes did get the better of him. He noticed that when he worried too much about his children or when he was working on an especially complicated job, his bowel problem would flare up, causing him significant stomach discomfort. Indeed, he frequently required medicine for relief.

In November 1993, George was not surprised by daily stomach pain while working on a difficult assignment in Portland, Maine. The fact that the pain was also in his chest didn't bother him too much—he figured it must be heartburn—but the severe discomfort in his shoulder disturbed him. By the time he finished up the job late one evening, he had decided to make an appointment to have his shoulder evaluated.

That night, while traveling home, he felt weak and nauseated, and his left shoulder was aching so badly he had trouble driving. "I must be getting the flu," he decided. His main reaction was annoyance—it was the worst time to get sick. His mother had just arrived for Thanksgiving and he had a service call in Berlin, New Hampshire, the next day that simply couldn't wait.

He arrived home at eleven that night, exhausted. Sharon took one look at him and said, "You can't go to Berlin tomorrow." George, however, insisted stubbornly that he had to go—he didn't want this call hanging over his head through the Thanksgiving holiday. Knowing her husband, Sharon didn't push the point, but told him matter-of-factly that she and his mother would be coming along for the ride.

Although he felt no better the next day, George did go to Berlin. Once there, however, the size of the job and his now extreme discomfort forced him to admit that he wasn't up to doing it. He told the hospital staff that he would need to order some parts and would return within a few days.

The next day, he called in sick. At noon, feeling slightly better, he made himself some lunch, but as he sat down to eat he was overcome by severe feelings of anxiety. Unable to identify the cause, he sat quietly for a few minutes but soon began sweating profusely. As the pain in his shoulder radiated to his left arm, it suddenly clicked—"I'm having a heart attack," he thought.

He asked his mother to call Sharon at work immediately. "Tell her I'm on my way to the emergency room," he said, putting on his jacket and picking up the car keys.

His mother was shocked. "Let me call an ambulance," she insisted, but George was adamant that he would drive himself. "What if I'm not having a heart attack?" he asked her. "I'd feel like an idiot calling an ambulance for nothing."

Somehow George made it to the hospital where he was quickly evaluated in the emergency room. Two tools are used to determine whether a person is having a heart attack: the electrocardiogram (ECG) and blood enzyme tests. The ECG measures changes in the electrical activity of the heart as it is beating. In the face of a heart attack, the ECG may be quite abnormal (unfortunately, it may also be totally normal).

The blood enzyme test is also problematic. When heart muscle cells are destroyed during a heart attack, they release their contents (enzymes) into the bloodstream. These can be measured to determine the extent of the damage. However, since it may be several hours before the enzymes can be detected by a blood test, the first readings are not always accurate.

George's ECG and first enzyme tests were, in fact, normal. But because of his symptoms, family history, smoking habit, and the fact that he was considerably overweight, the emergency room physician was not willing to rule out the possibility of a heart attack. He gave George two of the most commonly prescribed medications for the pain associated with a heart attack: morphine, which helped considerably, and nitroglycerine, which did nothing.

George, relieved of most of his pain, was embarrassed to hear that his test results were negative. "What an ass I am, wasting everyone's time this way," he thought. "I probably have the flu." Rather sheepishly, he asked about going home and was surprised to find that the doctor was not ready to release him. He explained to George the preliminary and fallible nature of the tests and that his history raised certain doubts which should be cleared before he returned home. He suggested that George relax until the next day, when further test results would be available.

In spite of his growing certainty that the whole thing was a big mistake, George agreed and let himself be moved to the coronary care unit (CCU). Feeling much better due to the morphine, yet surrounded on all sides by highly sophisticated machines, he felt more and more embarrassed by the situation. He was particularly upset at having traumatized his mother so badly. A very traditional man, he hated the idea of seeming weak or vulnerable to the women he cared about. By the next morning, he was convinced that there was nothing wrong with his heart and that what he really needed was a cigarette.

So when cardiologist Dr. Patrick Lawrence arrived in his room that day with the news that his second and third blood enzyme tests clearly indicated a heart attack, George was stunned. He listened in silence as Dr. Lawrence explained that although his heart attack appeared to be quite small, he would still need to make major changes in his life, including giving up smoking, exercising regularly, and drastically reducing the fat in his diet. His cholesterol values, obtained the day before in the emergency room, were also cause for concern.

	George's Level	Desirable Level
Total cholesterol	236 mg/dl	Less than 200 mg/dl
Triglycerides	600 mg/dl	Less than 150 mg/dl
HDL cholesterol	23 mg/dl	Greater than 45 mg/dl
LDL cholesterol	—	Less than 100 mg/dl

There was no reading for LDL cholesterol, because when the triglycerides are over 400 mg/dl, LDL values cannot be easily determined.

By now George was feeling overwhelmed. He had been told while in the service that his triglycerides were elevated, but he'd not realized by how much. He had also been unaware of how low his HDL was or of how important all these numbers were in determining his cardiac well-being.

Finally, Dr. Lawrence told him that it was important to get an idea of the extent of his heart disease. To do this, he wanted to have George undergo a cardiac catheterization a few days later. After explaining the procedure to him, he left George to rest.

Rest, however, was the last thing on George's mind. "How could this be happening?" he wondered. There must have been some mistake—maybe his blood test had been mixed up with someone else's? He just felt too good to be having a heart attack. But even as he worried and argued with himself, his chest pain began again. While not uncommon, this symptom is nonetheless worrisome since even more of the already-compromised heart muscle becomes at risk. The decision was made to bring George to the catheterization laboratory immediately.

Although he himself had installed dozens of X-ray procedure labs in hospitals all over New England, the thought of being a patient in one had never occurred to him. By nature a light-hearted person with a fine sense of humor, George was unusually quiet as Dr. Bob Dewey, Dr. Lawrence's partner, began the procedure. Sedated but conscious, he was soon aware that he was, in one critical sense, his father's son after all. He had inherited his father's heart.

Two of the major heart arteries, the left anterior descending (LAD) and the circumflex, had significant cholesterol blockages—95 percent and 75 percent, respectively. On the LAD, Dr. Dewey was able to perform a directional coronary atherectomy (DCA), a procedure in which a cholesterol deposit (plaque) is actually shaved off the wall of the diseased artery and removed from the body by an X-ray guided catheter. Within 90 minutes, George's deposit was reduced from 95 to 10 percent. The same procedure, unfortunately, was not possible for the circumflex artery, since the blockage was at a location unsuitable for the use of DCA. It was decided to tackle this blockage by means of balloon angioplasty. George was scheduled to return to the laboratory the following day.

That night, he had trouble sleeping. Everything had happened so quickly and dramatically that he still hadn't been able to take it all in. He examined the situation from every angle, trying to make some sense of it. How could it be possible? And how could he get his hands on a cigarette without anyone finding out?

The next day, however, he found he was much less nervous as he was wheeled into the catheterization lab. "Hey, Doc," he called across the room as Dr. Dewey walked in. "How come you guys are X-raying me on my competitor's equipment?"

"What do you mean, George?" Dr. Dewey asked

"Does this lab have pulse fluoro [a built-in radiation-reduction device]? You guys better not be cooking me in here!"

Dr. Dewey laughed. "Shall we transfer you to a hospital with one of your own labs, then?"

"Ah, but then I wouldn't have you, would I?" George was laughing, too.

The procedure went beautifully. In spite of some significant chest pain while it was going on (at one point, George asked, "Can you get this family of elephants off my chest?"), the result was outstanding—a plaque reduction from 75 percent to less than 10 percent.

The days that followed, however, were extremely difficult for George. Smoking was turning out to be a more serious addiction than he had imagined, and the prospect of giving it up disturbed him more than any of the other changes the doctor had told him would be necessary. While in the hospital, the strict no-smoking rule made compliance inevitable, but once he returned home, the choice was his.

His wife made her decision on the day he was discharged: she gave up her own 25-year habit that morning. George, however, had no interest in quitting—he was interested only in getting a cigarette. Unable to go out to buy his own, he turned in desperation to his 17-year-old son who had also been smoking for years. Chad initially refused, but George was insistent and was soon back up to a pack a day. Sharon was so furious she decided, in a fit of illogic, to go back to smoking herself.

A few days later, however, in a cooler mood, she reconsidered her decision. Maybe the best way to influence George would be by example. She quit again, with the help of the nicotine patch, and this time she stuck with it.

George didn't like to admit it, but her resolve impressed him. Even less did he like to admit how moved he was by her obvious concern for his well-being. Six weeks after his heart attack, George finally made up his mind that he was going to quit smoking. He went so far as to consult a hypnotist, but in the end, it was his own will that won the battle.

And a battle it was, fought at the beginning almost minute by minute. George discovered to his surprise just how much of his life revolved around smoking, and how important cigarettes were in helping him relax. This realization was useful to both George and Sharon—together they began new routines for relaxing which did not include smoking. Five minutes at a time, both of them got through the difficult first weeks. For Sharon, the break has been a welcome one; George continues to struggle with the smoke-free life, but both have stayed off cigarettes to this day.

George's first cardiac rehabilitation class coincided with a period he remembers as the blackest in his entire life. Lady, his beloved 10 ½-year-old dog, had been seriously ill for some time and finally had to be put to sleep. His grief for her was such that at one point he actually developed chest pain thinking about it.

But entering cardiac rehabilitation at this time was, ironically, the perfect solution. Emotionally devastated and physically weakened, George had no place to go but up. At first, he found the classes both intimidating and embarrassing. At age 38, he was ashamed of being so much younger than everyone else and still so out of shape. He was also afraid that he might just have another heart attack exercising on all of the complicated-looking equipment.

Lydia Crabtree, the exercise physiologist at his rehabilitation class, was reassuring. The whole point of the class, she explained, was that he would be able to exercise in a supervised setting. In the unlikely event that some problem did arise, people with cardiac expertise would be there to assist. More important, however, the class would enable him to develop a safe and appropriate program that he could continue for the rest of his life. Whatever he tried in class he could safely try at home.

After the initial awkwardness of settling in, George found cardiac rehabilitation a truly positive addition to his life. Because of his youth, he was able to get back into shape very rapidly, and he soon found himself looking forward to the class. Because he was not yet back at work, the program gave his day a structure and focus he had been missing. With the other members of the group, he developed a camaraderie that went beyond the typical exercise class esprit de corps—they had all been through a momentous life-and-death experience and the bonds that were created as a result were strong.

Most people in George's situation share the same experience. A good cardiac rehabilitation program is much more than just exercise. At The New England Heart Institute, for example, each participant receives private nutritional counseling from Mary Card, a registered dietitian, and attends lectures on the importance of cholesterol and stress reduction, blood pressure control, and quitting smoking. I give a lecture on cholesterol to every group that goes through the program.

I still remember the day I met George. After my lecture to his group, he was the first one to raise his hand with a question. He wanted to understand the subject thoroughly and he kept asking until he did. His lively spirit made him a clear favorite in the class, and I found his attitude infectious. He seemed determined to enjoy his life in spite of his cardiac disease, and from what I could see, he was succeeding.

At his first visit to my clinic, he charmed the entire staff when he insisted that our scale needed recalibrating as it made him weigh two pounds more than he actually did. This is a line we hear very often, but not usually from a professional. He was, of course, absolutely right. He recalibrated the scale and threatened to send me a bill.

George's cholesterol values at his first clinic visit confirmed the levels obtained at the time of his heart attack:

	George's Level	Desirable Level
Total cholesterol	234 mg/dl	Less than 200 mg/dl
Triglycerides	546 mg/dl	Less than 150 mg/dl
HDL cholesterol	23 mg/dl	Greater than 45 mg/dl
LDL cholesterol	—	Less than 100 mg/dl

Given his very strong family history of cardiac disease, I suspected that George suffered from Familial Combined Hyperlipidemia (FCH). FCH is the most common genetic cholesterol disorder, affecting roughly 1 out of every 100 Americans. It was discovered over 20 years ago by researchers at the University of Washington in Seattle. Investigation has shown that roughly one-half of the first-degree relatives of an FCH patient will have the same condition, and that such persons have a high risk of developing premature heart disease, as George did.

The designation "Familial Combined Hyperlipidemia" describes what is found in the lipid profiles of affected individuals. This could be a high total cholesterol level, a high triglyceride level, or both. In a family with FCH, one person may have a high total cholesterol, another high triglycerides, while a third might have both. All three would share an increased risk of developing early heart disease.

I explained to George the basic treatment plan, consisting of diet, exercise, weight loss and, if necessary, cholesterol-lowering medications.

When I asked George about his food preferences, he reminded me somewhat apologetically that he was from Baltimore. "We eat a lot of fried stuff down there," he said. "Face it—anything tastes good as long as it's deep fried." He admitted that he was very fond of sweets as well. In spite of these preferences, however, he said he had made a strong effort to stick to the diet Mary Card had worked out for him while in cardiac rehabilitation, but that he still hadn't lost much weight. He was clearly frustrated by the lack of results, but I saw things a bit differently. I pointed out that he had given up smoking since his heart attack and had managed not to gain any weight in spite of it. He had a right to be proud of himself.

He did, however, still need to lose a fair amount and he agreed to make a loss of five pounds his target for our next meeting one month later. Because an elevated triglyceride level was one of his specific lipid abnormalities, I was pleased to hear that he drank very little alcohol—triglycerides are dramatically elevated by fats, sugars, and alcohol.

We also discussed the importance of exercise, but here I was preaching to the converted. George was sold on the value of exercise, and although he had "graduated" from cardiac rehabilitation and no longer had the group to keep him on the straight and narrow, he still worked out three to five days a week.

One month later I met George again. He had not been able to lose any more weight, and when he saw his latest cholesterol levels, he was even more discouraged:

	George's Level	Desirable Level
Total cholesterol	235 mg/dl	Less than 200 mg/dl
Triglycerides	1396 mg/dl	Less than 150 mg/dl
HDL cholesterol	23 mg/dl	Greater than 45 mg/dl
LDL cholesterol	—	Less than 100 mg/dl

The triglyceride level was particularly alarming. I asked George if he had eaten any rich foods in the past few days, but he said he hadn't. Before coming to the clinic, in fact, all he had had was a cup of coffee with cream and sugar. I hated to have to tell him, but even that was enough to send his triglycerides through the ceiling. Indeed, anything other than water could do it. I explained to George that this was the reason we ask people to fast for 12 hours before coming to the clinic.

It was a dramatic realization for George. "Look," he said. "If I eat three meals a day and at least one or two snacks—does it mean my triglycerides are always this high?"

Unfortunately, that was exactly what it meant.

"Well, what's so bad about high triglycerides," George asked. He pointed out that all the media ever reported on was LDL—the bad cholesterol.

I told George that he wasn't alone in wondering whether high triglycerides were a bad thing. For years the medical community has debated this question. At first, it appeared that triglycerides were only a risk factor for the development of cardiac disease in women.

Recently, however, Dr. Melissa Austin has examined the results of many research studies. Taken together, they made clear that high triglycerides are a risk factor *for men as well as women*. Even more recently, Dr. Gerd Asserman, director of the very large PROCAM study in Germany, has conclusively proven that high triglycerides predict cardiac disease in men. It has now been shown that just as in the case of LDL cholesterol, triglycerides can be found in the plaques that block the heart arteries. I told George that if Dr. Dewey had sent the material he had removed from George's coronary artery to the lab we would have found triglycerides to be present.

To make matters worse, triglyceride elevation seems to be a marker for a whole host of metabolic abnormalities. For example, persons with high triglycerides tend to have high levels of clotting factors in their bloodstreams (which, in combination with arterial plaque, places them at high risk for a heart attack) and very low levels of the protective HDL cholesterol, which brings the LDL cholesterol back to the liver for processing.

Finally, high triglycerides tend to occur along with a particularly dangerous form of LDL called small dense LDL, which is very likely to cause plaque buildup within an artery. As a person with high triglycerides lowers his or her level of this blood fat, these related metabolic abnormalities tend to improve dramatically, especially the low HDL.

I reminded George of his very low HDL cholesterol level and explained that in individuals with his particular cholesterol abnormality—Familial Combined Hyperlipidemia—triglyceride reductions are essential. He didn't need any more convincing. Now all he wanted to know was how to bring his levels down.

I suggested that George begin a medication called gemfibrozol (Lopid). Given the extent of his cardiac disease, I thought it important to reduce his cholesterol rapidly. Once he had lost a considerable amount of weight, we might consider taking him off the medication to see if his levels remained normal. With Lopid, I told him I expected to see a significant drop in his triglycerides and a corresponding increase in his HDL. Since his triglycerides were so high, we had never been able to measure his LDL (bad) cholesterol, because it cannot be accurately determined when triglycerides are above 400 mg/dl. Thus, getting George below 400 would allow me to see if his LDL were a further risk factor. That day, he met again with Mary Card to review in more detail the components of a triglyceride-lowering diet.

George returned eight weeks later, beaming. He had lost 13 pounds and he was thrilled. It had been a major struggle: he still craved the rich foods he was so fond of and he felt hungry most of the time. But his hard work paid off, both on the recalibrated scale and in his lab report:

	George's Level	Desirable Level
Total cholesterol	218 mg/dl	Less than 200 mg/dl
Triglycerides	259 mg/dl	Less than 150 mg/dl
HDL cholesterol	30 mg/dl	Greater than 45 mg/dl
LDL cholesterol	136 mg/dl	Less than 100 mg/dl

Even though this was indeed a big improvement, it still wasn't good enough. George's LDL—which we could now measure accurately—was still too high, his HDL too low, and his total cholesterol divided by his HDL level (i.e., the total to HDL ratio) was very high at 7.3. In persons with cardiac disease, I aim to get this ratio below 4.0, with 3.5 being the ideal. George was eager to see if losing more weight would make an appreciable difference, since he wanted to avoid a second cholesterol-lowering medication if possible. He left my office determined to reduce his weight still further.

When George returned to my office about three months later, he was very discouraged because he had regained 5 pounds. Although still eight pounds lighter than when he had his heart attack, his weight gain was reflected in his lipid profile:

	George's Level	Desirable Level
Total cholesterol	292 mg/dl	Less than 200 mg/dl
Triglycerides	348 mg/dl	Less than 150 mg/dl
HDL cholesterol	43 mg/dl	Greater than 45 mg/dl
LDL cholesterol	179 mg/dl	Less than 100 mg/dl

Even though his ratio was actually slightly better at 6.7 (probably due to the Lopid-induced rise in his HDL), it was still too high. The increase in his LDL and triglycerides were likely the direct result of his weight gain. I told George I thought it was time to consider a second cholesterol-lowering medication aimed at reducing his LDL.

I explained that many studies had shown that reversal of existing coronary artery disease is possible when the LDL level falls below 100 mg/dl, but that at 179 mg/dl, his disease was not only unlikely to reverse, it was quite possibly worsening. Since he had already had a heart attack, I knew I didn't have the luxury of waiting any longer for diet to improve his levels. This did not mean, however, that he should stop his dietary or exercise efforts: his goal should be to come off the second medication as soon as possible.

I asked George to begin simvastatin (Zocor), a very powerful LDL-lowering drug. Zocor also has a modest effect on HDL and triglycerides. As George was now on two cholesterol-lowering medications which both worked in the liver, it would be very important that his liver function be monitored closely. If he did develop a problem, it would very likely be completely reversible if caught early.

When I saw George seven weeks later, he had lost a few more pounds and had taken both medications faithfully. He was happy to report that he had not noticed any side effects. We were both thrilled with his lab report:

	George's Level	Desirable Level
Total cholesterol	192 mg/dl	Less than 200 mg/dl
Triglycerides	226 mg/dl	Less than 150 mg/dl
HDL cholesterol	40 mg/dl	Greater than 45 mg/dl
LDL cholesterol	107 mg/dl	Less than 100 mg/dl

While not yet perfect, his ratio of 4.8 was a dramatic improvement on his initial ratio of 10.6. With the loss of a few additional pounds, he will be right where he wants to be.

George's battle with heart disease can be seen as a metaphor for his life. Nothing in his struggle for cardiac health has been easy. Giving up smoking, changing his diet, learning new ways to cope with anger and stress—all have been accomplished only with enormous effort and self-discipline. But where an observer sees the struggle, George sees the challenge. "It [heart disease] got the Irish in me up," he says. "I just decided it wasn't going to beat me."

Street smart and determined, George has managed not only to survive but to prosper in one tough situation after another. Heart disease, which is tough any way you look at it, has forced George to mobilize his resources most effectively: with the prize being his life, this is a battle he is going to win. Having worked with him now for two and a half years, I am as certain as he is that any setbacks along the way are only temporary. The victory will be his.

5

~~~~~~

Estrogen Replacement Therapy

and Your Heart: Sorting Out

the Risks and Benefits

Coronary artery disease (cholesterol blockages in the heart arteries) kills 250,000 American women each year. More women die from heart disease than from all cancers combined. The cancers most women worry about, breast and uterine, kill 45,000 and 5700 women, respectively, each year.

These cancers can be devastating, and I in no way want to diminish your justified concern about them. However, as a scientist (and woman), the statistics make it clear to me that the majority of postmenopausal women should be more concerned about their personal risk for developing heart disease. Even more important than understanding your own risk is the willingness to take steps to prevent it from occurring. Taking estrogen is one such step.

The average American woman begins menopause at the age of 51 (this figure is about a year earlier for smokers). At menopause, blood estrogen levels decline sharply and cardiac risk increases dramatically. Although menopause cannot be prevented, increased cardiac risk can be decreased by estrogen replacement therapy (ERT). Women who take estrogen after menopause are much less likely to have a heart attack than those who don't. Studies have shown that women who take estrogen reduce their risk for heart disease by 35 to 50 percent. If they already have heart disease and begin ERT, they can reduce their risk of a future cardiac event such as a heart attack, bypass surgery, or angioplasty by as much as 80 percent.

What You Should Know About Estrogen Replacement Therapy

Estrogen protects against heart disease in many ways:

1. It raises high-density lipoprotein (HDL), also known as the "good cholesterol," and lowers low-density lipoprotein (LDL), "bad cholesterol." These effects account for about 50 percent of estrogen's protection.

2. Estrogen decreases lipoprotein (a)—abbreviated Lp(a)—levels, one of the risk factors mentioned in Chapter 1. Lp(a) is a predictor of premature heart disease. Levels of Lp(a) are entirely genetically determined and do not seem to be modified by diet or exercise. To date, the only medications shown to reduce Lp(a) levels have been niacin and estrogen.

3. Estrogen is an antioxidant (much like vitamins E and C). In many studies, antioxidants appear to protect LDL from being oxidized. Oxidized LDL is the form of LDL that most easily enters the atherosclerotic plaque, which is a cholesterol deposit within an artery wall. Plaques have fibrous caps full of cholesterol and cellular debris. Plaques containing lots of cholesterol are likely to rupture, and when this happens, the body responds by forming a blood clot on top of the rupture. The combination of the plaque and the blood clot can be devastating, causing a complete blockage of the artery and an ensuing heart attack.

4. Estrogen is a powerful dilator of coronary arteries, and of course when an artery dilates, more blood can flow through it.

5. Finally, estrogen also seems to inhibit platelets, or blood-clotting cells, from clumping and leading to a blockage within the heart's arteries.

Despite these benefits, many women are still concerned about the side effects of estrogen. This is a very important matter because there are a number of side effects, some minor and others quite serious. Most women will experience breast tenderness when they begin ERT, while others will have headaches, nausea, and occasionally weakness or dizziness. Most of these side effects disappear or are greatly reduced in severity after several weeks of therapy.

It is a widely held belief that hormones cause weight gain; not uncommonly this is a woman's biggest concern. Is there any solid evidence for this? The answer is quite simply No. There is little doubt that during the first couple of months on hormone replacement many women do experience a sensation of bloating, but this goes away and does not cause weight gain.

In the recently published PEPI (Postmenopausal Estrogen Progesterone Intervention) study, women were divided into five groups—one group received a placebo (an inert pill that caused no effects), and the other four received different hormone preparations daily for three years. At the end of the study all groups, including the group receiving the inert pill, had gained exactly the same amount of weight. So it appears that women tend to gain weight with age regardless of whether or not they are taking hormones. With a sensible diet and exercise program, such as the one outlined in this book, this age-related weight gain may be totally avoided.

Women on estrogen have a very slight increase in the risk of gallbladder disease. If you have had previous gallbladder problems, it will be important to discuss this issue with your doctor prior to beginning estrogen.

When estrogen is taken alone, there is an increased risk of developing uterine cancer, but because of this, physicians should add progesterone to a woman's hormone regime. Its use either as a daily dose or for 12 days out of the month appears to eliminate excessive risk of uterine cancer.

There is also some concern that estrogen therapy might increase the risk of breast cancer, but most studies have found no increased risk when it is used for up to five to ten years. However, women using ERT for more than five to ten years may be at a slight increased risk for the development of breast cancer, though there is evidence that women who develop breast cancer while on estrogen replacement have a better chance of early detection and cure than women who are not on ERT.

The fear of cancer is terrifying. Many women for whom the benefits of ERT clearly and dramatically outweigh its risks are nonetheless unable to overcome this fear. In the near future, however, women may no longer find themselves in this cruel dilemma. Although it is too early to say for sure, exciting new research by Dr. Thomas Clarkson and his group at Bowman-Gray School of Medicine has come up with an estrogen derived from soybeans which may provide women with all of the cardiovascular benefits of ERT and none of the risks of uterine cancer. The data for breast cancer are a little more preliminary, but this research, too, looks promising.

Dr. Clarkson's studies have been conducted in monkeys so it is still too early to make conclusive statements about humans, but since women and female monkeys have similar reproductive cycles, these studies are very encouraging.

It is wonderful to see this research being done, and I look forward to the day when women will be able to protect themselves against cardiac disease, their number one killer, without having to agonize over their increased risk of cancer.

Aside from prevention of coronary artery disease, ERT has other benefits. Women on the therapy are at decreased risk for development of osteoporosis, which is a very important benefit because twice as many women die each year of complications resulting from hip fractures caused by osteoporosis than die of breast cancer. Those on ERT have improved sleep patterns, no longer have hot flashes, and may also have generally improved moods, increased concentration, and higher energy levels. In addition, ERT may restore sexual interest and it generally improves vaginal lubrication.

For women who have not had a hysterectomy (surgery to remove the uterus), estrogen must be combined with progesterone in order to prevent uterine cancer. Although scientists and physicians thought it probable that the combination of estrogen and progesterone would reduce the risk of cardiac disease, until recently there was little information regarding this question. But in January 1995, the PEPI study was published along with its findings. This national study found that women taking a combination of estrogen and progesterone do in fact experience significant improvement in cardiovascular risk factors. And in August 1996, results of a 16-year followup from a Nurses' Health Study were published in *The New England Journal of Medicine*. This study, participated in by over 59,000 nurses, found that the estrogen and progesterone combination was as effective against the development of cardiac disease as estrogen taken alone.

As you think about estrogen (and progesterone) replacement, it is very important to know that there are many different hormone preparations. Sometimes a woman will experience side effects with one medication but not with another. Estrogen can also be given either orally or through a patch worn on the skin. Although we try to use the oral form, for some women the patch may be the better option.

It is crucial that you work with your doctor to tailor your estrogen replacement regime to your personal needs. Use the list of different estrogen preparations at the end of this chapter to discuss your options and keep trying until you find the estrogen that is right for you.

Is Hormone Replacement Therapy for You?

If you are wondering whether hormone replacement therapy (HRT) is right for you, I urge you to discuss this issue with your primary care doctor, considering the following questions:

- Do I have heart disease, or am I at high risk for heart disease?
- Do I have osteoporosis, or am I at high risk for osteoporosis?
- Do I have a history of breast cancer, or a family history of breast cancer? (See the detailed discussion of this topic in the next section.)
- Do I have gallbladder disease or am I at high risk for gallbladder disease?

Finally, prior to beginning estrogen all women should obtain a complete cholesterol profile. As mentioned above, estrogen dramatically improves cholesterol levels. It can however, in certain circumstances, cause striking increases in another blood fat, the triglycerides. This situation typically arises when a woman's baseline cholesterol profile reveals a triglyceride level greater than 250 mg/dl. In such a case I recommend using an estrogen patch rather than a tablet. While the patch does not significantly improve the LDL and HDL levels, it provides the other cardiovascular benefits without causing triglyceride elevations.

So the research is clear: estrogen protects postmenopausal women from developing cardiac disease and can help prevent further complications for women who already have heart disease.

In Patricia's case, which follows, you will see how estrogen—and the lack of it—affected one young woman's life.

If You Have a History of Breast Cancer

Until recently, I would have said that if a woman had a history of breast cancer, estrogen replacement therapy was really out of the question. I was prompted to question this notion several months ago when, after giving a lecture on the topic of women and cardiac disease, I was approached by Nancy, the director of a support group for breast cancer survivors. Nancy asked, "In what situations can breast cancer survivors consider the use of postmenopausal estrogen?" I was embarrassed to admit I'd never thought about this question. But of course it made perfect sense. Postmenopausal women often experience unpleasant and even crippling symptoms related to declining estrogen levels, and breast cancer survivors are no exception. Among the immediate symptoms of menopause are hot flashes, night sweats, mood swings, and dryness of the vaginal tract which can lead to painful intercourse and urinary tract infections. These may be the symptoms women notice most, but they are also aware that estrogen has other benefits, among them protection against heart disease and bone loss.

I told Nancy I would research the question and get back to her.

The survival rate after treatment for breast cancer has been improving since 1979. To deny breast cancer survivors the use of postmenopausal estrogen might leave them in the situation of having beaten cancer only to die of heart disease or complications from a hip fracture. The chemotherapy used in the treatment of breast cancer often causes the ovaries to cease functioning (that is, stop producing estrogen). This means that premenopausal breast cancer patients may go through a very abrupt and early menopause. Because these women become estrogen deficient at an early age, they are at high risk for the eventual development of heart disease and osteoporosis.

Unfortunately, to date there are no published reports of large-scale trials evaluating the use of estrogen in breast cancer survivors. I did, however, review a number of articles that considered the pros and cons of this approach.

Of great concern is the theoretical possibility that long-term use of estrogen after being treated for breast cancer may increase the risk for cancer recurrence or even the development of a new breast cancer. Also troubling is the fact that estrogen use can increase the density of breast tissue, thus making it more difficult for a radiologist to find a recurrence or a new cancer on a mammogram.

Support for the notion that cancer may recur in these patients stems from data on healthy women in whom it appears that use of estrogen for more than five to ten years may increase the risk of breast cancer.

This concern has prompted the Breast Cancer Committee of the Eastern Cooperative Oncology Group to suggest the use of tamoxifen in conjunction with estrogen replacement therapy. Tamoxifen is a medication that has been proven to reduce the risk of recurrent or new breast cancers in women with a history of breast cancer. What's more, tamoxifen actually improves cholesterol levels.

Another concern voiced over the use of estrogen in breast cancer survivors is the possibility that it might activate quiescent or "sleeping" cancer cells and promote their rapid growth. Admittedly, this argument has several flaws: if this were the case, one would expect women diagnosed with breast cancer after menopause to fare better than premenopausal women because they do not have estrogen circulating in their bloodstreams to promote cancer cell growth. But quite the contrary is true: a woman's prognosis deteriorates if she is diagnosed following menopause. And women diagnosed with breast cancer while taking estrogen replacement therapy actually have an improved survival rate as compared to women not receiving hormone replacement therapy.

The bottom line is that at this point there is no firm evidence indicating harm from estrogen replacement following breast cancer and there are some possible advantages to its use—decrease in heart disease, decrease in bone fractures, and possible decreased risk of Alzheimer's disease. A woman who has had breast cancer and wants to consider estrogen replacement therapy needs to work closely with her personal physician to determine if the benefits in her particular situation outweigh the risks.

Estrogen Replacement Preparations

Brand Name	Dose	Oral versus Transdermal
Climara (estradiol)	0.05 to **0.1** mg/d	Transdermal Change weekly
Estrace (estradiol)	0.05 to **1**, 2 mg/d	Oral
Estraderm (estradiol)	0.05 to **0.1** mg/d	Transdermal Change biweekly
Estratab (esterified E)	0.3, **0.625**, 1.25, 2.5 mg/d	Oral
Menst (esterified E)	0.3, **0.625**, 1.25, 2.5 mg/d	Oral
Ogen (estropipate)	**0.75**, 1.5, 3 mg/d	Oral
Ortho-Est (estropipate)	**0.625**, 1.25 mg/d	Oral
Premarin (conjugated E)	0.3, **0.625**,* 0.9, 1.25, 2.5 mg/d	Oral
Vivelle (estradiol)	0.0375, 0.05, 0.075 0.1 mg/day	Transdermal Change biweekly
Combination Therapy		
Premphase (conjugated E + medroxyprogesterone acetate)	**0.625mg/5mg**	Oral
Prempro (conjugated E + medroxyprogesterone acetate)	**0.625mg/2.5mg**	Oral

*The highlighted doses are equivalent to 0.625 mg of Premarin. This dose of Premarin is thought to provide the greatest level of cardiovascular protection.

The Case of Patricia

Too Little Estrogen

One Friday evening in mid-September, after a long day and a longer week at work, Patricia, 39, a nurse, and her husband, Bob, set out from Salem, New Hampshire, with Danny, their 14-year-old, on an 85-mile trip to Freedom, New Hampshire, where they were to close their summer camp for the season. They arrived late at night, exhausted, and went immediately to bed.

They were up early the next morning, refreshed and ready to begin working. Bob got their boat on shore to prepare it for winterizing. Pick (Patricia's nickname) got Danny started on scrubbing the boat and then began working inside the camp, defrosting the refrigerator, cleaning out the cupboards, and putting things into storage. At intervals, she dashed down to the shore to help Danny with scouring, while Bob occupied himself with winterizing the engine.

By about 11 A.M., Pick began to feel nauseated. Blaming it on the oil fumes from the engine, she moved some distance from the boat and sat down on the ground, hoping the feeling would pass. Her shoulders began aching in a way she had never experienced before. She asked Bob to rub her back, but when this didn't help, she decided to go back to the camp and lie down. On the way she noted, with the clinical detachment that her nurse's training gave her, severe pain in her left arm. "I hope this isn't a heart attack," she thought, knowing this was certainly a pos-

151

sibility. A moment later, she felt pressure in her chest and began sweating profusely.

Luckily, Danny had followed her into the house. "Go get Dad," she told him. "Tell him I'm having a heart attack." Danny took one look at his mother and ran. Bob rushed in moments later, breathless and frightened, and the sight of Pick's ashen face did nothing to reassure him.

Because their camp was so secluded, they decided that rather than risk having the ambulance get lost looking for the place, they would drive to the ambulance stand themselves. Leaving Danny in the camp with strict instructions not to let anyone inside, they took off at 85 miles an hour for the eight-mile ride into town. To their dismay, however, the ambulance stand was vacant when they arrived. A neighbor's call to 911 brought a rescue squad volunteer within minutes, but the ambulance was still 25 miles away. The wait seemed endless. Although the volunteer put Pick on oxygen, she was having more and more trouble breathing and her chest pain had become almost unbearable. Bob stood by helplessly, with his own heart pounding uncontrollably as he watched his wife struggle.

Just as she was beginning to feel she wasn't going to make it to the hospital, the ambulance arrived and the trip into the city got underway. Enroute, the technicians attempted unsuccessfully to start an intravenous drip (IV), while Pick, an IV nurse, watched in frustration: "If only I had the energy, I could help them," she thought from somewhere at the end of a long tunnel. By then, she was too weak to even speak.

Following the ambulance in his truck, Bob was feeling much calmer, reassured by the fact that they were keeping to the speed limit. What he didn't know was that this was only because they were trying to start the IV—once they aborted their attempts, the driver surged ahead, throwing Bob into a terrible panic as he did his best to keep up with them.

Inside the ambulance, Pick was also very frightened, remembering all the young heart attack patients she had cared for as a nurse. She knew that younger people often fare poorly during their first heart attack because they have not had a chance to develop collateral vessels—the small blood vessels that sprout from undamaged heart arteries and help nourish portions of the heart served by the arteries that have become slowly blocked over a number of years. Collateral blood vessels are typically small and fairly tenuous, but certainly better than no blood flow at all.

By the time they arrived at the hospital, Pick's pain had intensified. In the emergency room a cardiogram was performed immediately, but unfortunately, as can sometimes happen, it failed to prove conclusively that Pick was in fact having a heart attack. As a result, she was not given the clot-dissolving medicine known as tissue plasminogen activator (TPA). Indeed, because of her age (she was only 39), and the fact that she had few obvious risks for the development of heart disease—she was a nonsmoker, and both her weight and blood pressure were normal—she was not even given nitroglycerin immediately. Nitroglycerin opens the heart's arteries, often relieving the pain of a heart attack. (It was eventually given to Pick, alleviating much of her chest pain.)

By this time, a cardiologist had arrived. Although he agreed that Pick's cardiogram was nondiagnostic, he knew that a heart attack could not be ruled out because Pick did, in fact, have a major cardiac risk factor: at 39 she had already been through menopause. Ten years earlier, at the age of 29, severe endometriosis had led to her having a total hysterectomy.

What is it about going through menopause that suddenly increases a woman's risk for developing cardiac disease? The most likely explanation is that at the time of menopause a woman's ovaries cease production of the female hormone, estrogen. Estrogen appears to protect women from cardiac disease prior to menopause in many ways. In fact, now it seems that almost weekly new such reports appear in scientific journals verifying its important role.

It has long been known that estrogen supplementation favorably affects a woman's cholesterol profile, lowering the low-density lipoprotein cholesterol (LDL) level, or "bad cholesterol," and raising the high-density lipoprotein cholesterol (HDL) level, or "good cholesterol."

Recent evidence also indicates that estrogen not only lowers the LDL level in the bloodstream but may additionally also prevent it from being deposited into the artery wall. Estrogen also seems to allow the heart arteries to dilate, leading to improved blood flow to all portions of the heart. Finally, additional evidence suggests that estrogen blocks platelet clumping. Platelets are small blood cells that tend to clot together. When such a blood clot forms within a coronary artery and blocks it, heart cells downstream from it are deprived of oxygen. If not quickly reversed, this situation can lead to a heart attack.

Pick had started on estrogen replacement therapy immediately following her hysterectomy, but soon afterward developed a severe allergic reaction. Her allergist identified the estrogen as its cause and, on his advice, she stopped taking it. For nearly 10 years, then, she had been deficient in estrogen.

A heart attack can be diagnosed in one of two ways: either through a cardiogram or by the use of a blood test which can determine whether the heart's muscle cells have been damaged. It was the blood test that finally spelt it out for Pick—she had in fact had a heart attack.

It was then decided that a catheterization should be performed to determine the location and size of the blockages in her coronary arteries. Pick's doctor decided to stabilize her over the weekend and then transfer her to a larger medical center for the procedure.

She was moved to the coronary intensive care unit, where she was put on blood thinners and IV nitroglycerin. For Bob, who had no medical background, the experience had a sort of nightmarish quality to it: everywhere he stood, he seemed to be in the way, and although he longed to reach out to Pick and offer her some reassurance, he was afraid that he might end up causing her more pain.

Everyone on the hospital staff knew exactly what to do, while he stood on the side, feeling more and more helpless. He wanted to understand the situation, but he didn't know where to begin or even what questions to ask. When Pick suggested that he call the family to let them know, he went immediately to a phone in the hall, happy to be doing something, however small.

When he tried to dial, however, he found to his dismay that he couldn't remember his own number, let alone anyone else's. He returned to Pick's bedside where she patiently recited the numbers he needed. For Bob, there was no more telling proof of how much he relied on her in his life.

"She's got to get through this," he kept repeating to himself as he went back to make the calls. "She's got to."

When Bob returned to her room, Pick was comfortable enough for the nurse to suggest that he go out to the camp to get Danny. Relieved to be doing something positive, he set out at once.

Danny, who had been alone all day, imagining the worst, was frightened and upset. In spite of Bob's reassurances, he remained withdrawn, not speaking a word during the entire ride to the hospital. When they arrived at Pick's bedside, Danny stood still, staring at the floor. She spoke to him gently, telling him that she would be alright and that he could give her a hug. Suddenly he broke down and rushed toward her, sobbing. As she held him, Pick's eyes met Bob's. Although no words were spoken, both resolved then that they would do whatever it took for Pick to make it.

After they left, Pick began what seemed like the longest night of her life. Nitroglycerin, while radically reducing chest pain, can also cause severe headaches. For the next 12 hours, Pick suffered from this side effect so intensely that she felt almost blinded by pain. She vomited so many times she lost track of the number, and after a few hours her chest pain returned.

This time she was given morphine to alleviate it, but this narcotic is so powerful she often wasn't sure where she was. During her brief coherent moments, however, one thought kept recurring with disturbing regularity: "It's possible I may not make it home." At last she asked that a priest be called. The nurses tried to reassure her, but her professional training made her realize that things could easily turn sour.

Sunday was a blur of continued chest pain, headaches, nausea, and vomiting. Pick's mother and their two older children, Rob and Laurie, had arrived but, unlike the day before, family visits were now limited to three minutes. Bob took this to mean that her condition had deteriorated, but was too afraid to ask anyone about it.

The next morning at 7 A.M., Pick was transferred to Catholic Medical Center in Manchester, New Hampshire. Bob arrived a few minutes later, alone. He had insisted that all three children attend school and had declined the company of other family members, confident that he could manage on his own. The moment he entered the hospital, however, he felt bewildered and overwhelmed. The woman at the information desk sensed his anxiety and quickly found out where Pick had gone. A moment later, Bob was being escorted to the cardiac care unit (CCU).

When he arrived, he found that Pick had already been taken to the catheterization lab where she would have to wait in line for her turn. Unfortunately, there were many emergencies that day and, since Pick was relatively stable, her procedure was postponed until later in the day. It was three o'clock before she finally returned to the ward. Bob spent that time in the waiting room with the families of other patients undergoing similar procedures.

He quickly realized how new to the game he was—everyone else seemed to know so much more than he did. They casually traded terms like "balloon angioplasty" and "coronary bypass" and asked him questions about Pick's condition that he couldn't begin to understand, let alone answer.

When he met Pick at three o'clock in the cardiac stepdown unit, both were physically and emotionally exhausted. Bob sat with her until the evening, hoping that when the cardiologist came he would be able to get some answers, but in the end, anxious to get back to the children, he had to leave before Dr. Bob Dewey arrived.

When he did come, quite apologetic for being so late—he had been in the catheterization lab for 12 straight hours—he explained to Pick that one of her main heart arteries, the left anterior descending (LAD), had a 50 percent cholesterol blockage. This puzzled Pick, as she knew from her training that such a blockage is rarely enough to cause a heart attack.

Dr. Dewey explained that it was likely that her blockage (or plaque) had become "unstable" and developed a blood clot on top, which completely blocked the artery. He went on to tell her that this combination of blood clot and cholesterol plaque is the cause of most heart attacks.

At any rate, coronary artery balloon angioplasty would not be required (for more information on this procedure, see Glossary). Balloon angioplasty, Dr. Dewey explained, is generally performed only on blockages of 70 percent or greater. Angioplasty of a smaller blockage can actually make matters worse.

Pick thought that having survived the catheterization, the worst was over. But late that evening, when she was allowed to get up to wash her face and brush her hair, the pain began all over again, and she was moved back to the CCU for closer monitoring. When her cardiogram began showing signs of inadequate blood flow, another catheterization was performed. Ultimately, after a second hellish night, she was stabilized with medications.

The following day, Pick turned the corner. Her condition improved dramatically, and a few days later, she was able to exercise for nine minutes without chest pain or worrisome changes on her cardiogram.

With each passing day, Pick became more confident that she could do whatever was required to prevent a second heart attack. Her cardiologists agreed. Before her discharge, she had a long discussion with them in which they told her that, because her exercise performance had been so encouraging, she would be able to begin a cardiac rehabilitation program and would probably be able to return to work and routine activities within a few months. Bob, unfortunately, was not present for this discussion.

Pick was determined to start in a cardiac rehabilitation group as soon as possible. Such a group provides a structured exercise program as well as an educational component in which participants are taught about low-fat diets, stress management, and ways to quit smoking.

Before joining the group closest to her home, she had to meet the program director, a meeting she insisted that Bob attend with her, so that he could hear for himself how well she was doing and perhaps learn to relax a bit about her health.

But her plan backfired. The director focused on the negative, stressing that because of her substantial heart damage, Pick would always be limited in how much she could manage. While it is true that many people do experience limitations following a heart attack, most lead very active lives, especially when they are as young as Pick.

She was furious that the director failed to focus on her progress and even more determined now to prove him wrong. Bob, however, now felt justified in his solicitude and did his best to protect her from even the smallest exertion. Pick found that the children, picking up on Bob's fears, were also treating her differently. Bob's mother, who was living with them at the time of Pick's heart attack, began to take over many of the household tasks, even refusing to let Pick lift a laundry basket.

In cardiac rehabilitation, Pick had begun to feel more and more like her old self, but at home she felt smothered and incompetent. She knew she had a chance of beating the spectre of heart disease, but she also knew she couldn't do it unless her family was behind her. Her illness was everyone's problem—in fact, it was consuming them. Everyone in the house was living daily with the fear that Pick was going to have another heart attack.

She decided it was time for a family meeting. Before calling everyone together, she mentally prepared a list of her cardiac risk factors, and the solutions with which she proposed to tackle them. Many of her solutions required substantial commitments from her husband, mother-in-law, and children, and she tried to be as clear as possible in spelling out what she was asking of them.

1. *Stress at work*: Pick's job just prior to her heart attack had involved a lot of overnight travel and lecturing. Although she was very well paid, she was always in fear of a layoff, making for a tense work atmosphere.

    Solution: She decided to leave this job, reasoning that although finding a new one would not be easy, her health was the most important thing at this point.

2. *Stress at home*: After a long day at work, it was Pick's habit to come home and prepare dinner, clean the house, run errands, and perform the thousand and one tasks that keep a home running smoothly. Although neither Bob nor the kids were unwilling to help, it simply had never occurred to her to ask them to offer.

    Solution: Everyone would be asked to pull their weight. Pick was pretty sure they would all actually feel better about themselves if they were contributing in a positive way.

3. *Lack of exercise*: Before the heart attack, Pick just couldn't find the time to exercise. Now, as far as she was concerned, finding the time had become a question of survival.

Solution: Cardiac rehabilitation had given her the confidence she needed to begin; the family helping out at home would give her the extra time she needed to continue. She also planned to encourage the rest of the family to join her—after all, the children shared her genes. She wanted them to reduce their own risk of cardiac disease in the future.

4. *High-fat diet*: Although Pick had never been overweight, she did enjoy high-fat foods, especially red meat.

   Solution: In cardiac rehabilitation, she had learned the importance of a low-fat, low-cholesterol diet. She had already purchased several books with information, menus, and recipes. She knew that the only way for her to stick to such a diet would be to ask the whole family to participate: having to prepare two separate meals would just not be practical.

5. *Cholesterol abnormalities*: Since her complete hysterectomy at the age of 29, Pick's cholesterol profile had been abnormal. She knew that this was largely due to her body's sudden lack of estrogen.

   Solution: Pick's cardiologist had recommended that she be evaluated at the cholesterol clinic to determine the best treatment for her situation. Pick decided to make the appointment, knowing that while exercise and diet would improve her cholesterol levels, they were never likely to completely normalize without estrogen replacement therapy.

6. *Family history of cardiovascular disease*: Pick's maternal grandfather had suffered his first heart attack in his fifties.

   Solution: Since she couldn't change her family history, Pick made up her mind to work even harder in the areas she could control.

When Pick presented this information to her family, she was delighted by their enthusiastic and positive response. Everyone had the chance to voice their fears and concerns, but by the end of the meeting, all had promised to make cardiac health a family goal.

The next day, they began to work as a team. Bob and Pick started grocery shopping together, reading labels and counting fat grams, then preparing meals as a couple. The children became much more responsible about cleaning their rooms and helping around the house. Everyone began exercising and they often found time for family walks.

About a month into her cardiac rehabilitation, Pick came to see me at the cholesterol clinic. After taking her history and doing a full physical, I considered her estrogen allergy closely. The bottom line was that she needed estrogen to protect her against future heart disease. Given the fact that studies have shown that in women with a history of heart disease, estrogen replacement reduces the risk of a future cardiac event by as much as 84 percent and that estrogen allergies are extremely rare, I decided to have her reevaluated by another allergist.

Dr. Helen Hollingsworth, who was at the time a professor at the University of Massachusetts Medical School, reviewed Pick's case and found, through the painstaking detective work for which allergists are famous, that each time Pick was thought to have had an allergic reaction to estrogen, she had also eaten at a particular sandwich shop. Her conclusion was that the allergy was more likely to have been caused by something in the sandwiches she had eaten—such shops, for example, often treat lettuce with meta-bisulfites, which are well known to cause allergic reactions.

We decided to give estrogen replacement therapy a trial. Pick did beautifully. Her HDL (the good cholesterol) rose from a low of 29 mg/dl to 38 mg/dl, while her LDL (the bad cholesterol) fell from 110 mg/dl to 72 mg/dl. Although her lipid profile is still not absolutely perfect, she is at much lower risk for another cardiac problem than she was before beginning estrogen.

In the two years since I met Pick, she has continued to exercise daily, and her low-fat diet has become her way of life. She has found a less stressful job that she enjoys immensely, and the changes her family made during her rehabilitation period have become permanent. Bob told me that Pick's heart attack forced them all to look at their harried lives and to reassess what was really important to them. As a result, he believes they have become much closer to each other. And, in case you are wondering, they decided to sell their boat.

6

∿∿∿∿∿∿∿∿∿∿∿∿∿∿∿∿∿∿∿∿∿

Reducing Stress

in Your Life

As a young physician, I read two books which surprised me: *Diet, Stress and Your Heart* by Dr. Dean Ornish and *Is It Worth Dying For?* by Dr. Robert Eliot. Both books explore the relationship between stress and the development of cardiovascular disease. This idea was quite new to me at the time and to test it out, I began asking my patients in the Cardiac Intensive Care Unit what they saw as the major cause of their heart disease. I expected them to identify their high-fat diets, lack of exercise, elevated cholesterol levels, smoking, obesity, or bad family histories as the primary source of their trouble. To my amazement, the majority offered none of these factors as the main one. To them, the real culprit was stress.

But when I asked what they planned to do about it once they were discharged, very few had any concrete plan in mind. They had new diets, exercise prescriptions, medications, and the will to quit smoking, but almost no one had a way to deal with stress.

Luckily, the hospital where I was then working, the University of Massachusetts Medical Center, offered an outstanding stress reduction and relaxation program, an eight-week course designed by Dr. Jon Kabat-Zinn to help people learn to cope with stress and pain that may be the cause of physical and emotional difficulties. One of Dr. Kabat-Zinn's primary tools is "mindfulness meditation," which helps create, as he explains in his book on the subject,* "moment-to-moment awareness. It is cultivated by purposefully paying attention to things we ordinarily never give a moment's thought to. It is a systematic approach to developing new kinds of control and wisdom in our lives, based on our inner capacities for relaxation, paying attention, awareness, and insight."

Not everyone to whom I suggested the program took it, but among those who did, I found even more surprises. I noticed, for example, that people who really took the course to heart were far more likely to be successful at quitting smoking, developing an exercise program, and losing weight. Of course, when I thought about it, it made perfect sense: these people were no longer wasting their best energy wrestling with inner demons. They were focused on their real goal of cardiac health.

In spite of my efforts on behalf of my patients, however, it was quite some time before I began to look at my own life and how I myself was dealing with stress. As a new doctor, I often worked a 36-hour shift without a moment's rest. When I did go home, exhausted as I was, I often had trouble sleeping, knowing the next day I had to tell one patient she had terminal cancer or another that his heart wasn't strong enough to withstand bypass surgery. Since I could do nothing to change the intense nature of my work, I decided to follow my own advice and take Dr. Kabat-Zinn's program.

It wasn't until I caught myself worrying about meeting one of my patients in the course that I realized that my true feelings about reducing stress were complicated and ambivalent. I recommended the course and talked a good line about its importance in cardiac rehabilitation, but what I really thought was that joining it was a sign of weakness and that I, a physician, was above such things. However, I did manage to get myself to the first class and that was all it took to put my worries to rest. People from all walks of life were there, including many who were highly successful and, to all appearances, very well adjusted. I soon began experiencing the same benefits of meditation that I had observed in my patients.

In the beginning, I was regular and disciplined about meditating. After about a year, however, something happened which I guess I should have anticipated. I was feeling wonderful, so good, in fact, that meditation no longer seemed such a necessity. Every now and then, I would skip a session, reasoning that I really didn't need it that much anymore. I also became pregnant and began to crave sleep more than anything

*Full Catastrophe Living: Using the Wisdom of your Body and Mind to Face Stress, Pain and Illness (New York: Delacorte/Dell, 1990)

else in life. It had been my habit to meditate first thing in the morning, but now I found that I just couldn't get up early enough. Rather than make time later in the day, I simply stopped meditating altogether.

Midway through my pregnancy, my husband, Tom, and I took jobs at Johns Hopkins Hospital in Baltimore, Maryland. What with getting ready for our first baby, moving to another city, and beginning new jobs, I believed I didn't have a moment to spare. And anyway, everything seemed to be going smoothly. If I had paused for breath, I might have noticed the tightrope I was walking, but who had time to stop?

In the end, it was my baby (who hadn't learned yet what a busy, important mother he had) who pulled me up short. Patrick, who was delivered by cesarean section, was born with a rare internal birth defect which made it impossible for him to eat. I was still dazed from my own surgery when Tom and I signed the consent form and our baby, whose face we barely knew, was whisked into the operating room for surgery that would last six hours.

During the procedure, I was unable to concentrate. My heart pounded wildly, I was nauseated, and my body trembled uncontrollably. Tom was my anchor, steady, sure, and somehow able to maintain his composure.

Although the surgery went beautifully, Patrick suffered four weeks of postoperative complications and on several occasions we believed we would lose him. My mental state was totally dependent on the kind of day Patrick had. If he did well, without the insertion of yet another tube or talk of a blood transfusion, I felt good. But if there were problems, I couldn't speak without crying.

I slept very little during his first month. After I was discharged myself, I commuted to the hospital daily and even felt guilty about the 15 minutes I snatched to run down to the cafeteria for lunch. Tom came every evening after work, and we stayed until we were almost too exhausted to drive home.

But somehow, with the support of our families, friends, and the wonderful hospital staff, we got through that horrific month. Today, though it seemed unimaginable then, Patrick is a sturdy six-year-old. Thank God, his little brother Liam, now age three, arrived in the world with much less commotion.

Soon after Patrick's operation, I began keeping a journal of the whole experience—a ritual that took on enormous importance to me. I told myself that I would give it to Patrick when he was old enough to understand, and I think this helped me believe that he was actually going to make it.

After Patrick came home, I continued writing the journal for several months, but I just didn't have the courage to go back and read what I had written earlier. I was in a state of almost constant tension, living with the fear that something could still happen to Patrick. In fact, when my maternity leave ended, I found myself unable to return to work. My boss, Dr. Alain Joffe, a wise and insightful man, suggested that I try coming back part time for a few months and then reevaluate the situation.

With great trepidation, I took his advice, but the toll on my nerves was enormous. Although we had a very competent sitter, I tortured myself the entire time I was away with visions of Patrick choking. I couldn't concentrate on anything while I was at work and even at home, with Patrick right in the same room, I was constantly on edge, unable to relax and enjoy his infancy. At night, sleep eluded me as I lay awake, my body tense, straining for the slightest sound of labored breathing from his crib. I was literally making myself sick.

The idea that stress can adversely influence our health is not new. Phrases like "worried to death" and a "nervous wreck" are part of our language because they reflect a reality that people intuitively understand. As far back as 1939, Dr. Franz Alexander, a Chicago psychiatrist, made the then controversial statement that many chronic disturbances were not caused by the commonly accepted agents of disease such as germs or chemicals, but by the "continuous functional stress" of simple everyday life.

Several years later, Dr. Walter Cannon, a physiologist at Harvard Medical School, traced the connection between the hypothalamus (a part of the brain) and the adrenal gland. He found that under certain stressful conditions, the hypothalamus directs the adrenal gland to release the powerful chemicals epinephrine (adrenalin) and norepinephrine (noradrenalin) into the bloodstream, producing many of the bodily sensations we associate with stress: increased heart and respiratory rate, higher blood pressure, an increased blood flow to the muscles, a faster blood clotting time, and the release of fats and sugars into the bloodstream.

Since then, Dr. Hans Syles, an organic chemist at McGill University in Montreal, found that under stress the adrenal gland also produces corticosteroids, powerful hormones with the potential to suppress the body's ability to fight disease.

Why should our bodies respond to stress in such self-destructive ways? At one time in our evolution, this stress response, often referred to as the "fight-or-flight response," was perfectly appropriate and at times even lifesaving. We didn't always buy our food in grocery stores.

Our ancestors lived in the wild and must have been often confronted by predators of all kinds, both animal and human.

The fight-or-flight response maximized a person's chance of survival in the face of a physical threat. The hyperaroused stress state allows for peak physical performance: blood is diverted to the muscles, allowing greater speed in running; the blood clots faster, preventing excessive bleeding in the event of injury; and fat stores are released, providing a ready source of energy.

These days, with very few of us likely to meet tigers in the bushes, the fight-or-flight response seems outmoded, at best. But while stress in the 1990s is more apt to be the result of emotional or intellectual conflicts (being stuck in traffic, an argument with one's spouse or child, financial difficulties, work pressure), as far as the brain is concerned, the enemy is out there, poised for attack. The body tenses, prepared for the on-slaught that never comes. If the stress is chronic, a state of continuous hyperarousal may develop, leading ultimately to serious medical complications, including cardiac disease, hypercholesterolemia (excess cholesterol in the blood), high blood pressure, fatigue, anxiety, and depression, to name a few.

While it is impossible to control all the things that may cause you stress, you do have the power to determine how your body responds to them. In the process of evolving beyond the fight-or-flight response, we have developed our minds to such an extent that we can now deliberately control much of what goes on in our bodies.

In Eastern cultures, meditation techniques have been practiced for centuries and are prescribed for many ailments. Here in the West this understanding came later, but is now documented in over 1200 scientific publications. Meditation has been found to result in many physiological changes, including reductions in cholesterol, blood pressure, heart rate, oxygen consumption, respiration, and muscle tension.

People who meditate regularly have been shown to be healthier than those who don't. In one study, 2000 meditators were compared to 60,000 nonmeditators with regard to their use of medical services over a five-year period—all had the same insurance carrier. Meditators had far fewer outpatient visits and fewer hospital admissions for a wide range of problems, including tumors, heart disease, and mental illness. When they were admitted to the hospital, they spent less time there.

Finally, it appears that it's never too late to benefit from meditation: in a study of elderly nursing home residents, those who began meditating were less likely to die over the three-year study period than those who did not.

In the early 1970s, Dr. Herbert Benson, a cardiologist at Harvard Medical School, introduced his patients to the "relaxation response." He found that through the practice of transcendental meditation (TM) many were able to achieve a relaxation response, resulting in a dramatic reduction in blood pressure. Some patients were even able to safely discontinue their medications. TM is a form of concentration meditation which involves placing the mind's attention on a single object and returning to it whenever the mind wanders.

In 1979 Dr. Jon Kabat-Zinn began the first stress reduction and relaxation program in the United States based on mindfulness meditation. This type of meditation is inherently different from other forms. It seeks to develop a calm, objective, nonjudgmental, neutral attitude of sustained alert attention. Although initially certain daily time periods must be devoted to developing mindfulness, eventually the habit can be brought to bear on each moment of life. Through its use, one can begin to recognize the root causes of stress, rather than simply using it as a quick fix for the symptoms of stress.

Dr. Kabat-Zinn's program is now well known internationally and to date over 7000 people have attended it at the University of Massachusetts Medical Center. Most recently, it was featured on Bill Moyers' Public Broadcasting System (PBS) television program "Healing and the Mind."

Although many people find it helpful to attend a formal stress reduction course, this is not essential. If you are sincerely interested, you can develop your own program at home. Not every meditation technique works for everyone—you may like to experiment a bit with the different ideas described here to find the one that works for you, remembering that no one approach is better than another. The general guidelines are meant to be used with all the different techniques. Don't be disturbed by a little frustration or restlessness as you begin meditating—these are common experiences and pass gradually as you continue practicing. The more you keep at it, the deeper and more lasting will be the benefits.

Each of the eight techniques I want to share with you will help your mind develop the habit of sustained attention. Eventually you will be able to allow thoughts, judgments, and opinions to simply pass through your awareness as a bird flies through the sky. You will see the mind-object, but only as a passive, nonjudgmental observer. It continues on its way while you bring your attention back to the technique you are using. Another way to understand this process is to see the distraction as a momentary event that has as much power as you choose to give it. With this perspective, you can develop a quality of mind that can be described as tranquil but alert.

Stress Management Techniques

The eight techniques commonly used in stress reduction programs are the body scan, breathing meditation, mindfulness meditation, self-hypnosis/creative visualization, hatha yoga, progressive muscle relaxation, exercise, and music. Each of these will be explained in detail. There are some general guidelines to follow to maximize your stress reduction experience and minimize the frustration commonly felt by beginners.

General Guidelines and Information

1. Find at least 30 minutes during which you will not be interrupted.
2. Wear loose comfortable clothing.
3. Keep the lights dim and the background noise low.
4. Position yourself comfortably, with your entire body supported.
5. Choose a time of day when you are most awake and alert; the idea is *not* to fall asleep.
6. Falling asleep is, nonetheless, common in the beginning, so be sure your head is supported.
7. Practice the techniques daily.
8. Simply follow the directions as described, finding your own breathing rhythm. You may follow the instructions on your own, make an audiocassette of the particular technique that you find most useful, or order a premade audiocassette (audiocassette list and mail order address on p. 177).
9. *Be kind to yourself.* It is very common for your attention to wander frequently during the early stages of practice. When you realize that your mind has wandered, simply return to the instructions for whatever technique you are using, letting go of whatever distraction pulled your attention away.
10. People tend to like one technique more than the others. Begin by practicing several different techniques until you find the one you are most comfortable with. As you become more proficient at stress reduction, you may find it helpful to alternate among several techniques.
11. Each time you practice one of the techniques, your experience will be different. It is important to begin each session without expectations and simply work with the way you are feeling at that moment.
12. Many people are surprised and often discouraged when they see how easily their attention wanders. *Remember that few things worth*

having come easily. Be patient and persevere, and you cannot help but succeed.

13. As your attention grows and distractions lessen, you will notice increasing calmness and relaxation.

All the stress reduction techniques that follow will help you to develop sustained attention. It is okay and inevitable that you will have passing thoughts, judgments, and opinions but try not to dwell on them. Simply observe them and let them pass. Then bring or return your attention to the technique you are using. The quality of mind that develops can be called *tranquil but alert.*

The Body Scan

This technique will guide your attention through your body. You will begin with your right foot and move systematically through the rest of your body. Throughout the exercise you should direct your breath to each body part, channeling calmness and relaxation with each in-breath and breathing out any stress, muscle tension, or distracting thoughts. Feelings of lightness, warmth, or numbness are common. These are signs for some people that their body has become deeply relaxed. Other experiences that can occur with any of the techniques include feeling as though your body is floating (which indicates that your muscles are so relaxed that they become like fluid, with your bones no longer firmly held in place by tense muscles); feeling that your mind is leaving your body (also a result of deep relaxation—this state is sometimes called "depersonalization"); and the recalling of past personal events from anytime in your life that may have been suppressed or repressed (discussed in more detail in the section on "Mindfulness Meditation").

As you work with this technique, you will become better able to quickly induce a state of relaxation in your body as well as your mind. You should plan to spend 30 minutes practicing the body scan. In that much time, your body can relax enough to allow for the necessary physiological changes to bring about the antistress effect.

Begin by placing yourself in a supported, comfortable position. If you like, slowly close your eyes. Focus your attention on your breathing, and feel your breath as it enters and leaves your body. Once you feel grounded in your breathing, direct the next breath down to the big toe of your right foot, sending calmness and relaxation to the toe and breathing out any tension, stress, or distracting thoughts. Do this for several minutes. You may also spend time feeling any sensations that may be present at the big toe: for example, the texture of clothing, the toe's position in space, or any sensations in the toe itself.

After several minutes, expand your attention to include all of your right foot and follow the same procedure. After several minutes on the right foot, continue with the body scan in the following order, following the same instructions as with the big toe: the right lower leg from the knee to the foot . . . the right upper leg from the hip to the knee . . . the entire right leg from the hip to the toes . . . the left big toe . . . the left foot . . . the left lower leg from the knee to the foot . . . the left upper leg from the hip to the knee . . . the entire left leg from the hip to the toes . . . the pelvic region including the buttocks . . . the abdomen—feeling any movement there as you breathe . . . the chest wall—feeling it expand and relax with each in-breath and out-breath . . . the back from the bottom of the neck to the buttocks . . . both the shoulders . . . the right hand . . . the entire right arm . . . the left hand . . . the entire left arm . . . the neck . . . the face, including the mouth, tongue, nose, cheeks, eyes, forehead, ears, and scalp . . . the entire head . . . the entire body, from the top of the head to the tips of the toes, feeling the breath move through the entire body . . . when you feel ready, slowly open your eyes, and bring the relaxation you attained into the rest of your day.

Breathing Meditation

This technique helps to develop one-pointed awareness, otherwise known as attention. Although we may believe that we are always paying attention, most people are surprised at how easily their attention drifts off to something "more interesting" than the breath. The instructions for this technique are simply to direct your attention to the in-breath and out-breath; *not* controlling the breath, but simply observing it as you might observe some object in nature, like a cloud passing by or a bird in the sky. When your attention wanders, simply let the distraction go with the next out-breath and redirect your attention to the breath, *with no judgment regarding the ease of distraction.*

Beware of the temptation to keep looking at your watch or clock. In the initial stages of practice, it may be helpful to set a watch alarm for the desired time: when the temptation to look at the time presents itself, simply observe this as another thought passing by and return your attention to the breath. It sounds easy, until you try it. It is truly a learning experience to watch, *nonjudgmentally*, how clever the thinking mind is at distracting your attention from such a simple task as watching your breath.

It often makes sense to start just by watching your breath for 5 to 10 minutes, and gradually increasing the time up to 30 to 45 minutes. Initially, you can combine this technique with one of the others to practice your full 30 minutes each day. As you feel more comfortable with the breathing meditation, you can gradually increase your time practicing it.

Later, as your mind and body begin to associate breathing with relaxation, you can direct your attention to your breath for just a few seconds anytime and anywhere to reach that place inside yourself that is always calm, relaxed, and fully present to whatever is happening.

The following scenario demonstrates what often happens during the early stages of breathing meditation: You begin in a relaxed, comfortable position. Allow your eyes to gently close and direct your attention to the in-breath, out-breath, experiencing the breath as it enters and leaves your body with its own rhythm, simply noting "in-breath and out-breath." Thoughts, feelings, emotions, memories, sounds, smells, bodily sensations, and anything else you can imagine will begin to intrude into your focus on the breath, often successfully distracting your mind's attention away from the breath. When, *not if*, this occurs, as soon as you realize that your attention has wandered from your breath, let the distraction leave with the next out-breath, *without judgment*, and return to paying attention to your breath.

For example, you are watching your breath and you hear a car drive by outside; your mind grabs onto this distraction and begins the following dialogue with itself: "Car, my car, I need to get an oil change soon, do I have enough money to do that this week? Oh yeah, Tom still owes me that $50 that I lent him last month. Boy, am I angry at him, he said he would pay me back in a week ... but we're such good friends he must have just forgotten ... it's nice to have such a good friend ... that television show had that unfortunate person in it who trusted his friend, while all along this friend was having an affair with his wife ... wait a minute ... I'm supposed to be watching my breath ... okay ... let the thought go ... in-breath ... out-breath ... in-breath ... out-breath ... in-breath ... out-breath ... in-breath ... out-breath ... [a dog barks outside] ... dog ... my dog ... I have to get some dog food, we are almost out of it ... grocery store ... I forgot to make a list of what we need ... let's see ... what's in the refrigerator? We need juice, fruit, salmon, potatoes, carrots, kale ... do I have enough money in my checkbook to buy all that stuff ... I forgot to balance my checkbook last month ... I hate balancing my checkbook ... wouldn't it be nice to win the lottery ... no more worries about money ... wait a minute ... I'm supposed to be watching my breath ... boy, how my mind can wander ... okay ... let me   clear   my   mind . . . in-breath . . . out-breath . . . in-breath . . . out-breath," . . . and so the process goes.

During the early stages of breathing meditation, you will likely spend more time away from your breath than with it. This is what commonly happens. The challenge is not to get frustrated but to continue to practice breathing meditation. Over time, you will find it easier and easier to return to your breath and stay with it—and reap the benefits of calmness and relaxation that accompany the practice of this technique.

Mindfulness Meditation

The breathing meditation is a natural lead-in to mindfulness meditation. With mindfulness practice, it is usually helpful to begin with 5 or 10 minutes of breathing meditation to develop the qualities of calmness and attention. Once grounded in those qualities, one seeks to develop an attitude of "free attention" or "choiceless awareness," in which you quietly observe what is happening both within and around you *without feeling any need to either judge or act.*

Dr. Kabat-Zinn defines mindfulness meditation as "paying attention, on purpose, to the present moment, in the service of self-understanding." Mindfulness meditation involves developing the capacity to observe nonjudgmentally whatever object comes to mind. Common mind-objects include thoughts, feelings, sensations, emotions, and memories, some of which are pleasant, unpleasant, and neutral.

The challenge of mindfulness is to observe all the different parts of ourselves with an open mind, without constant self-justification, denial, entitlement, or self-criticism. One result of this process is learning who we really are, and then making choices as to who we want to become. Mindfulness holds the potential for us to see deeply ingrained patterns of belief and behavior which often have their roots in childhood when we innocently internalized family and cultural beliefs. Some of these beliefs and behaviors may be the source of our deepest anxieties. Shining the light of awareness onto them holds the possibility of breaking their grip on us, freeing ourselves from the stress they provoke.

Another way of viewing mindfulness is that we leave the common Western mind-set of *becoming,* and begin to allow ourselves the experience of *being.* We enter into the here and now with our full presence. Instead of existing in the "object mode" of relating to the environment around us, we enter the "receptive mode," whereby we become part of the environment with no barrier of mind separating us from it.

Using your breath as the anchor to the present moment, when you feel grounded and ready, observe without judgment the various distractions that arise as you meditate. Ideally, these distractions can be used to begin to understand who you are and what fills your mind. Initially, what is commonly observed is the mind's chatter about recent events or about things that you feel you should be doing rather than meditating. But as the mind quiets down from this superficial chatter, deeper patterns will present themselves for neutral observation and inquiry.

A common experience of the practitioner of mindfulness meditation is remembering unconscious material previously suppressed or repressed. Fond memories or emotions from our childhood may be relived with all their original clarity and intensity. For some individuals, the unveiling of traumatic memories or emotions may actually create quite painful emotional states and turbulence of mind, in rare cases requiring psychiatric intervention.

For this reason, anyone beginning to practice any stress management technique should be informed of this unlikely but possible risk. If you have recently experienced a significant loss or severe emotional turmoil, mindfulness meditation should probably be postponed to a time when you are feeling more centered and grounded.

The potential power of mindfulness practice is that you can begin to understand how your mind works rather than getting lost in its contents. One tool that is very helpful in this regard is called *noting*. If you are practicing mindfulness and you find yourself thinking over and over again about some injustice that was done to you, and feel your anger getting stronger and stronger, simply note "angry mind" and begin to explore the bodily sensations accompanying your state of mind. How do your muscles feel? What is happening to your heart rate and your breathing? Do you enjoy being in this state? In this way, instead of getting lost in the circle of thought that propagates the angry mind, you begin to understand what anger really is, and what situations evoke anger in you (they are usually different for everybody, depending on past experience).

If, on the other hand, you find yourself thinking about some pleasing event and feel content and happy, simply note "content mind" or "happy mind." Explore your mind and body when you are in this state. How do your muscles feel? What is happening to your heart rate and breathing? Is this a mind-state that you enjoy? Do you want it to last forever? If so, note "wanting mind" and deepen your understanding that even though we want blissful mind-states to last forever, they will not.

A guaranteed law of the universe is change, and this applies to mind-states. We are not any one mind-state but rather a series of ever-changing states. When you realize that the blissfulness will not last forever and feel disappointed, simply note "disappointed mind" and explore disappointment.

If you find yourself getting caught up in thinking rather than in noting or experiencing, simply return to your breath, following your in-breath and out-breath until you once again feel anchored in the present moment. Then return to the instructions for free attention or choiceless awareness, using the noting technique if you find this useful.

The power of mindfulness is that as you practice it more and more, you begin to understand yourself in a deeper way and begin to have choices about what to do in different circumstances. Put another way, you can begin to respond rather than react and to disentangle yourself from automatic thoughts and behaviors of which you may not previously have been aware. This understanding opens the door to positive change, and with it, decreased stress.

Self-Hypnosis and Creative Visualization

Hypnosis is a poorly understood concept. Fundamentally, it uses directed attention to alter one's state of consciousness. Self-hypnosis can be used to develop states of calmness and a relaxed state of mind. Creative visualization uses the imagination to create an inner experience that can alter one's state of mind. A combination of the two techniques can be a powerful tool, allowing the practitioner to enter a state of mind in which the effects of stress can be reversed.

It is often useful to begin self-hypnosis and creative visualization with a brief body scan, lasting approximately five minutes; in other words, a shortened version of the body scan described previously in this chapter. This technique helps your body to relax and be more receptive to the self-hypnotic and creative visualization exercises. The situation created for you here is only an example. Please feel free to invent your own images—your imagination is your only limitation.

Once you are relaxed, close your eyes, and continue with deep, steady breathing. When you are ready, picture yourself alone in a magic elevator. Try to imagine it in vivid detail, remembering that you are the creator of this scene: What color are the walls? What sounds can you hear? What can you smell?

Now imagine the elevator on the hundredth floor and traveling slowly down. As you descend, level by level, you will become more and more relaxed, tranquil, and at peace with yourself. The elevator can exist in any type of environment, because it is magic. It may be in a large redwood tree so that when you reach level one, you will be in a quiet, peaceful forest. It may be in intergalactic space, so that level one will find you in the stillness of the infinite universe. Or you may descend to a deserted, beautiful beach with the sound of the waves in the background, further deepening your relaxation. You might want to create a special space of your own that does not in fact exist in your real world.

Once you reach level one, use all your five senses (seeing, hearing, smelling, tasting, and sensing) to experience the soothing qualities of this place. For example, if you are at the beach, you can imagine the pleasant warmth of the sun shining down on your body. You can hear the waves gently breaking against the shoreline and watch a seagull flying across the brilliant blue sky. You can smell the salt in the air and feel the sand against your skin. Looking out over the horizon, you may be able to let yourself drift across the water, floating endlessly in a sea of tranquility.

After spending 20 minutes or so in your special place, you can begin the ascent in your magic elevator, slowly returning to your awake, alert, and fully present state of mind at level 100, but carrying your calmness and relaxation through the rest of your day. The more you practice this technique, the faster you will be able to achieve deep states of relaxation.

Hatha Yoga

Hatha yoga, commonly used in stress reduction programs, is a series of exercises that stretch different muscle groups, holding each posture for at least 20 seconds before relaxing, enabling a deeper relaxation than before. Breathing is an integral part of this approach to exercise and relaxation. There are many books, audiocassettes, and videocassettes that teach these exercises, and most major cities offer hatha yoga classes. While practicing hatha yoga, it is important to focus your attention and breathing on the muscle group you are working on, since developing the ability to maintain an alert presence of mind is fundamental to all stress reduction techniques. An excellent book on developing an individual program is *Stretching* (Bob Anderson, published by Shelter Publications).

Progressive Muscle Relaxation

Progressive muscle relaxation is another common technique used in stress reduction and is especially useful for people with chronic muscle tension. It is similar to hatha yoga in several ways. First, you should place yourself in a relaxed and fully supported position and ground yourself with a few deep slow breaths.

Next, go systematically through each muscle group, contracting the muscles for about 10 seconds, and then relaxing them as deeply as you can. You can go through the entire sequence two or more times in the same order.

One common approach is to start by contracting the muscles of both feet and legs and then relaxing them. Then proceed through the body as with the body scan, the major difference being the active contracting and relaxing of each major muscle group, and working with both sides of the body simultaneously. After spending 10 seconds in an active contraction, spend at least 20 seconds in passive relaxation.

As with the rest of these techniques, plan to spend a solid 30 minutes practicing progressive muscle relaxation. At the end of the exercise, spend a few minutes observing how your body feels as compared to how it felt beforehand.

Exercise

Exercise can be used as a stress reduction technique as well as for providing a good cardiovascular workout (see Chapter 3). The exercising itself can become the object of meditation. Rather than letting your mind wander or chatter endlessly, as it enjoys doing so much, focus your attention on the movements of your body and your respiratory rate as you exercise. This helps develop the one-pointed awareness so crucial to any stress reduction technique.

Mending with Music

Music can also be used as a form of stress reduction. Follow these guidelines, and if you are comfortable, allow your eyes to close.

- Choose soothing music with *no lyrics*.
- Focus your attention exclusively on the sound your ears are hearing.
- As with all the other techniques, if your mind becomes distracted, simply let the distraction go and return your attention to the music.
- Possibilities include classical or new age music, sounds of nature, or any other type of music that you find particularly soothing.

Maybe you have read this chapter dutifully, shaking your head somewhat at the idea of hatha yoga or mindfulness meditation and thinking it's all a bit of a joke: How is self-hypnosis going to help me cope with the fact that my husband has cancer or I've just lost my job?

I have to admit that there was a time when I shared that skepticism. Meditation was all very well when I was "stressed out" as a young resident, but when the life and death crisis of my baby's illness occurred, meditation was the first thing to get tossed out the window. I was too busy worrying to waste time being mindful.

It was my husband who brought me back to my senses. One evening, when Patrick was just a few months old, he watched me writing in my journal. "Mary," he said casually. "You write in that book every night. Why don't you put your pen down and read it?" Somehow I steeled myself and went through it from beginning to end with clinical detatchment. I was able to see a woman who seemed to have everything anyone could want: a wonderful husband, a beautiful son, a loving family, great friends, an understanding boss, and an exciting job at a prestigious university hospital but who was, in spite of all that, just barely hanging on.

Tom and I had been married for six years. We had gone through medical school and residency together, we had just been through the most traumatic period of our lives, and we were both now struggling with the sleep deprivation of new parenthood. I was falling apart and Tom was managing beautifully.

Given our long and intense relationship, I thought I knew everything there was to know about him. Half joking, since I "knew" he didn't meditate, I asked him how he managed to stay so calm. His answer was a revelation to me: he said that whenever he felt himself getting too upset about something, he could clear his mind simply by concentrating on his breathing. It was a technique he had developed in high school while running on the track team and it was now second nature to him. He had been meditating all along but just hadn't given it a name.

Obviously, Patrick's illness would have been a difficult time for me, no matter what I did to cope, but I can't help thinking that I made it worse for myself than it needed to be.

Most of the people I see in my cholesterol clinic have heart disease and have faced the prospect of life-threatening illness. Confronted as they are with possible death, one would think they would find it easier to make the lifestyle changes their cardiac problems require.

This may sound logical, but human beings are not always interested in being logical. It is extraordinarily difficult to change a way of life, to give up habits and activities we may have engaged in for decades. People with heart disease are often asked to make many big changes all at once. In addition to the enormous strain of suddenly becoming a person with a life-threatening condition, they are also expected to give up smoking, lose weight, stop eating all their favorite foods, make time for exercise, and oh, by the way, reduce the stress in their lives. It is hardly surprising that the stress level of the average heart patient usually increases after his or her problem has been diagnosed and that depression and erratic mood swings are very common.

It is easy to focus solely on the physical aspects of cardiac rehabilitation, to put all of one's energy into losing weight and getting the cholesterol levels down. The problem with this strategy, however, is that one comes to see oneself as little more than a series of numbers: How much do I weigh? What does the lab report say? Failures and setbacks, which for most people are inevitable, take on a larger than life aspect: if I've gained five pounds, I'm a terrible person; if I smoked a cigarette after quitting, I must really be a hopeless case.

It is important, actually essential, to accept and love yourself *as you are today* before beginning to think about making changes. You are not your habits, your weight, your cholesterol level. The more you focus on these factors as the sum total of your personality, the more difficult it will be to do something about them.

How can you begin? I think the first thing to do is to observe yourself. Look at the various areas of your life, the different roles you play, the work you want to accomplish, the tasks you set yourself. Write down all the things you do on a typical weekday, a typical weekend. Do you have a hobby? Are you sleeping well? Are you happy with the important relationships in your life: with your spouse or partner, your children, parents, friends, and co-workers? Do you find your work fulfilling? Do you have a close friend you can really confide in?

In this chapter, with the assistance of my good friend, Dr. John Miller, I have given you the tools you need to develop a personal stress reduction and relaxation program. This program will not make your problems disappear, but it will help you to find within yourself the patience, balance, and wisdom to cope with whatever difficulties life presents you.

But at the outset, we really need to realize that stress reduction and relaxation are lifelong processes. Stress is not some foreign body which can be dug out and gotten rid of once and for all. Like brushing your teeth, feeding your body, and watering your plants, keeping an inner balance is a daily commitment.

And when you are feeling good, don't take it as permission to slow down on the meditating. See it for what it is: evidence that your program is working. When parents see their baby thriving, they don't conclude that she no longer needs milk. They go right on feeding her, knowing that this is what is making her growth possible. So make the commitment to take care of your inner life and to continue doing it, especially when crises come (for they do keep coming). Your ability to remain calm and centered will enable you to face them with equanimity and balance— even in the darkest night, you will have at least a memory of the dawn.

Audiocassette Order Form

Body Scan and Breathing Meditation tape
Side one: 30-minute guided body scan
Side two: 30-minute guided breathing meditation

To purchase tape send $10.00 to:
John J. Miller, MD.
Harris Street Associates, Inc.
44 Merrimac St.
Newburyport, MA 01950

The Case of Bill

~~~~~~

Diabetes, Stress,

and the Heart

Bill is an unusual man. Meeting him for the first time, it is instantly apparent that he is an enormously successful person. His self-confidence and inner security are reflected in the way he moves, the way he connects with the people he meets. At the same time, however, one is struck by his essential gentleness. His soft blue eyes say more about his personality than does his imposing six-foot frame. And although it is easy to imagine him in a three-piece suit at a board of directors meeting for some large corporation, it is equally easy to picture him soothing a frightened child or giving words of encouragement to a young person just starting a career.

Perhaps all this has to do with the fact that Bill had to become responsible very young—his father died of a stroke at the age of 36. This early and devastating loss made him keenly aware of life's tenuousness, and he determined to provide for his own family both emotionally and financially.

Bill and his wife Kate had three children—Kevin, Bruce, and Karen. While the children were young, Bill did his best to maintain a balance between work and home. Throughout his career in the computer industry, he made it a special point to keep physically fit. An avid racquetball player, at the time of his retirement in 1984, he was still able to keep up with young men 30 years his junior.

His motivation had two sources: the first was the understanding that, in his field, youth and energy are highly valued—anyone who wants to succeed in the computer industry has to be able to keep up with the young crowd that dominates it. The second was more personal: he knew that the better his physical condition, the less likely he was to follow in his father's footsteps. He couldn't imagine his children growing up without a father or Kate managing without a husband. He was determined not to let it happen.

If he had one weakness, it was his fondness for sweets. Kate was an excellent cook and the kitchen was always well stocked with cakes, cookies, and other treats. Although never very overweight, in middle age he did carry a few extra pounds.

In 1984, Bill retired and he and Kate moved from New Hampshire to North Carolina, where they built a beautiful home and settled in to enjoy a more leisurely life. But in spite of reveling in the beaches, the golf courses, and frequent family visits, they found they missed day-to-day involvement with their children, who had remained in Concord, New Hampshire, where they were raising their families.

In 1989, they returned to the state and bought a house in a condominium development not far from where Kevin and Bruce lived (Karen had moved to California). For the first time since he had owned a home, Bill was not responsible for cutting the lawn or shoveling the snow—and he loved it.

Unfortunately, the dream house slowly began to turn into a nightmare. Shortly after moving in, Bill and Kate received a sinister and very frightening letter suggesting that they move out of the neighborhood immediately. This was followed by phone calls and more letters, each more graphic than the last. When the letters began containing pictures of guns and thinly veiled threats, they called the police. They were closely questioned about their past associations: Was there anyone—a disgruntled employee, perhaps, or an unstable relative—who might want to settle some old score? Try though they did, Bill and Kate could come up with no one who might hate them so much, and they spent many agonizing months in fear and confusion, wondering when and where the blow would strike.

Finally, although many questions remained unanswered, it became clear that Bill and Kate had nothing to do with what was going on—they were simply pawns in a bitter real estate battle being waged within the condominium development. The harassment ultimately ceased, but not without a heavy cost.

Bill, who had always prided himself on being able to meet any crisis with composure, found himself terrified in his own home. In an attempt to shield Kate from many of the worst letters, he had generally managed to reach the mailbox before she did, and as a result, he carried much of the burden of fear alone. While it was going on, he noticed that he was becoming increasingly short of breath—even the slightest activity left him feeling winded.

In late October 1992, he woke with chest pain—a heavy feeling and sweating that lasted several minutes. Later that day his family doctor examined him and performed a cardiogram, which failed to reveal any abnormality. He was told to continue with his routine activities and to return should the chest pain recur.

When it became obvious that Bill's shortness of breath and chest pressure were not going away, his doctor recommended that he have an exercise (stress) test. It was soon clear that Bill did have heart disease—the only question was how severe.

Bill called a physician friend who referred him to a cardiologist, Dr. Beatty Hunter. Dr. Hunter told Bill that his exercise test did suggest the presence of cardiac disease and gave him two treatment options: first, to try to relieve his chest pressure and shortness of breath with cardiac medications alone, and to consider a cardiac catheterization procedure should his symptoms continue despite the medications; second, to perform the catheterization straightaway to determine if his condition required immediate therapy, such as an angioplasty or bypass surgery.

Although he had no medical background, Bill was convinced that this problem should be tackled in the same way he had tackled so many others in his business career: first get the facts. He had always found that he could deal with almost anything as long as he knew exactly what was involved. Because he wanted to know just how big his blockages were and where they were located, he requested Dr. Hunter to proceed with the second option, a catheterization. The procedure was scheduled for a few days later.

In the meantime, Bill did his best to understand the factors which had brought him to this point. Dr. Hunter spent a lot of time going over the risks with him: some—like being a male over 45 and having a family history of heart disease—he could do nothing about. Others, however, were more modifiable, and given his family history, it was imperative that he take them seriously.

The first was a borderline problem with his blood sugar level, a condition consistent with people who eventually develop diabetes, while the second concern was a somewhat depressed HDL level (HDL is the good or protective cholesterol). Bill brought up the issue of stress himself, describing the torturous time they had just been through and his own belief that this had been a contributing factor to his heart disease. Although he felt that in general he handled stress well and was quite sure that the situation which had caused him so much anxiety would not be repeated, he was still interested in the idea of stress reduction. His physician advised him to look into a cardiac rehabilitation program that included a course in stress reduction. At the same time, he referred him to my cholesterol clinic for special advice on raising his HDL level.

The blood sugar problem had been a surprise to Bill. In spite of his passion for sweets, his weight—175 pounds at six foot one inch—was just right. He had always thought only overweight people developed diabetes. Although his blood sugar was only 123 mg/dl, and did not meet the strict criterion for the diagnosis of diabetes (that is, a fasting blood sugar above 140 mg/dl), studies have shown that anyone with a level greater than 100 mg/dl is at risk for developing symptomatic diabetes within the next five years. The symptoms include increased urination and thirst, in addition to fatigue and weakness.

Bill was right in assuming that diabetics are usually overweight. This is not always the case, however, as his own example proves. Diabetics also have a greater tendency toward cholesterol abnormalities and are at high risk for the development of cardiac disease. Indeed, most diabetics die not from elevated blood sugar levels, but from the cardiac complications of their condition.

For Bill, the advice given to diabetics to improve both cholesterol profiles and blood sugar levels was not too difficult to follow:

1. Exercise
2. Avoid concentrated sweets
3. Lose weight or maintain an ideal body weight
4. Avoidance of alcohol

Since the only thing on this list that he wasn't doing was avoiding sweets, Bill made up his mind then and there to cut back drastically.

He approached his catheterization, then, already well prepared mentally for the new life ahead of him. The procedure revealed two large blockages in his left anterior descending (LAD) artery, both of which were successfully angioplastied the same day.

When he was released from the hospital the next day, he felt fine, but by the fifth day, he again began experiencing shortness of breath and chest pressure. Remembering his doctor's warning that 30 percent of all angioplasties fail within the first six months, he returned to the hospital. There a repeat catheterization showed that he had developed a blood clot at the site of one of the angioplasties and a recurrent blockage at the other. Once again, he underwent angioplasties for both—this time, he remained free of symptoms for nearly three weeks.

Although yet another angioplasty was possible, Dr. Hunter was less inclined to continue with this treatment plan, explaining that repeat angioplasties frequently fail and that people with depressed HDL are statistically more likely to have early problems with the procedure. For these reasons, he now advised bypass surgery as a more sensible option. The next day, Bill was operated on and within a week he was back home.

His whole family gathered to support him during this difficult time; his sons, who lived close by, made daily visits, while Karen came cross country to be with her father. Bill was deeply moved by the strong and steady love they showed him, but at the same time he was strangely disinclined to see anyone. His emotions seemed totally out of his control and he felt on edge and easily upset. A person who never cried in public, he suddenly found himself in tears at the slightest provocation. He was also troubled by an inability to begin exercising and was hiding a deep fear that his chest pain would recur and virtually immobilize him.

But after about a week, he remembered what Brian, a cardiac rehabilitation nurse, had told him while he was in the hospital. He had suggested that when Bill first began exercising he should remain in his own house, where help would be close at hand. He had also taught Bill how to take his own pulse and given him a target heart rate to work toward.

Bill decided to follow Brian's advice. Exercising gently around the house, he was gratified to find that he didn't experience any chest pain. As he gained strength, his former confidence in his body began returning, and his spirits rose proportionately.

It wasn't until he joined a cardiac rehabilitation program, however, that he really began to feel like himself again. In fact, for a time, the program was the focus of his whole life, the one place he felt safe. Surrounded by health professionals, he knew he could push himself while exercising, thus testing his limits. Once he felt comfortable with his ability to exercise without difficulty while at the program, he began repeating the exercises at home.

One very important aspect of cardiac rehabilitation for Bill was the camaraderie the program offered—he loved meeting so many different people from so many different backgrounds, all sharing a common commitment to fight heart disease. As he progressed in the program, he found he was developing a whole new lifestyle: he learned about nutrition, stress reduction, and other ways to develop a healthy heart. By the end of his program he was healthier, both physically and emotionally, than he had been for years.

I first met Bill the day before his bypass surgery. His cardiologist had asked me to review his cholesterol profile and develop a plan to improve his levels. His profile looked like this:

	Bill's Level	Desirable Level
Total cholesterol	172 mg/dl	Less than 200 mg/dl
Triglycerides	107 mg/dl	Less than 150 mg/dl
HDL cholesterol	36 mg/dl	Greater than 45 mg/dl
LDL cholesterol	115 mg/dl	Less than 100 mg/dl

Although his profile wasn't too bad, neither Bill nor I was satisfied with anything less than perfection. We decided to concentrate on the two areas that needed work: lowering his LDL and raising his HDL. His total cholesterol to HDL ratio was 4.9—a desirable level, but not 4.0 or lower as recommended.

I explained to Bill that although his numbers were good, a person with documented cardiac disease needs every possible advantage. If he were able to lower his LDL to below 100 mg/dl, for example, many studies have documented that at that level cholesterol deposits in the arteries can be reduced, thereby reducing the risk of a future heart attack. As for total cholesterol to HDL ratio, the lower the better, with 4.0 the target, though even lower is desirable.

We discussed diet and exercise at length, as well as the importance of restricting sweets, considering his borderline blood sugar level. Although he was already at his ideal weight, I told him that losing a few more pounds wouldn't hurt and might also serve to improve his HDL. Even though weight loss may transiently lower HDL, the ultimate effect is to raise the good cholesterol.

I saw Bill again eight weeks later. He had already made significant improvements in his diet, which had normalized his blood sugar and brought his weight down by a pound. His cholesterol profile was nearly perfect:

	Bill's Level	Desirable Level
Total cholesterol	158 mg/dl	Less than 200 mg/dl
Triglycerides	87 mg/dl	Less than 150 mg/dl
HDL cholesterol	38 mg/dl	Greater than 45 mg/dl
LDL cholesterol	103 mg/dl	Less than 100 mg/dl

His total cholesterol to HDL ratio was 4.1. With increased exercise and a few more dietary changes, I was confident that Bill would reduce his cardiac risk even further. I told him that it was very unlikely that he would ever require cholesterol-lowering medications.

A few weeks later, Bill and Kate left to spend the winter in Florida. We sent him off armed with a new diet and a recommendation to join the community phase of cardiac rehabilitation down south and to supplement this with daily walks and tennis.

When he returned in the spring, he looked wonderful. His weight was down to 163, his blood sugar had remained normal and his cholesterol profile was like a dream:

	Bill's Level	Desirable Level
Total cholesterol	133 mg/dl	Less than 200 mg/dl
Triglycerides	83 mg/dl	Less than 150 mg/dl
HDL cholesterol	43 mg/dl	Greater than 45 mg/dl
LDL cholesterol	74 mg/dl	Less than 100 mg/dl

His total cholesterol to HDL ratio was now 3.1.

Although he was now slightly underweight, he seemed to be thriving. I asked him not to lose any more, and recommended extra bagels, cereal, and potatoes should the weight loss continue.

Over the past two years Bill has been able to maintain his excellent program of diet and exercise. He says he has never felt better and that the idea of being "on a diet" never occurs to him: "This is my life," he says simply.

He and Kate recently returned from a Bermuda cruise. In the past, going on such a trip almost guaranteed that he would return 5 to 10 pounds heavier, feeling sluggish and a bit bloated. This time, because he called ahead and arranged for low-fat meals, he returned well rested, fit, and, because he exercised so much on board, a pound lighter.

Bill's methodical problem-solving approach to his heart disease has been an inspiration both to me and to his colleagues in cardiac rehabilitation. The skills that served him so well during his many years in business have been put to excellent use in the more important task of saving his own life. And those of us who have been able to observe him in action have learned a great deal in the process.

7

~~~~~~~~~~~~~~~~~~~~~~~~~~~~~~~~~~~~~~~

Elevated Blood Pressure:

What Can You Do to

Lower Your Level?

The United States launched a national high blood pressure education program in 1972. Since then, many more people have been made aware of and are receiving treatment for hypertension (high blood pressure). In 1972, only 51 percent of persons with this condition had been told about it by their physician. Worse yet, only 16 percent had brought their blood pressure under control. This seeming neglect came about because at that time the medical community simply had insufficient information on the devastating effects high blood pressure can have on the human body.

By 1991, however, 84 percent of those with hypertension had been alerted to their condition, and 55 percent had taken corrective measures. While this is a tremendous improvement, it is not enough. Looked at another way, 45 percent of the 50 million Americans with hypertension are not being treated for their potentially deadly condition.

Blood pressure (BP), which is measured in millimeters (mm) of mercury (Hg), is the force with which blood pushes against the walls of the arteries. When the heart beats, it pumps blood into the blood vessels and the pressure peaks. This is the systolic blood pressure, the top number of a blood pressure reading. As the heart relaxes between beats, blood pressure falls to its lowest level. This is known as the diastolic blood pressure, the bottom number.

When your blood pressure is consistently above 140/80, it becomes more difficult for your heart to pump effectively and, over time, it increases the risk of your developing cardiac disease. Drug therapy is certainly one way to control BP, but lifestyle changes such as salt restriction, exercise, weight loss, reduction in the use of alcohol, and increased potassium intake are preferable.

For many people, however, lifestyle changes are insufficient and blood pressure–lowering medications are required. This chapter details lifestyle changes aimed at blood pressure control; for a full discussion of blood pressure medications, see Chapter 8.

What can you do for yourself to make sure your blood pressure is not putting you at risk for the development of heart disease and stroke? The first step is knowing your blood pressure. Make sure your doctor checks it regularly and tells you your reading.

Sometimes a person has an elevated reading only in the doctor's office. You have probably heard about this, and it even has a name: white-coat hypertension. But before you dismiss your blood pressure problem as simply that, you should realize that many people whose blood pressure soars at the doctor's office have the same experience when they find themselves in the wrong line at the bank or grocery store, when they're stuck in traffic, or when they're involved in a heated discussion.

Through the use of ambulatory blood pressure monitoring,* scientists have shown that people with white-coat hypertension experience many more elevations of blood pressure throughout the day than do persons who have normal blood pressure in the doctor's office. If this is your situation, at the very least you should do as much as you can to lower your blood pressure through lifestyle changes.

At present, it is not clear if people with white-coat hypertension benefit from the use of blood pressure medications; but it is certain that no one has ever experienced adverse side effects from decreased salt intake, a doctor-approved exercise program, weight loss, reduction in alcohol consumption, and increased potassium intake.

What About Salt?

Americans love salt, and I cannot deny that it can add much to the flavor of many foods. The average American adult consumes about 3900 milligrams (mg) a day, and in the United States and in other countries with high-salt intakes, blood pressure increases steadily as a person ages.

---

* This monitoring involves wearing a blood pressure cuff for a 24-hour period. The cuff inflates periodically and records blood pressure readings.

Many studies have shown that salt restriction not only lowers blood pressure in the short term but also prevents age-related increases in blood pressure. The Food and Drug Administration has established 2400 mg per day as an acceptable daily allowance.

However, for many Americans, the problem is not the salt shaker but rather the processed foods in their diets that contribute greatly to their daily intake of sodium, the major chemical in salt. The following list includes some of the major sources of dietary sodium:

Canned soups
Canned vegetables, unless labeled "no salt added" or "low sodium"
Processed meats—luncheon meats, hot dogs, ham, sausage
Broth or bouillon, unless labeled "low sodium"
Meat tenderizers
Seasoned salts
Soy sauce
Pickles, relish, olives
Sauerkraut
Frozen dinners
Fast foods
Cooking wines

If these products are your downfall, look for reduced-salt versions of your favorite foods and make sure to read food labels to determine your daily intake of sodium. What can you expect when you reduce your salt intake? For salt-sensitive persons, a reduction in dietary sodium can drop their systolic blood pressure (the top number) by 5 to 10 mm/Hg and the diastolic blood pressure (the bottom number) by 3 to 5 mm/Hg. This might not sound like a lot, but when it is coupled with weight loss, exercise, and alcohol restriction, it may mean the difference between requiring and not requiring medications.

Not everyone can lower blood pressure by restricting salt intake. People who can are called salt-sensitive. Although it is impossible to predict exactly who will be responsive to salt restriction, most studies have found African Americans and the elderly to respond better than other groups to salt restriction.

What About Exercise?

Sedentary people with normal blood pressure have a 20 to 50 percent greater chance of developing high blood pressure than do their active friends.

If you already have high blood pressure, take heart, the situation can be reversed. In a classic study of untreated middle-aged hypertensive males, it was found that exercising on a stationary bike for 45 minutes three times a week for six weeks led to an 11 mm/Hg drop in systolic and a 9 mm/Hg drop in the diastolic blood pressure.

When the same experiment was repeated with participants exercising seven instead of three times per week, the fall in blood pressure was even more dramatic: a 16-point drop in the systolic and an 11-point drop in the diastolic.

I tell my patients that exercise is as good as many blood pressure medications and has virtually no adverse side effects. However, I do recommend that before beginning any exercise program you discuss it with your personal physician. Once you are cleared to exercise, use Chapter 3 as a guide.

What About Weight Loss?

If you are overweight, weight loss is very important. Often the loss of as little as five or ten pounds will lead to a substantial reduction in blood pressure. Daily exercise will help you begin to lose weight, but most people will also require a diet that restricts calories. Chapter 2 will arm you with a diet that will not only help you lose weight, but will also lower your blood pressure and cholesterol. The "Recipes" section at the end of the book offers you a selection of tasty dishes that will help you stick to your diet.

What About Alcohol?

Alcohol can also dramatically affect your blood pressure, with as little as two drinks per day leading to significant elevations. In fact, it is estimated that 5 to 10 percent of hypertension in American males is directly caused by alcohol consumption. Blood pressure medications often fail to work effectively in individuals who consume more than two drinks per day.

When I was an intern, I had a patient whose blood pressure I simply could not get under control. I evaluated him for a group of rare disorders that can cause very high blood pressure, but he tested negative for all of them. He lost 10 pounds and began an exercise program, but even with these changes he required three medications to control his blood pressure.

While I was treating him, I attended a lecture given by Dr. David

Clive, a professor of nephrology at the University of Massachusetts Medical Center. I was stunned to hear him casually mention that when a hypertensive patient does not respond to conventional treatment, one should question him or her closely about alcohol intake, since more than two drinks a day may make it almost impossible for the medications to work.

It suddenly hit me that I had never asked Michael how much he drank. I called him the same afternoon and he very matter-of-factly told me that he had five drinks a day. I told him that this might be causing his blood pressure problem and asked him if he thought he could cut down to two drinks a day. He was sure he could, but I had my doubts: at that level of consumption, it seemed pretty certain that he was addicted.

Two weeks later, Michael called from work to tell me he was feeling dizzy. I asked him to have his BP evaluated by the nurse at his plant, and she reported that it was 100/60. No wonder he was dizzy! He told me he had tapered his alcohol consumption over the course of one week, and now had stopped altogether, adding that he really didn't miss it. Within a year, I was able to stop his BP medications completely, since he was able to maintain a normal reading of 135/78 on his own.

Drinking, he said, had been a rut he had gotten into without even realizing what he was doing to himself. Once he stopped, he was able to exercise more and still feel rested and alert. He was thrilled with his new reserves of energy and grateful to me for having figured out his problem. I just wished it had occurred to me sooner.

What About Potassium?

Over the past few years, more and more evidence has indicated that a diet rich in potassium can protect against the development of high blood pressure. The exact mechanism by which potassium protects against the development of hypertension is not known. For most people this means increasing their intake of fruits and vegetables. Many foods contain a rich supply of potassium, including bananas, cantaloupes, oranges, tomatoes, prunes, and white potatoes. And like most other nutrients, it appears that potassium from food sources is more effective than from nutritional supplements.

What About Medications?

Some people, however, do require medications to control their blood pressure, regardless of what other lifestyle changes they make.

They should be aware that some blood pressure medications have an adverse effect on blood sugar and cholesterol levels, while others lead to favorable changes in both. If you have high cholesterol or diabetes in addition to high blood pressure, it will be very important to make sure that the drug your doctor chooses to treat your blood pressure will not aggravate or create a new cardiac risk factor.

Take the drugs known as beta-blockers, for example. While they do normalize blood pressure and have been shown to prolong life after a heart attack, they also adversely affect both blood sugar and cholesterol levels. It is crucial for you and your doctor to be aware of the various side effects of any drug you are taking and for him or her to prescribe your medications accordingly. You should therefore never hesitate to ask your doctor why a particular drug has been prescribed. Chapter 8 will review the various classes of blood pressure medications in detail.

Guidelines for Lowering Your Blood Pressure

If you have high blood pressure, there are several lifestyle changes you can make that can dramatically reduce it.

- Restrict salt intake to 2400 mg per day.
- Develop a regular exercise program.
- Try to achieve your ideal body weight—as little as five to ten pounds will make a difference.
- Limit alcohol intake.
- Be sure your diet includes foods rich in potassium.

If you do need blood pressure medications, be sure your doctor is aware of all other medications you may be taking.

The Case of Jim

Sometimes Diet and Exercise Can Do It All

"Don't disturb Daddy," his mother warned him. "He's not feeling well." Jim was only eight and the temptation to disobey was strong. He peeked in anyway and saw his father lying quietly in bed. He seemed fine. But a few hours later, he was rushed to the hospital. Within a week, he was dead. He was 52 years old, the victim of a heart attack.

Overnight, Jim took on the role of the head of the family. Whether it was true or not, in his eight-year-old mind, he was now responsible for the safety and well-being of his mother and three younger sisters. He grew up quickly, even to the extent of waking in the middle of the night to add wood to the first-floor stove that heated the house. In spite of the difficulties of life, Jim remembers his abbreviated childhood without resentment. His family's religious faith gave his life the stability and courage he needed to adjust to the difficult circumstances. When he was 20, Jim's mother died, also of a heart attack. The writing seemed to be on the wall. Jim knew that if he ever did have children, he'd better have them early.

After high school Jim, however, studied six years for the priesthood at St. Charles Seminary outside Baltimore. But eventually he decided not to continue to ordination and instead joined the army during the Korean conflict, after which he attended graduate school at the University of Maryland. He received a doctorate in history and became a professor at Keene State College in New Hampshire.

At the age of 30, Jim married and within a year Eleanore gave birth to Christopher, their first son. Angela was born the next year, and Michael five years later. Jim was fully immersed in the challenges of fatherhood and his work at the college.

In the early seventies he took a sabbatical leave for study in England. In preparation for the trip, the entire family had full physical exams, as a result of which Jim learned that his total cholesterol was 253 mg/dl.

At that time, a total cholesterol of 260 mg/dl was considered average, and one of 300 only moderately high. Viewed by today's standards, this is, of course, quite amazing. In addition, in the 1970s, getting an HDL cholesterol (the protective cholesterol) reading was virtually unheard of. We now know that the total cholesterol divided by the HDL gives us a number which is one of the single best predictors of cardiac risk. Given Jim's later readings, it is likely that his HDL in the seventies was very low, probably only in the twenties.

A total cholesterol of 253, coupled with such a low HDL, made Jim, to use an unfortunate image, a walking time bomb. It is likely that his total cholesterol divided by his HDL (often referred to as the total to HDL ratio) was over 10, whereas a desirable ratio is less than 4. To illustrate the importance of HDL, imagine a person with a total cholesterol of 253, but an HDL of 63. In spite of having the same total cholesterol as Jim, this person's ratio would be a perfect 4. This recognition has prompted the National Cholesterol Education Program's Expert Panel to recommend that all Americans over the age of 20 have both total and HDL cholesterol measured and, if necessary, brought under control.

This was all far in the future, however. Jim flew off to England quite unconcerned about his health and unaware of any need to make changes in his diet or activity level. Indeed, given his work and involvement with his children, he wouldn't have felt he had time for exercise.

Soon after returning from his sabbatical abroad, Jim's doctor told him that his blood pressure was too high. The news jolted him. "It made me feel old," he recalls. "It made me feel like my father." High blood pressure was well known at the time to be associated with strokes and heart attacks, and Jim made up his mind to bring his down.

He began biking to and from the college, reasoning that exercise and losing weight would reduce his blood pressure without medications. A few weeks later, however, an episode of dizziness while cycling landed him in the doctor's office again. This time, he was given a drug prescription to normalize his blood pressure.

Jim's aversion to medication amounted almost to an obsession. Although he agreed reluctantly to taking the prescribed medicine, he resolved to get off it as soon as possible. He plunged into a vigorous running program and soon had his weight down to its ideal level. When he was able to discontinue his medication, he felt both triumphant and confident: "Maybe I'll be the one in my family who lives to see his grandchildren," he told his wife.

For years Jim's weight and blood pressure remained stable. He found that his exercise level allowed him to eat exactly what he chose without gaining any weight—but what he chose was plenty of red meat, ice cream, butter, and cheese.

In the spring of 1985, Jim began having chest pressure while running. Gradually, over the course of several weeks, he began to slow down until finally, without making a conscious decision, he stopped running altogether. With exams and final papers to grade in the history department, he had no time to wonder about the discomfort he was experiencing. Since it never occurred while at rest, he assumed it was just a pulled muscle. The time "saved" through not running he gratefully put into his work, making a mental promise to get back to his routine once school let out.

Just a few weeks after Jim's chest pain had begun, he and Eleanore attended a party at the home of the college president, their first stop on an evening that was to end with Jim's giving a lecture at his church. It had been a difficult and tumultuous day. He had made a difficult personal decision about someone in his department. Anxious and upset, he arrived at the president's party feeling tense and distracted.

He told himself he was feeling better as he greeted the president and his wife, and he had even begun to believe it as he mingled with the other guests in the living room. But as he settled in with a group of his own close friends in one corner of the room, he noticed an odd sensation in his back. Shifting positions didn't improve the situation, and soon the strange feeling had extended all the way down to his right hand. It was as if his whole arm were numb. A slow wave of nausea kept passing through his body.

In spite of his discomfort, he managed to make it to the church where he delivered an excellent lecture. By the time he got home, however, he had to admit he was unwell. Assuming it was just indigestion, he suggested to Eleanore that they go for a walk. They covered three miles before returning home, but by then Jim was feeling far worse. Uneasy and restless, he actually took a sleeping pill, something unusual for him.

This brought him only a few hours of troubled sleep. When he woke, he took two sleeping pills, hoping that whatever was bothering him would just go away.

An hour or so later, Jim woke to a chest pain so severe he knew something was seriously wrong. He woke Eleanore and they set out for the emergency room. A cardiogram performed there confirmed what Jim most feared: he was indeed having a heart attack. An injection of morphine worked almost magically to relieve his pain, and his condition soon stabilized.

Jim remained in the hospital for 10 days while his doctor puzzled over the best treatment plan to recommend. Except for his family history and the fact that he was a male, Jim seemed to have no cardiac risk factors: his weight was perfect, his blood pressure was normal, he was a nonsmoker, he didn't have diabetes, and at 168 mg/dl, his total cholesterol was impressively low. When he was discharged, he was left with the impression that he now had a clean slate: the heart attack had been just an aberration. It was not even suggested that he attend a cardiac rehabilitation program.

What his doctor apparently didn't realize is that following a heart attack (or indeed, any severe stress), cholesterol levels artificially fall. It is not until about eight weeks later that a true reading can be obtained. More important, even in 1985, HDL levels were not routinely measured. Had Jim gotten an accurate and detailed cholesterol report, I am sure he would have had a better understanding of his situation.

As it was, he left the hospital with about as much knowledge of his heart condition as he had when he was admitted. Not only was he ignorant about what had taken place in his body, but he felt powerless to prevent it from happening again. Within two days of his discharge, he was back again. This time he was reassured that his chest pressure was caused by anxiety. "Just relax," the emergency room physician told him. "Go home and take it easy."

Jim went home, but he didn't relax. He couldn't. Memories of his parents and their early deaths began to haunt him. Getting through each day became more and more of an effort, and as the summer wore on (Jim was on vacation, but the rest of his family was working), he found himself relying on his son Michael's dog for security and companionship. He took him for long walks, every day increasing the distance they would cover. Whenever he felt too anxious, he would pet the dog—the repetitive motion had a calming effect on him.

With lots of activity, Jim was able to get through his days. The nights were another story. Lying in bed, the thoughts and fears he had worked so hard to suppress came flooding into his mind, making sleep difficult. Had it not been for Eleanore, Jim wonders how he would have made it. Many nights she took him in her arms as she had their children when they were frightened or hurt. She rubbed his back for as long as it took for him to relax enough to fall asleep. Thus day by day, night by night, Jim went on with his life.

But it wasn't long before the role of passive victim became too much of a burden. Jim began educating himself about cardiac disease. Together, he and Eleanore made modest changes in their diet, switching to margarine and cutting back on red meat. Without a complete understanding of the importance of fat in the diet, however, Jim's commitment to really significant change was not what it needed to be.

He resumed his college duties, but found, however, that the additional time required for daily exercise and extra rest meant that he had no time to relax and little time for Eleanore. He switched to a parttime schedule. Only 58 years old, this much of a concession to his health was difficult to make, but his exhaustion, both emotional and physical, left him with no other option. And once the change was made, he found his anxiety diminished considerably.

Jim resumed an exercise program, but couldn't find the energy to get back to running and as a result his weight increased. By 1991, he found himself more and more tired. One of his most disturbing memories is of needing a full three days of rest to recover from an afternoon helping his oldest son prune the trees in his yard.

As the year progressed, he began having chest pressure again while walking. Once more, his response was to limit his exercise and avoid the real issue. He purposely arrived early at work to give himself the extra 15 minutes he knew he would need to recover from the one and a half block walk from his car to the office. A consultation with his physician didn't help much—he was started on medications whose effect was only marginal. Switching doctors didn't help either: his new physician juggled the medications only slightly, leaving him in about the same condition.

It was a situation he was no longer able to tolerate. He had begun to feel like a prisoner in his own home. Now unable to walk even half a block without pain, he felt forced to confine himself to his yard and house. Eleanore finally convinced him that things could not go on as they were. His primary care physician had been recommending bypass surgery for some time, and Eleanore began a subtle campaign to persuade him to do it. "You can't go through life as an invalid," she argued. "You've got to fight for your health, fight for your right to a happy and productive life."

In January 1992, Jim finally agreed. He entered Dartmouth's Mary Hitchcock Medical Center where, after a series of evaluations and tests, his bypass surgery was successfully performed. Jim was amazed. Within weeks he felt better than he had in years. He and Eleanore were delighted with the changes they discovered in the medical community and its approach to cardiac health. While still in the hospital, Jim attended a series of classes designed to benefit his heart, and after discharge, he enrolled in a cardiac rehabilitation program.

In the program he developed a moderate (three days a week) exercise routine and started looking seriously at his diet. On the basis of the book *Dr. Dean Ornish's Program for Reversing Cardiac Disease*, he cut his fat intake to only 10 percent of his total calories. Unfortunately, focusing exclusively on fat, he neglected to cut calories and his weight remained pretty much the same. Nonetheless, an important step had been taken. For the first time, Jim was in part able to understand the basis of his heart disease and empowered to do something to prevent another attack.

In January 1993, Jim joined a cardiac support group. Although at this point he felt no particular need for such a group, it was being started by several friends and he wanted it to be a success. In addition to providing emotional support and trading exercise and nutrition ideas, the group met occasionally for a potluck dinner. One of my patients, Dr. Edna Katz, was a founding member of the support group. She invited me to come and speak to it on cardiac risk factors. Before the lecture, we met at Wayne and Sarah's (see Wayne's case) for dinner, and it was there that I first met Jim.

He told me briefly about his history and mentioned that his doctor had told him cholesterol was not his problem. Concerned that he might not have had as complete an evaluation as he should have, I suggested that he come to my laboratory for a blood test. It took many months for him to decide to do it, but when he did, his problem was immediately apparent.

His former physician had been measuring only Jim's total cholesterol, which at 181 mg/dl, was just fine. A complete breakdown, however, revealed a very different picture. At his first appointment, his values were as follows:

	Jim's Level	Desirable Level
Total cholesterol	181 mg/dl	Less than 200 mg/dl
Triglycerides	247 mg/dl	Less than 150 mg/dl
HDL cholesterol	25 mg/dl	Greater than 45 mg/dl
LDL cholesterol	106 mg/dl	Less than 100 mg/dl
Lp(a)	19 mg/dl	Less than 20 mg/dl

Jim's total to HDL ratio was elevated at 7.2. I explained that a depressed HDL cholesterol is a strong risk factor for the development of cardiac disease, and that his goal should be to achieve a ratio of 4.0.

Although a number of nondrug therapies would probably improve his HDL, in the end I was fairly sure he would require medication. To begin with, though, we needed to look at the drugs he was already on. Lopressor, which is a beta-blocker known to protect the heart, also lowers HDL cholesterol substantially. After a careful evaluation of Jim's cardiac status and his blood pressure (Lopressor also lowers blood pressure), we decided that we should wean him off this medication.

A second area of concern was his weight. At five feet nine inches and 189, Jim was about 25 pounds overweight. Related to this problem was an elevated triglyceride level, which was in turn connected to his depressed HDL. Concentrated sweets and alcohol, which Jim admitted enjoying, cause both weight gain and elevated triglycerides. Since triglycerides and HDL are metabolically related, as one rises the other falls. Jim suddenly saw the interconnectedness of the many different aspects of his life. Improvement in one area would necessarily bring about improvement in others.

It was in this positive frame of mind that Jim met with Mary Card to review his diet and design a new program aimed at weight loss and an improved lipid profile.

Finally, I asked Jim to increase his exercise. I suggested walking three miles a day, seven days a week, and Jim agreed. One of his main motivations, both in diet and exercise, was his strong desire to avoid medications. My own belief was that lifestyle modifications, important as they were, would not alone be able to bring his lipid profile into the normal range. I agreed, however, to wait eight weeks before prescribing anything.

Eight weeks later his weight was down by 14.5 pounds and his cholesterol profile was significantly improved.

	Jim's Level	Desirable Level
Total cholesterol	188 mg/dl	Less than 200 mg/dl
Triglycerides	193 mg/dl	Less than 150 mg/dl
HDL cholesterol	34 mg/dl	Greater than 45 mg/dl
LDL cholesterol	115 mg/dl	Less than 100 mg/dl

Although his LDL was up slightly, his total to HDL ratio was much better at 5.5. But since it was still too high, and since it seemed unlikely that Jim would lose any more weight, I suggested that he consider niacin, which would improve all his lipid levels.

Jim was still sure that with more dietary adjustments, he could make even more of a difference. To my surprise, he also admitted he was still taking Lopressor. He had been on it for so long that he just couldn't wean himself off it. This time he wanted three more months to prove himself. Reluctantly, I agreed, certain that in that much time he would have to see reason.

One week before Christmas he returned. Although his weight was now down by an additional two pounds, his cholesterol levels were awful—an accurate reflection of his attendance at many holiday parties.

	Jim's Level	Desirable Level
Total cholesterol	207 mg/dl	Less than 200 mg/dl
Triglycerides	251 mg/dl	Less than 150 mg/dl
HDL cholesterol	31 mg/dl	Greater than 45 mg/dl
LDL cholesterol	109 mg/dl	Less than 100 mg/dl

Disappointed as I was with his results, I was glad that at least now he would have to concede defeat. Anyone could see that diet alone couldn't possibly get his levels to where they should be. But Jim was stubborn as ever. He was philosophical about his results: he admitted to overindulging at Christmas parties and said he had been expecting his comeuppance in the lab reports. "Numbers don't lie," he explained sagely. He was also, he confided without a hint of guilt, still taking Lopressor. I was baffled: here he was moving heaven and earth to avoid cholesterol-lowering medication, while simultaneously refusing to give up Lopressor. It just didn't make sense.

I could hardly believe my ears when he said he wanted more time: he was certain that with renewed commitment to diet and exercise and a firm determination to get off the Lopressor, he would achieve the desired levels.

I was even more amazed to hear myself agreeing yet again to this proposal. "This guy must have been the captain of his college debating team," I thought to myself. Being a bit of a debater myself, however, I wasn't content to give up quite so easily. Before he left my office I made him promise that if his numbers weren't normal or nearly so in three months, he would give niacin a try. This time I was all but certain he would have to do it my way.

Three months later, it was time for humble pie. Jim had further reduced his Lopressor dosage, he weighed 165 pounds, and his cholesterol profile was almost perfect:

	Jim's Level	Desirable Level
Total cholesterol	169 mg/dl	Less than 200 mg/dl
Triglycerides	104 mg/dl	Less than 150 mg/dl
HDL cholesterol	39 mg/dl	Greater than 45 mg/dl
LDL cholesterol	109 mg/dl	Less than 100 mg/dl

His current ratio is 4.3, so close to normal that I believe once he is off Lopressor entirely, his profile will be perfect.

I learned a great deal working with Jim. In over 10 years in medicine I have never seen such a dramatic improvement in HDL without the use of medications. I have also never met a patient so stubbornly insistent about not taking cholesterol-lowering drugs. When I questioned Jim about it, he said that Mary Card and I had shown him so many new ways to improve his diet and exercise that he just had to try them all before resorting to the chemical route. His confidence in our approach has increased my own, while his success has made me a bit more flexible regarding drug therapy in general.

I shouldn't have been surprised at Jim's tenacity, of course. He is well known around here as a man with the courage of his convictions. Just last year he organized a local campaign to save a forest that had been targeted for destruction to raise revenue for the municipality. The battle was a tough one, but Keene, New Hampshire, is a greener place because of his efforts. I have no doubt that Jim will be around to enjoy that forest for many years to come.

$\mathscr{8}$

vvvvvvvvvvvvvvvvvvvvvvvvvvvvvvvvvvvvvvvv

The Crucial Role of Medications

in Lowering Cholesterol

and Blood Pressure

In some cases in spite of one's best efforts, diet, exercise, and weight loss cannot completely normalize cholesterol or blood pressure levels. This chapter is divided into two parts. The first part is devoted to cholesterol-lowering medications and the second part to blood pressure medications.

Cholesterol-Altering Medications

While lifestyle changes are important in determining your cholesterol level, they are not the only factors. In some people the liver simply over-produces cholesterol. While a good diet and plenty of exercise will help, without medication, cholesterol levels are unlikely to completely normal-ize. Being on a cholesterol-lowering drug does not mean you are a failure, just that you need a little more help than diet and exercise can deliver.

Being on medication does not mean you should abandon your efforts, however. By continuing to exercise and eat well, you will be able to take the lowest dose possible. In fact, in one study published in the *Journal of the American Medical Association*, only 50 percent of people taking a cho-lesterol-lowering drug alone reached their cholesterol goals, whereas 80 percent who followed a diet and faithfully took their cholesterol-lowering medication reached their cholesterol goals.

Many people do not realize that cholesterol-lowering medications are a life-long proposition. Unlike antibiotics which may require only 10

200

days of therapy, cholesterol-lowering drugs work only as long as you are taking them. Once discontinued, cholesterol levels will increase.

Taking your medication correctly and faithfully can greatly reduce your risk of having a heart attack or requiring bypass surgery. Studies have shown, however, that drug therapy must continue for at least one year before you will see a substantial decrease in the risk of death or illness due to cardiac disease. In other words, to reap the benefits of your cholesterol-lowering medications, you must be in it for the long haul.

This being so, it is important to figure out how to incorporate your medication into your daily routine. It doesn't do you any good to have a medication that you forget to take. Since there are many cholesterol-lowering medications, all with different dosing requirements and side effects, it is essential to discuss your schedule with your doctor as you determine which medication is right for you.

Many people worry about the possible side effects of cholesterol-lowering medications. The fact of the matter is that these medications are very safe. Nonetheless, it is important for you to know the side effects of any drug you are taking.

The most common concern my patients voice is the fear of liver toxicity. The liver is one of the few organs in the body that can repair itself, but only if the injury is caught quickly. With careful monitoring of liver function through simple blood tests, it is very rare for any cholesterol-lowering medication to cause an irreversible complication. When a cholesterol-lowering medication is initiated, a blood test of liver function is obtained. This is repeated six weeks later, and then periodically (in general, every three to six months) thereafter. Liver toxicity, which is often accompanied by nausea, fatigue, and abdominal discomfort, can typically be reversed by stopping the medication for several days. In many cases the medication can be restarted and continued at a lower dose.

The most important thing for you to remember is that regular followup visits to your doctor are essential.

Some cholesterol-altering medications lower LDL cholesterol (the bad cholesterol) and others lower triglycerides. In general, medications that lower triglycerides will also improve HDL cholesterol (the good cholesterol). I give written information to anyone I start on a cholesterol-altering medication.

In this chapter I list the major medications used in treating heart disease along with brand name and generic designations, how the medication works, and the best way of taking it.

The following table lists the cholesterol-altering medications I discuss at length.

Cholesterol-Altering Medications

Class of Drug	Drug Name*
LDL-LOWERING MEDICATIONS	
Bile acid sequestrant	Cholestyramine (Questran)
	Colestipol (Colestid)
Niacin	Nicotinic acid
HMG CoA reductase inhibitor	Lovastatin (Mevacor)
	Simvastatin (Zocor)
	Pravastatin (Pravachol)
	Fluvastatin (Lescol)
	Atorvastatin (Lipitor)
TRIGLYCERIDE-LOWERING MEDICATIONS	
Fibric acid	Gemfibrozil (Lopid)
	Clofibrate (Atromid-S)
Niacin	Nicotinic acid

* The first drug name given is the generic designation; the second one in parentheses is the brand name. Probucol (Lorelco) has now been taken off the market.

Questran or Questran Light

Mode of Action Questran binds bile acids (which are made from cholesterol) within the intestine and excretes them into the stool. In addition, Questran increases the number of special LDL-removing
receptors on the liver cell.

What Is It For?   Questran is used to lower your LDL cholesterol
level. It is used as a supplement to a low-fat, low-
cholesterol diet and is not a substitute for that diet.

How To Take It: The usual starting dose of Questran or Questran
Light is one packet or scoopful (4 grams) twice a
day. Some people may require as much as two packets or scoops, three times a day.

When To Take It: It is best to take this medication just before a meal.
However, since Questran can interfere with the ab-
sorption of other medications, it is best to take the
other medications two hours before or four to six
hours after taking Questran.

How To Prepare:	1. Dissolve one packet or scoop in 4 to 6 ounces of water or juice (never take the medication in dry form).
	2. Let the mixture stand without stirring for one to two minutes.
	3. Stir until it is completely mixed (it will not dissolve), and drink slowly; this will minimize belching.

Side Effects: The most common complaint is constipation. This can be minimized by slowly increasing the dose of Questran and by increasing daily fiber and water intake (see Chapter 2 on diet for ways to increase fiber). Other less-common side effects include nausea, gas, and diarrhea.

Other: Since Questran can interfere with the absorption of folic acid and possibly other essential nutrients, I recommend taking a daily multivitamin.

Questran can raise triglycerides, and as such, should generally not be used if triglycerides are elevated.

Since Questran is not absorbed into the blood, there is no risk of liver toxicity.

Effect: Depending on the dose, Questran can lower LDL cholesterol by 15 to 30 percent.

Colestid (Powder)

Mode of Action: Colestid binds bile acids (which are made from cholesterol) within the intestine and excretes them into the stool. In addition, Colestid increases the number of special LDL-removing receptors on the liver cell

What Is It For?   Colestid is used to lower your LDL cholesterol level. It is used as a supplement to a low-fat, low-cholesterol diet and is not a substitute for that diet.

How To Take It: The usual starting dose of Colestid is one packet or scoopful (5 grams) twice a day. Some people may require as much as two packets or scoops, three times a day.

When To Take It: It is best to take this medication just before a meal. However, since Colestid can interfere with the absorption of other medications, it is best to take the other medications two hours before or four to six hours after taking Colestid.

How To Prepare: 1. Dissolve one packet or scoop in 4 to 6 ounces of water or juice (never take the medication in dry form).
2. Let the mixture stand without stirring for one to two minutes.
3. Stir until it is completely mixed (it will not dissolve), and drink slowly; this will minimize belching.

Side Effects: The most common complaint is constipation. This can be minimized by slowly increasing the dose of Colestid and by increasing daily fiber and water intake (see Chapter 2 on diet for ways to increase fiber). Other less-common side effects include nausea, gas, and diarrhea.

Other: Since Colestid can interfere with the absorption of folic acid and possibly other essential nutrients, I recommend taking a daily multivitamin.
  Colestid can raise triglycerides, and as such, should generally not be used if triglycerides are elevated.
Since Colestid is not absorbed into the blood, there is no risk of liver toxicity.

Effect: Depending on the dose, Colestid will lower LDL cholesterol by 15 to 30 percent.

Colestid (Tablets)

Mode of Action: Colestid binds bile acids (which are made from cholesterol) within the intestine and excretes them into the stool. In addition, Colestid increases the number of special LDL-removing receptors on the liver cell.

What Is It For?   Colestid is used to lower your LDL cholesterol level. It is used as a supplement to a low-fat, low-cholesterol diet and is not a substitute for that diet.

How To Take It: The usual starting dose of Colestid is two tablets (2 grams) twice a day. Some people may require as much as 16 tablets a day. It is important to drink at least 8 ounces of water with each dose.

When To Take It: It is best to take this medication just before a meal. However, since Colestid can interfere with the absorption of other medications, it is best to take the other medications two hours before or four to six hours after taking Colestid.

Side Effects: The most common complaint is constipation. This can be minimized by slowly increasing the dose of Colestid and by increasing daily fiber and water intake (see Chapter 2 on diet for ways to increase fiber). Other less-common side effects include nausea, gas, and diarrhea.

Other: Since Colestid can interfere with the absorption of folic acid and possibly other essential nutrients, I recommend taking a daily multivitamin either two hours before or four hours after taking Colestid.

Colestid can raise triglycerides, and as such, should generally not be used if triglycerides are elevated.

Since Colestid is not absorbed into the blood, there is no risk of liver toxicity.

Effect: Depending on the dose, Colestid will lower LDL cholesterol by 15 to 30 percent.

Niacin (Nicotinic Acid)

Mode of Action: Although all the actions of niacin are not known, it is clear that niacin lowers the liver's production of VLDL cholesterol. Since VLDL cholesterol is triglyceride rich, triglycerides fall, and because VLDL cholesterol is ultimately converted to LDL cholesterol in the bloodstream, LDL levels also fall with niacin. Niacin can also dramatically increase HDL levels, but the mechanism for this action is less well described.

What Is It For? Niacin will lower LDL, Lipoprotein (a), and triglyceride levels. It will also lead to increases in HDL.

Dose:	Niacin must be taken in high doses to lower cholesterol levels. The target dose is typically 1.5 to 3 grams per day. The usual starting dose is 250 milligrams (mg) three times a day for two weeks followed by 500 mg three times a day for six weeks. At this point your cholesterol levels will be reevaluated and your dose adjusted as necessary.

How To Take It:

1. Always take niacin with meals.
2. To minimize flushing, take an aspirin or ibuprofen prior to each dose. I typically suggest taking an aspirin, followed by eating a meal, followed by taking the niacin. This gives the aspirin a chance to work prior to taking the niacin.
3. Avoid hot beverages or hot showers for at least an hour after taking niacin, as this too will cut down on flushing.

Side Effects:	Flushing, itching, and nausea.
Precautions	Although niacin is an excellent medication, it does have a number of possible serious side effects. It can worsen diabetes, cause gout, and may increase the occurrence of peptic ulcer disease.
Followup:	While on niacin it is important to have followup blood tests to evaluate your cholesterol response, liver function, blood sugar, and uric acid (a predictor of the risk of developing gout). I typically measure these blood tests within two months of beginning niacin and then every three to six months thereafter.
Other:	Niacin is a vitamin that can be purchased over the counter. A derivative of niacin called nicotinamide is also freely available. It is important for you to know that only niacin (nicotinic acid), and not nicotinamide, lowers cholesterol.

Please be careful not to take slow release (no flush) niacins as they increase the risk of liver toxicity. |

Effect:	Depending on the dose, niacin will lower LDL cholesterol by 15 to 30 percent, triglycerides by 30 to 40 percent, and Lp(a) by 15 to 30 percent and will raise HDL by 15 to 25 percent.

One additional word on niacin. Since niacin is a vitamin and can be purchased over the counter without a prescription, there are no strict quality control regulations regarding its formulation. It has been my experience that people are safest with niacin purchased from large drug store chains. I personally recommend Niacor-B3, a brand of niacin made by a drug company called Upsher-Smith. Twin Labs and Bronsen Pharmaceuticals also make reliable niacin preparations.

In closing, niacin is a drug. In high doses it can and will lower cholesterol levels, but because of its potential to cause liver toxicity, it should never be taken without the guidance of your physician.

Mevacor

Mode of Action: Mevacor partially blocks the liver enzyme HMG CoA reductase. This enzyme regulates the production of cholesterol. The net result is a profound reduction in total and LDL cholesterol, a small reduction in triglycerides, and a slight increase in HDL.

Dose:	10 to 80 mg/day
How To Take It:	Mevacor should be taken with your evening meal. At higher doses it must be taken twice a day, in which case it should be taken with breakfast and your evening meal. If you miss a dose, take it as soon as you remember. If it is almost time to take your next dose, skip the missed dose and go back to your regular schedule. Do not take a double dose.
Side Effects:	The side effects of Mevacor are typically mild and do not last. Possible side effects include constipation, diarrhea, abdominal cramps, nausea, headache, and muscle aches.
Followup:	While on Mevacor you will need to have your cholesterol profile and liver function tests followed. These should be checked at six and 12 weeks after starting Mevacor and then every six months.
Precautions:	If you develop fever, muscle cramping, and weakness while on Mevacor, you may have a rare com-

plication of this drug called myositis. Of course, these symptoms may simply be the flu. In such a case your doctor will run a blood test to evaluate your muscle function. If you do have myositis, your doctor will ask you to stop the Mevacor. In general, you will be back to normal within two to three days of stopping the medication.

Effect: Depending on the dose, Mevacor will lower LDL cholesterol by 25 to 40 percent.

Zocor

Mode of Action: Zocor partially blocks the liver enzyme HMG CoA reductase. This enzyme regulates the production of cholesterol. The net result is a profound reduction in total and LDL cholesterol, a small reduction in triglycerides, and a slight increase in HDL.

Dose: 5 to 40 mg/day

How To Take It: Zocor should be taken in the evening with or without food. If you miss a dose, take it as soon as you remember. If it is almost time to take your next dose, skip the missed dose and go back to your regular schedule. Do not take a double dose.

Side Effects: The side effects of Zocor are typically mild and do not last. Possible side effects include constipation, diarrhea, abdominal cramps, nausea, headache, and muscle aches.

Followup: While on Zocor you will need to have your cholesterol profile and liver function tests followed. These will be checked at six and 12 weeks after starting Zocor and then every six months.

Precautions: If you develop fever, muscle cramping, and weakness while on Zocor, you may have a rare complication of this drug called myositis. Of course, these symptoms may simply be the flu. In such a case your doctor will run a blood test to evaluate your muscle function. If you do have myositis, your doctor will ask you to stop the Zocor. In general, you will be back to normal within two to three days of stopping the medication.

Effect:	Depending on the dose, niacin will lower LDL cholesterol by 15 to 30 percent, triglycerides by 30 to 40 percent, and Lp(a) by 15 to 30 percent and will raise HDL by 15 to 25 percent.

One additional word on niacin. Since niacin is a vitamin and can be purchased over the counter without a prescription, there are no strict quality control regulations regarding its formulation. It has been my experience that people are safest with niacin purchased from large drug store chains. I personally recommend Niacor-B3, a brand of niacin made by a drug company called Upsher-Smith. Twin Labs and Bronsen Pharmaceuticals also make reliable niacin preparations.

In closing, niacin is a drug. In high doses it can and will lower cholesterol levels, but because of its potential to cause liver toxicity, it should never be taken without the guidance of your physician.

Mevacor

Mode of Action: Mevacor partially blocks the liver enzyme HMG CoA reductase. This enzyme regulates the production of cholesterol. The net result is a profound reduction in total and LDL cholesterol, a small reduction in triglycerides, and a slight increase in HDL.

Dose:	10 to 80 mg/day
How To Take It:	Mevacor should be taken with your evening meal. At higher doses it must be taken twice a day, in which case it should be taken with breakfast and your evening meal. If you miss a dose, take it as soon as you remember. If it is almost time to take your next dose, skip the missed dose and go back to your regular schedule. Do not take a double dose.
Side Effects:	The side effects of Mevacor are typically mild and do not last. Possible side effects include constipation, diarrhea, abdominal cramps, nausea, headache, and muscle aches.
Followup:	While on Mevacor you will need to have your cholesterol profile and liver function tests followed. These should be checked at six and 12 weeks after starting Mevacor and then every six months.
Precautions:	If you develop fever, muscle cramping, and weakness while on Mevacor, you may have a rare com-

plication of this drug called myositis. Of course, these symptoms may simply be the flu. In such a case your doctor will run a blood test to evaluate your muscle function. If you do have myositis, your doctor will ask you to stop the Mevacor. In general, you will be back to normal within two to three days of stopping the medication.

Effect: Depending on the dose, Mevacor will lower LDL cholesterol by 25 to 40 percent.

Zocor

Mode of Action: Zocor partially blocks the liver enzyme HMG CoA reductase. This enzyme regulates the production of cholesterol. The net result is a profound reduction in total and LDL cholesterol, a small reduction in triglycerides, and a slight increase in HDL.

Dose: 5 to 40 mg/day

How To Take It: Zocor should be taken in the evening with or without food. If you miss a dose, take it as soon as you remember. If it is almost time to take your next dose, skip the missed dose and go back to your regular schedule. Do not take a double dose.

Side Effects: The side effects of Zocor are typically mild and do not last. Possible side effects include constipation, diarrhea, abdominal cramps, nausea, headache, and muscle aches.

Followup: While on Zocor you will need to have your cholesterol profile and liver function tests followed. These will be checked at six and 12 weeks after starting Zocor and then every six months.

Precautions: If you develop fever, muscle cramping, and weakness while on Zocor, you may have a rare complication of this drug called myositis. Of course, these symptoms may simply be the flu. In such a case your doctor will run a blood test to evaluate your muscle function. If you do have myositis, your doctor will ask you to stop the Zocor. In general, you will be back to normal within two to three days of stopping the medication.

Effect: Depending on the dose, Zocor will lower LDL cholesterol by 25 to 41 percent.

Pravachol

Mode of Action: Pravachol partially blocks the liver enzyme HMG CoA reductase. This enzyme regulates the production of cholesterol. The net result is a profound reduction in total and LDL cholesterol, a small reduction in triglycerides, and a slight increase in HDL.

Dose: 10 to 40 mg/day

How To Take It: Pravachol should be taken in the evening with or without food. If you miss a dose, take it as soon as you remember. If it is almost time to take your next dose, skip the missed dose and go back to your regular schedule. Do not take a double dose.

Side Effects: The side effects of Pravachol are typically mild and do not last. Possible side effects include constipation, diarrhea, abdominal cramps, nausea, headache, and muscle aches.

Followup: While on Pravachol you will need to have your cholesterol profile and liver function tests followed. These will be checked at six and 12 weeks after starting Pravachol and then every six months.

Precautions: If you develop fever, muscle cramping, and weakness while on Pravachol, you may have a rare complication of this drug called myositis. Of course, these symptoms may simply be the flu. In such a case your doctor will run a blood test to evaluate your muscle function. If you do have myositis, your doctor will ask you to stop the Pravachol. In general, you will be back to normal within two to three days of stopping the medication.

Effect: Depending on the dose, Pravachol will lower LDL cholesterol by 20 to 32 percent.

Lescol

Mode of Action: Lescol partially blocks the liver enzyme HMG CoA reductase. This enzyme regulates the production of cholesterol. The net result is a *modest* reduction in total and LDL cholesterol, a small reduction in triglycerides, and a slight increase in HDL.

Dose:	20 to 80 mg/day
How To Take It:	Lescol should be taken in the evening with or without food. If you miss a dose, take it as soon as you remember. If it is almost time to take your next dose, skip the missed dose and go back to your regular schedule. Do not take a double dose.
Side Effects:	The side effects of Lescol are typically mild and do not last. Possible side effects include constipation, diarrhea, abdominal cramps, nausea, headache, and muscle aches.
Followup:	While on Lescol you will need to have your cholesterol profile and liver function tests followed. These will be checked at six and 12 weeks after starting Lescol and then every six months.
Precautions:	If you develop fever, muscle cramping, and weakness while on Lescol, you may have a rare complication of this drug called myositis. Of course, these symptoms may simply be the flu. In such a case your doctor will run a blood test to evaluate your muscle function. If you do have myositis, your doctor will ask you to stop the Lescol. In general, you will be back to normal within two to three days of stopping the medication.
Effect:	Depending on the dose, Lescol will lower LDL cholesterol by 20 to 30 percent.

Lipitor

Mode of Action: Lipitor partially blocks the liver enzyme HMG CoA reductase. This enzyme regulates the production of cholesterol. The net result is a profound reduction in total and LDL cholesterol. This is the one drug in this class that also lowers triglycerides quite substantially. A small increase in HDL can also be expected.

Dose:	10 to 80 mg/day
How To Take It:	Lipitor may be taken at any time of day with or without food. If you miss a dose, take it as soon as

you remember. If it is almost time to take your next dose, skip the missed dose and go back to your regular schedule. Do not take a double dose.

Side Effects: The side effects of Lipitor are typically mild and do not last. Possible side effects include constipation, diarrhea, abdominal cramps, nausea, headache, and muscle aches.

Followup: While on Lipitor you will need to have your cholesterol profile and liver function tests followed. These will be checked at six and 12 weeks after starting Lipitor and then every six months.

Precautions: If you develop fever, muscle cramping, and weakness while on Lipitor, you may have a rare complication of this drug called myositis. Of course, these symptoms may simply be the flu. In such a case your doctor will run a blood test to evaluate your muscle function. If you do have myositis, your doctor will ask you to stop the Lipitor. In general, you will be back to normal within two to three days of stopping the medication.

Effect: Depending on the dose, Lipitor will lower LDL cholesterol by 41 to 60 percent and will lower triglycerides by 30 to 45 percent.

Lopid

Mode of Action: Lopid increases the activity of lipoprotein lipase, the enzyme responsible for breaking down triglyceride-rich particles, and increases the amount of cholesterol excreted into the bile. Lopid also appears to slow the production of triglycerides within liver cells.

What Is It For?   Lopid is a drug used to lower elevated triglycerides. It may also cause an increase in HDL (the good cholesterol).

How To Take It: The usual dose is 600 mg twice a day taken before the morning and evening meals. The dose is reduced to 300 mg twice a day in people weighing less than 100 pounds and in those with liver or kidney disease.

Side Effects:	Lopid is generally very well tolerated; however, the following side effects may possibly occur: nausea, diarrhea, abdominal cramping, dizziness, blurred vision, skin rash, and muscle aches.
Followup:	While on Lopid your doctor will want to check your liver function tests and run a complete blood count periodically.
Precautions:	It is possible that prolonged therapy with Lopid may increase your risk of developing gallbladder disease. If you are taking blood thinners (e.g., warfarin [Coumadin]), your doctor will want to closely monitor your prothrombin (PT) when you begin Lopid therapy. It is quite likely that your dose of warfarin will be reduced while you are on Lopid.
Effect:	Depending on the dose and baseline triglyceride levels, Lopid will lower triglycerides by 25 to 60 percent and raise HDL by 15 to 25 percent.

Atromid-S

Mode of Action: Atromid-S increases the activity of lipoprotein lipase, the enzyme responsible for breaking down triglyceride-rich particles, and increases the amount of cholesterol excreted into the bile.

What Is It For?	Atromid-S is used to lower elevated triglycerides. It may also cause an increase in HDL (the good cholesterol).
How To Take It:	The usual dose is 1000 mg twice a day taken before the morning and evening meals. The dose may be reduced in individuals with liver or kidney disease.
Side Effects:	Atromid-S is generally very well tolerated; however, the following side effects may possibly occur: nausea, diarrhea, abdominal cramping, dizziness, blurred vision, skin rash, and muscle aches.
Followup:	While on Atromid-S your doctor will want to check your liver function tests and run a complete blood count periodically.
Precautions:	It is possible that prolonged therapy with Atromid-S may increase your risk of developing gallbladder

disease. If you are taking blood thinners (e.g., warfarin [Coumadin]), your doctor will want to closely monitor your prothrombin (PT) when you begin Atromid-S therapy. It is quite likely that your dose of warfarin will be reduced while you are on Atromid-S.

Other: Atromid-S fell out of favor as a cholesterol-lowering agent in the United States after the results of a World Health Organization study were published. Although Atromid was found to reduce cardiac risk, it was associated with an increased risk of death from causes other than cardiac disease. I very seldom use this medication.

Effect: Depending on the dose and baseline triglyceride levels, Atromid-S will lower triglycerides by 25 to 60 percent and raise HDL by 15 to 25 percent.

Drugs on the Horizon

Before a medication can be released for use in this country, extensive safety and effectiveness studies must be performed. In the next few years, a number of new cholesterol-lowering medications are likely to become available which are currently being tested. If you have been troubled by side effects from any of the cholesterol-lowering medications previously mentioned or have had an insufficient response, don't despair: it is quite possible that one of the new drugs about to be released will be the answer.

Approved by the Food and Drug Administration (FDA) in December 1996 and now available by prescription, atorvastatin (Lipitor) is a new drug in the same family as Mevacor, Zocor, Pravachol, and Lescol. Like them, atorvastatin lowers LDL cholesterol, but even more dramatically. It also lowers triglycerides significantly. Research trials suggest that atorvastatin will be very useful in the treatment of familial hypercholesterolemia and familial combined hyperlipidemia. My cholesterol clinic is currently participating in a "compassionate-use trial" of atorvastatin. In this trial people who have not lowered their cholesterol sufficiently with currently available medications receive atorvastatin free of charge from the manufacturer (Parke-Davis) on an experimental basis. I have been impressed with the results of this drug and would like to tell you how two of my patients have benefited.

Susan was a 36-year-old director of a busy daycare center when her primary care physician referred her to me because of an astronomical cholesterol level. When Susan first came to our lipid clinic, this is what her cholesterol profile looked like:

	Susan's Level	Desirable Level
Total cholesterol	427 mg/dl	Less than 200 mg/dl
Triglycerides	128 mg/dl	Less than 150 mg/dl
HDL cholesterol	35 mg/dl	Greater than 45 mg/dl
LDL cholesterol	366 mg/dl	Less than 100 mg/dl

While her family history and physical exam indicated that she had familial hypercholesterolemia (FH), her symptoms varied from the classic pattern for FH women of her age. Typically, such women do not experience clinical symptoms of cardiac disease until they are postmenopausal (assuming they have no other cardiac risk factors). Susan, however, described almost daily chest discomfort and extreme fatigue that were clearly coming from her heart.

It didn't take long to figure out. At the age of 23, Susan had undergone a hysterectomy, and for the next thirteen years, she had not had any estrogen replacement therapy. Her blood vessels were behaving as though she was in her fifties or sixties, and her heart was protesting. That day I started Susan on estrogen replacement, and a powerful cholesterol-lowering medication. I also suggested that she take a daily aspirin and begin a beta-blocker to reduce her symptoms of chest pain and pressure.

Three weeks into this new regime, Susan returned for a stress test and the results were troubling: cardiac disease was definitely present. The only question was how much. She then underwent a cardiac catheterization which revealed one completely blocked artery (right coronary) and one with a 50 percent blockage (left anterior descending).

We decided to treat her with medicines to lower her cholesterol and prevent further blockages from developing, as well as to reduce her chest pain. In addition, she began an aggressive diet and a moderate exercise program. At the end of three months, her cholesterol levels had reduced considerably and her chest pain was also less frequent.

	Susan's Level	Desirable Level
Total cholesterol	370 mg/dl	Less than 200 mg/dl
Triglycerides	180 mg/dl	Less than 150 mg/dl
HDL cholesterol	28 mg/dl	Greater than 45 mg/dl
LDL cholesterol	306 mg/dl	Less than 100 mg/dl

Improved as these numbers were, however, it was only in relative terms. Susan's cholesterol levels were still far too high. If they remained as they were, a heart attack was only a question of time. More had to be done, and it was clear that we had come to the end of the line where conventional treatments were concerned.

Because atorvastatin was not yet approved by the FDA, I applied for "compassionate use" of this drug for Susan. She was quickly approved and started on a daily dose of 40 mg. She continued to take estrogen, but discontinued all other cholesterol-lowering medications. One month later this was her lipid profile.

	Susan's Level	Desirable Level
Total cholesterol	223 mg/dl	Less than 200 mg/dl
Triglycerides	158 mg/dl	Less than 150 mg/dl
HDL cholesterol	43 mg/dl	Greater than 45 mg/dl
LDL cholesterol	148 mg/dl	Less than 100 mg/dl

Obviously, we were thrilled with such a rapid improvement. My goal, however, was to bring her levels into the desirable range. At this point, Susan is taking 80 mg of atorvastatin each day, and she continues to work on her diet and exercise program.

If her levels improve even a little bit more, I believe there is a distinct possibility that Susan's existing cholesterol deposits may begin to reduce. At the very least, I am confident that the combination of atorvastatin, estrogen, diet, and exercise will prevent any progression of Susan's cardiac disease.

The more experience I gain with atorvastatin, the more convinced I am that it is going to help some of the most difficult to treat patients in my practice. Ed is a patient whose cholesterol levels have made me feel like a failure. I first met him in 1993, when at the age of 45 he had suffered his second heart attack, his first having been ten years earlier. At that time his cholesterol levels looked like this:

	Ed's Level	Desirable Level
Total cholesterol	358 mg/dl	Less than 200 mg/dl
Triglycerides	180 mg/dl	Less than 150 mg/dl
HDL cholesterol	41 mg/dl	Greater than 45 mg/dl
LDL cholesterol	283 mg/dl	Less than 100 mg/dl

Despite two cholesterol-lowering medications and a relatively good diet and exercise program, Ed's cholesterol levels never came close to normalizing. In 1995, he suffered a stroke from which he thankfully recovered completely. But given his uncontrolled cholesterol levels, Ed and I both knew that it was simply a question of time before he had another stroke or heart attack. With a family to support, this was a frightening prospect.

As soon as I had access to atorvastatin on a compassionate-use basis I called Ed. While on two powerful cholesterol-lowering medications, this is what his levels were before beginning atorvastatin:

	Ed's Level	Desirable Level
Total cholesterol	322 mg/dl	Less than 200 mg/dl
Triglycerides	99 mg/dl	Less than 150 mg/dl
HDL cholesterol	40 mg/dl	Greater than 45 mg/dl
LDL cholesterol	262 mg/dl	Less than 100 mg/dl

One month after stopping his other cholesterol medications and beginning atorvastatin at 40 mg per day, his cholesterol levels looked like this:

	Ed's Level	Desirable Level
Total cholesterol	174 mg/dl	Less than 200 mg/dl
Triglycerides	129 mg/dl	Less than 150 mg/dl
HDL cholesterol	43 mg/dl	Greater than 45 mg/dl
LDL cholesterol	104 mg/dl	Less than 100 mg/dl

Both Ed and I feel we witnessed a miracle, and a well-deserved miracle, at that. Nothing in Ed's life has come easily, so his response to atorvastatin is truly a gift. These numbers have made Ed believe, for the first time in many years, that he will see his children graduate from college and that maybe he will never have another heart attack or stroke. I have to admit we were both on the brink of tears the day we saw these levels. I think I now know (and I'm sure Ed feels the same way) what it feels like to win the lottery.

As mentioned earlier, atorvastatin was approved by the FDA in December 1996 and became available in January 1997. It is likely to make a huge difference to the many people who until now have not been able to fully normalize their cholesterol levels. It is known by the brand name Lipitor.

ACAT (acyl coenzyme A, or cholesterol acyltransferase) inhibitors are still another class of cholesterol-lowering medications that are currently undergoing extensive testing. ACAT is an enzyme that is involved in the development of atherosclerosis at three distinct sites: the intestine, where ACAT helps in the absorption of cholesterol from the diet; the liver, where ACAT helps in cholesterol production; and cells of the artery wall, where ACAT seems to be involved in the deposition of cholesterol into the cells of the artery wall, leading to the formation of cholesterol plaque.

The ACAT inhibitors appear to lower LDL cholesterol by about 20 percent. The fact that this drug works by a totally different mechanism than the Mevacor family of drugs may allow it to be used in conjunction with this class of drugs, with an additive or even synergistic effect. We will be beginning some early trials on a very promising ACAT inhibitor in the near future.

Squalene synthase inhibitors are a third class of drugs that show great potential in the area of LDL reduction. These drugs act primarily by blocking cholesterol production in the liver. It is possible that a drug of this class may become available in the next few years. The major difficulty with squalene synthose inhibitors has been gastrointestinal toxicity. This will need to be significantly improved before FDA approval.

As mentioned earlier, the bile acid resins (cholestyramine [Questran] and colestipol [Colestid]) tend to cause bloating and are relatively unpleasant to take. This is unfortunate because these are among the safest cholesterol-lowering medications available. They are frequently given to children and are even safe in pregnancy. If they could be made more palatable they would be the ideal drug, either alone or in combination with another cholesterol-lowering medication.

Enter GelTex Pharmaceuticals, Inc. of Boston, Massachusetts. GelTex has developed a gelcap bile acid resin called CholestaGel that has no unpleasant side effects. I have recently spoken to Dr. Steven Burke of GelTex who tells me that early studies demonstrate a 15 to 30 percent reduction in LDL cholesterol with CholestaGel. The company is now working on formulations for delivering the drug. For children, the formulations being discussed are gelcaps and low-fat chocolates (the chocolate would contain the drug and about 1 to 2 grams of fat). For adults, the delivery system would most likely be a tablet. Of course, I suppose adults could eat the chocolates too, but they will have to decide if this is the way they want to spend their daily fat gram allowance. We typically allow children 40 grams of fat per day so a chocolate could more easily be worked into their diet. Since CholestaGel is in the early stages of development, much of what you just read could change; but I think you should be hearing more about CholestaGel in a year or two.

In addition to the cholesterol-lowering medications that are currently undergoing testing, there are a number of well-tested, triglyceride-lowering medications that are available in Europe. These may someday be available in the United States and include fenofibrate, bezafibrate, and ciprofibrate.

Finally, in 1998 look for a concentrated form of fish oil in capsules called Omacor. These have the potential to lower triglycerides by as much as 35 percent. Omacor was approved for the treatment of hyper-triglyceridemia in Norway in 1994, and in France, England, Germany, Austria, and Greece in 1996.

For people who require cholesterol-lowering medicines, the next few years will provide greater choice and hopefully greater success in nor-malizing high-cholesterol levels.

Blood Pressure–Lowering Medications

As with high cholesterol, sometimes lifestyle measures—diet, exercise, weight loss, increased potassium intake, salt and alcohol restriction—are insufficient to completely normalize blood pressure. And as is the case with cholesterol-lowering medications, in order to be on the lowest pos-sible dose of a blood pressure medication, it is crucial to implement life-style changes and stick with them.

Once the decision has been made to use an antihypertensive (a blood pressure-lowering medication), there are literally hundreds to choose from. Because some antihypertensives may have undesirable side effects (e.g., an increase in blood sugar and cholesterol levels, asthma, gout, abnormalities in blood potassium levels, and impotence), your medical history helps direct your doctor toward the antihypertensive that is right for you. But you too should be aware of the possible side effects. Do not hesitate to question your physician if he or she suggests a medication that you feel might be problematic.

Not every blood pressure medication works for every person. Al-though your physician will be guided by experience and an under-standing of potential side effects, it often takes patience to find a drug that lowers blood pressure and has no unacceptable side effects. It may sometimes take six months to a year to achieve perfect blood pressure control.

Because there are so many antihypertensives, I have divided these medications into three major classes: (diuretics, adrenergic inhibitors, and vasodilators. And as in the previous section, I have described how each class of drugs works and follow this with information on dosing, side effects, and necessary followup by your doctor while you are on the drug. Because there are truly hundreds of blood pressure medications, I have listed only a few from each class. If you do not see your drug listed, ask your doctor which general class it falls under.

Diuretics

Mode of Action: These drugs initially work by causing a reduction in total body fluid (this is why there is an increase in urination when a diuretic is initiated). This is followed by a decrease in resistance in the blood vessels throughout the body; in other words, they become more relaxed.

Most Commonly Used Drug in This Class: Hydrochlorothiazide (HCTZ)

Other Drugs in This Class:
Chlorthalidone (Hygroton)
Indapamide (Lozol)
Benzthiazide (Exna)

Dose of HCTZ: The usual dose is between 12.5 and 50 mg per day. Because one of its major side effects is an increase in urination, it is crucial to take this drug in the morning.

Other Side Effects: Diuretics have many negative side effects, including
1. Increase triglycerides (by as much as 14%)*
2. Increase LDL cholesterol (by as much as 10%)*
3. Increase blood sugar
4. Increase blood uric acid level (this may lead to gout)
5. Decrease blood potassium level (this can lead to heart arrythmias)

Drug Interactions:
1. For persons taking lithium, diuretics can increase the blood level of this drug into the toxic range. This does not mean a person on lithium may not take a diuretic; it just means that lithium levels will require very careful monitoring and dose adjustments may be necessary.
2. Aspirin and other anti-inflammatory medications can reduce the blood pressure–lowering effect of diuretics.

Followup: Aside from having blood pressure evaluated regularly, persons beginning diuretics should have their blood levels of triglycerides, LDL cholesterol, sugar, uric acid, and potassium measured before and soon after beginning this class of medications.

* The diuretic Indapamide (Lozol) seems to have less of an adverse effect on triglycerides and LDL cholesterol. In my clinic, because so many of my patients have both high blood pressure and elevated cholesterol levels, Lozol is my first choice as a diuretic.

Note: Although I use diuretics very sparingly (because of their bad effects on cholesterol and blood sugar), they are very good at lowering blood pressure and in some situations are the only medication that will work.

Adrenergic Inhibitors

Within this general class there are three subclasses of blood pressure–lowering medications, including beta-blockers, alpha-blockers, and alpha-beta-blockers. Even though they all fall under the same class they have slightly different modes of action. I will review one agent from each subclass.

Beta-Blockers

Mode of Action: These drugs decrease the work that the heart does by slowing it down. As you begin taking a beta-blocker, you will see that your pulse rate goes down considerably (generally to the 60 range). Beta-blockers also have many other effects, including preventing the release of substances such as renin and norepinephrine, both of which can increase blood pressure.

Example of a Beta-Blocker: Atenolol (Tenormin)

Other Commonly Used Beta-Blockers:
Metoprolol (Lopressor)
Metoprolol (long acting) (Lopressor)
Propranolol (Inderal)
Propranolol (long acting) (Inderol)
Nadolol (Corgard)
Pindolol (Viskin)

Dose of Tenormin: 25 to 100 mg once a day

Side Effects: Beta-blockers have both negative and positive side effects.

Negative Side Effects
1. May cause an increase in triglycerides (by as much as 30 percent).
2. May cause a reduction in HDL cholesterol.
3. May aggravate asthma in susceptible people.
4. May cause an increase in blood sugar.
5. May cause a decrease in circulation to the extremities, resulting in cold fingers and toes.

6. May cause a dramatic reduction in the heart rate called heart block.
7. May cause impotence.

Positive Side Effects
1. Beta-blockers may reduce the frequency and severity of angina (chest pain or pressure that results when the heart muscle gets too little blood flow as a result of cholesterol blockages in the heart's arteries).
2. Certain beta-blockers have been shown (in large studies) to improve survival significantly after a heart attack.
3. In a person with frequent migraine headaches, beta-blockers can reduce their occurrence.

Drug Interactions: Certain drugs, such as the anti-inflammatories rifampin and phenobarbitol, may decrease the ability of beta-blockers to lower blood pressure, whereas other drugs, such as cimetidine and quinidine, may enhance their ability.

Followup: Aside from regular blood pressure checks, persons on beta-blockers should have their triglycerides, HDL cholesterol, and blood sugar levels reevaluated soon after beginning this class of drugs.

Notes: Some beta-blockers (e.g., Pindolol) may have lesser effects on triglycerides and HDL cholesterol.

If for any reason you should need to discontinue your beta-blocker, remember that this is one class of medications that must be tapered off, generally over a period of one to two weeks. Failure to do this can result in marked elevations in blood pressure and in feeling absolutely awful.

Alpha-Blockers
Mode of Action: These drugs cause the blood vessels to dilate (open up).

Example of an Alpha-Blocker: Doxazosin (Cardura)

Other Commonly Used Alpha-Blockers:
Prazosin (Minipress)
Terazosin (Hytrin)
Dose of Cardura: 1 to 16 mg once a day

Side Effects: Alpha-blockers have few adverse side effects. The only troubling one is their ability to cause postural hypotension (a marked decrease in blood pressure with a change in position, such as when moving from lying down to standing up). This side effect seems to be most common with Minipress and much less of an issue with Hytrin and Cardura. Postural hypotension occurs most frequently with a person's very first dose of an alpha-blocker or immediately following a dose increase.

Positive Side Effects
1. Alpha-blockers improve all aspects of the lipid profile:
   Triglycerides—fall by as much as 8 percent
   LDL cholesterol—falls by as much as 13 percent
   HDL cholesterol—increases by as much as 5 percent
2. Alpha-blockers may also improve control of diabetes.

Followup: Routine blood pressure measurements are necessary.

Alpha-Beta-Blockers

The major drug in this class is *Labetalol,* which is a twice a day medication used at a dosage of 200 to 1200 mg per day.

As an alpha-beta-blocker it combines the effects of both the alpha- and beta-blockers and all the side effects and precautions noted above, for both those blockers apply to labetalol. Because it is a combination drug, it has little effect on cholesterol profiles, since the positive effects of the alpha-blocker cancel out the negative effects of the beta-blocker.

Vasodilators

The two classes of antihypertensive agents that fall under this category are angiotensin-converting enzyme inhibitors (ACE inhibitors) and calcium channel blockers. Such drugs are very widely prescribed.

Angiotensin-Converting Enzyme Inhibitors

Mode of Action: These drugs inhibit the conversion of the prohormone (inactive hormone) angiotensin I to the active angiotensin II. Angiotensin II is an extremely powerful vasoconstrictor. Vasoconstrictors work to make the blood vessels clamp down or become smaller in caliber (diameter), leading to blood pressure elevations. In addition to effects on blood vessels, angiotensin II has many other metabolic properties. ACE inhibitors block all actions of angiotensin II, not just its effects on blood vessels.

Example of an ACE Inhibitor: Enalapril (Vasotec)

Other Commonly Used ACE Inhibitors:
  Captoril (Capoten)
  Benazapril (Lotensin)
  Fosinopril (Monopril)
  Lisinopril (Prinivil, Zestril)
  Quinapril (Accupril)
  Ramipril (Altace)

Dose of Vasotec: 5 to 20 mg per day (either once or twice a day)

Side Effects: ACE inhibitors have both negative and positive side effects.

Negative Side Effects:
1. Cough: The most common side effect reported with the use of ACE inhibitors is cough, a dry nagging cough. In fact, such a cough is the most common reason people discontinue their ACE inhibitors.*
2. Loss of kidney function: This is a very rare and thankfully a reversible side effect of ACE inhibitors. It occurs in people who have undiagnosed blockages in the arteries leading to both kidneys.
3. Elevated potassium levels: In persons with abnormal kidney function, ACE inhibitors may raise potassium levels.

Positive Side Effects:
1. No negative effects on the cholesterol profile.
2. Improves control of diabetes.
3. Scientific research suggests that ACE inhibitors protect the artery wall from developing cholesterol deposits.
4. In diabetics with reduced kidney function, ACE inhibitors may prevent the loss of protein in the urine (proteinuria). This is one of their most beneficial side effects.

---

* The dry nagging cough seen in some people on ACE inhibitors can result in discontinuation of this class of medicines. This is a shame, because most people in this situation have achieved excellent blood pressure control on the ACE inhibitors. If you have a persistent cough, discuss switching to one of the new angiotensin receptor blockers with your doctor. These drugs don't actually block the conversion of angiotensin I to angiotensin II; instead, they block the action of angiotensin II on blood vessels only, thus preventing constriction. The result is that these medications do not cause cough.

In 1995 our clinic participated in a study comparing the first angiotensin receptor blocker, losartan (Cozaar), with other blood pressure medications. Persons who had intolerable side effects with other blood pressure medications (especially persons troubled by coughing while on an ACE inhibitor) were invited to participate in this study. Its design was such that approximately half the participants were started on Cozaar. We were very pleased with the results: Cozaar was very effective in lowering blood pressure and our patients were cough free.

5. In persons with heart failure (inability of the heart to pump adequately), ACE inhibitors have been shown to improve survival. For this reason, even in the absence of hypertension, many physicians prescribe these inhibitors for persons with mild heart failure.

Drug Interactions: Anti-inflammatories and antacids may decrease the blood pressure–lowering effect of ACE inhibitors. ACE inhibitors may also increase blood lithium levels; thus these levels should be closely monitored when first beginning an ACE inhibitor regime.

Followup: In addition to closely monitoring blood pressure, potassium levels and kidney function should be checked with a blood test soon after beginning ACE inhibitors.

Calcium Channel Blockers

These medications have become very controversial over the past few years. The controversy revolves primarily around the short-acting calcium channel blocker (CCB) nifedipine. Since sustained release (long-acting) forms of CCBs were introduced, the short-acting forms have rarely been used. In 1995 one small study linked an increased risk of heart attack with use of the short-acting forms. A more recent study in a group of elderly patients also raised concerns that the risk of developing cancer was higher if a study participant's blood pressure was being treated with a short-acting CCB as compared with any other blood pressure medication.

These studies are of concern and deserve to be carefully considered. However, it is important for you to recognize that they are very preliminary and center around the short-acting CCB, which is rarely used today. You may be asking yourself "What could possibly be so different between a short-and a long-acting CCB?" The short-acting CCBs generally need to be taken three times a day, which results in large swings in their concentration in the user's blood. Many scientists feel that it is the high (peak) blood levels of these medications that increase the risk of complications. The long-acting forms of CCBs behave quite differently, since they are formulated for a slow and steady release of medication and provide more consistent blood levels and better blood pressure control.

In the next five to ten years, we will have more detailed information on the merits and drawbacks of this class of blood pressure medications. I am aware of at least five major ongoing trials in the United States and Europe, all examining the risks and benefits of long-acting forms of CCBs. The two major trials in the United States are the Antihypertensive and Lipid-Lowering Treatment to Prevent Heart Attack Trial (ALLHAT),

which is using amlodipine (Norvasc), and the Controlled Onset Verapamil Investigation of Cardiovascular Endpoints (CONVINCE), using a timed-release preparation of verapamil called Covera-HS. We are currently enrolling many of our clinic patients in the Covera-HS trial. I personally believe that these studies will prove the long-acting CCBs to be safe and effective.

However, even before the results of these trials are available, it is important to remember that we already know that lowering blood pressure leads to a dramatic reduction in the risk of stroke, heart attack, and death. There are currently 50 million people with hypertension in the United States, and many have not achieved full blood pressure normalization. My own view is that if you are on one of the long-acting varieties of CCBs and have achieved good blood pressure control, you should remain on that medication. If you have questions about the safety of your medication, please do not stop taking it without first discussing such a move with your personal physician.

Mode of Action: These drugs block the inward movement of calcium into the blood vessel cells, leading to relaxation of the blood vessel.

Example of a Calcium Channel Blocker: Amlodipine (Norvasc)

Other Commonly Used Calcium Channel Blockers:
Diltiazem (Cardizem)
Diltiazem (long acting) (Cardizem CD, Dilacor)
Verapamil (Calan, Isoptin, Verelen)
Verapamil (long acting) (Covera HS)
Felodipine (Plendil)
Isradipine (Dynacirc)
Nifidepine (Procardia)
Nifedipine (long acting) (Procardia XL)
Nicardipine (Cardene)

Dose of Norvasc: 2.5 to 10 mg once a day

Side Effects: As a class, calcium channel blockers are very well tolerated. Some agents cause more side effects than others.

Negative Side Effects:
1. Fluid build up in the legs
2. Constipation
3. Headache
4. Dizziness
5. In rare circumstances some calcium channel blockers may interfere

with the heart's conduction system, leading to a reversible but dramatic slowing of heart rate (pulse)

Positive Side Effects:
1. No adverse effects on blood sugar or cholesterol levels
2. Can dramatically decrease the occurrence of angina
3. May prevent the development of cholesterol plaques within the artery by a direct effect on the artery wall

Drug Interactions: Some seizure medications (carbamazepine, phenobarbitol, and phenytoin) may act to decrease the amount of calcium channel blockers in the blood, thereby decreasing their ability to lower blood pressure. On the other hand, cimetidine, used for the prevention of stomach acid, can increase the blood level of calcium channel blockers. Some calcium channel blockers can increase the blood levels of theophylline, a drug used for asthma, and quinidine, a drug used in the treatment of heart arrhythmias.

Followup: If you are on a calcium channel blocker, your blood pressure and pulse should be monitored regularly.

The Case of Hans

^^^

The Importance of Knowing
All Your Risk Factors

Hans Johann was born in Switzerland in 1951. Like most Swiss citizens, he was raised on a rich and plentiful diet. Good food in his family meant cheese fondue, thick sausages and steaks, elegant egg-laden cakes, plenty of butter, and coffee with lashings of cream. Hans was fortunate in his metabolism—in spite of an enormous appetite, he stayed lean and trim. Worrying about his weight never occurred to him. Of course it helped that he was a long-distance runner. Running, however, was not a conscious devotion to exercise—it was just something he loved to do. It was his passion, as natural to him as breathing.

Hans graduated from trade school in 1970. After working for two years in Switzerland, he was offered a position in the United States. In addition to having to learning a new language, Hans's work responsibilities in the States were extensive and his free time became more limited. Exercise was one of the first casualties of his new life in America—he just couldn't fit it into his day. He did, however, manage to create American versions of his favorite rich foods and, to make matters worse, almost as soon as he arrived in the United States, he took up smoking. In almost no time, his weight began to increase.

Two years after his arrival in the United States, Hans switched companies. He also fell in love. His new job was a more demanding one and his romance with Susan, a nurse from Philadelphia, kept him even busier than before. There was just no time to consider his health. Susan, in spite

227

of knowing that Hans's smoking and sedentary habits were dangerous, reasoned that at age 24, there wasn't much to worry about. He had no family history of heart disease, and the high-fat diet they both enjoyed was not, in the late seventies, considered to be a major cardiac risk factor.

In 1977, when Hans was 26, his father developed cardiac disease. Through letters and phone calls, Hans kept track of his efforts to change his life—his father gave up smoking, modified his diet, took up exercise, and began taking cardiac medications. However, the distance between the two men and Hans's continued belief in his own youth and invulnerability allowed him to ignore the risk factors they shared. At that time, he didn't even know what cholesterol was—it certainly never occurred to him to have his checked.

Several years after his marriage to Susan in 1978, Hans accomplished his lifelong ambition of owning his own company—an automatic screw machine shop that he based in New Hampshire. Susan left her nursing job to work full-time with him, and the two of them threw themselves into the task of building a successful business. Their goals were financial independence and an early retirement.

The stress of Hans's previous life as an employee was nothing compared to the never-ending responsibilities of a CEO. With virtually no tolerance for error, Hans found it impossible not to get involved in every aspect of his company. With Susan also fully involved, going home provided no real escape. Although he loved his work and was proud of the company's success, looking back, he admits that it almost consumed him.

In 1989, two major events brought him up short. In early March, his uncle died at the age of 50—the victim of a massive heart attack. His uncle had worked hard and was very successful. Hans found himself wondering: What was the point of it all? What was the good of money if you had to kill yourself to get it?

It is easy now for Hans to see that the fact his uncle had died of heart disease should have made him look seriously at his own cardiac health. But his relative youth—in 1989, he was only 38—gave him a false sense of security and actually allowed him to ignore his own risk factors: along with his family history, he was overweight, inactive, and like his uncle, a smoker.

The second event happened in December. His best friend was diagnosed with pancreatic cancer. Hans sat at his hospital bedside and watched grief-stricken as a man he loved dearly died a painful death. In the weeks that followed, as he tried to adjust to life without his friend, one thought kept intruding: no one is immune.

Soon after his friend's death, Hans began noticing pain in both arms.

At first, he thought he had pulled a muscle, perhaps in moving some of the heavy equipment at work. But when the pain got bad enough to wake him at night, he began to wonder if something more serious might be going on. Susan, also concerned, persuaded him to check things out with his doctor.

A cardiogram obtained while he was experiencing the arm pain suggested that the problem was with his heart, although evidence of an actual heart attack could only be gotten through more extensive tests for which Hans was admitted to the hospital.

The tests determined that although he had not, in fact, had a heart attack, some level of heart disease was present. To better understand the extent of the problem, Hans's physician suggested a catheterization, for which he would have to be transferred to another hospital.

Never having been a patient before, Hans found the speed with which decisions were being made regarding him overwhelming and disorienting. He had barely got used to the idea of having heart disease when he was expected to make intelligent choices regarding procedures he'd never heard of. By nature a pragmatic, methodical person, he began collaring doctors and nurses whenever he got the chance, asking them to explain matters to him. Finally, after a long discussion with Susan, he decided that a catheterization would give him the information he needed: Just how bad was his condition?

The procedure revealed cholesterol deposits in most of his coronary arteries: the right coronary artery (RCA), a very small vessel, had a 90 percent blockage; the left anterior descending (LAD), 60 percent; and the circumflex, 70 percent. When the cardiologist came to review the results with him, Hans's first reaction was "The numbers look awful—what exactly do they mean?"

Fortunately, the cardiologist was able to offer some encouragement. The RCA, which had the largest cholesterol deposit, was a small blood vessel, doing very little work in the heart. It was best left alone.

The other two, the circumflex and the LAD, were critically important arteries, which did have significant blockages. However, chances were good that with radical lifestyle changes and some cardiac medication, neither surgery nor angioplasty would be necessary for the time being. Bypass surgery in younger people is avoided whenever possible for the simple reason that bypass grafts don't last forever—on average, 10 to 15 years— and that only if a person is careful and disciplined. In 10 years, Hans would only be 49. Also angioplasties are not typically performed on blockages of 70 percent or less because in such cases the blockage may recur, and when it does, the situation is often worse than before.

The cardiologist's recommendation to Hans was a combination of cardiac medication and a radical lifestyle restructuring. Hans already knew that he would have to give up smoking, begin an exercise program, and follow a low-fat diet. What he hadn't known was how high his cholesterol level was: at 240 mg/dl, he now realized that he had to lower it.

Once he left the hospital, he decided to tackle things one at a time. The first task he set for himself was to quit smoking. When cold turkey didn't work, he tried the gradual approach. Within a few months he had succeeded. His pride at this accomplishment gave him the courage to go on to the next item on his list.

Slowly he cut back on the obvious high-fat foods in his diet and simultaneously developed a walking program. Soon the changes became so much a part of his life that he no longer thought about them. Chest pain occurred, but rarely, and it was easily controlled with a little extra medicine. Hans relaxed, sure that he had overcome the disease.

On August 1, 1993, Swiss Independence Day, Hans and Susan were getting ready to leave for the Swiss Club in Harvard, Massachusetts. Since their move to New England, they had never missed its annual Independence celebration. Hans was waiting for Susan by their pool when he noticed an odd sensation in his left arm. He twitched his shoulder and shifted in his seat, assuming the discomfort was due to his position. Instead, its intensity increased. Minute by minute, it got worse. As he sat, frozen in horror and fear, it quickly became almost unbearable.

Simultaneously, he began feeling dizzy and nauseous. When two tablets of nitroglycerine (the medication which typically relieved his infrequent episodes of chest pain) initially only made things worse, Hans panicked. He called out to Susan. She took one look at him and called 911. Waiting for the paramedics to arrive, Hans had a clear vision of dying. By the time they arrived, however, the nitroglycerine had begun to take hold and Hans, feeling much better, questioned the need to go to the hospital at all. The expression on Susan's face, however, told him that was exactly where he was going, like it or not.

In the emergency room, tests established that the incident had been a warning, not a heart attack. But the warning was timely: a repeat catheterization showed a serious deterioration in the condition of his heart. His arteries were now so badly blocked that angioplasty was no longer an option. Hans could hardly believe what he was hearing when the cardiologist suggested bypass surgery. Bypass? Hadn't he quit smoking, started exercising, cut back on fats, and taken his medications faithfully?

Hadn't he just been told he hadn't had a heart attack after all? How could he be a candidate for a bypass?

"For about five or six hours, I was angry and even desperate," Hans remembers. "But after calming down and analyzing the situation, I realized that the best thing I could do was to go into the surgery with a positive attitude. I knew I couldn't live the rest of my life in fear of the next episode of pain. I decided to go through the surgery and then work even harder at changing my life."

During his hours of reflection, Hans had been very honest with himself. He knew he could cut back further on the high-fat foods and certainly he could exercise more. He even knew suddenly why he had slacked off: certain that he had won the battle against heart disease, he figured he could afford to relax. But within six hours of hearing the cardiologist's recommendation, Hans had, in his own words, "done an emotional 180-degree turn." He had confronted his past and considered his future. He was ready to plan for the rest of his life.

When I met him the day before his surgery, I was amazed at his ability to analyze what was a highly emotional situation. I was sure that with his thorough and rational approach, he would be able to ride out the difficult first weeks after surgery. We made arrangements to meet eight weeks later, at which time I would be able to get an accurate picture of his cholesterol values. Cholesterol values, I explained to Hans and Susan, plummet following surgery (any kind of surgery) but return to baseline within about eight weeks.

Within a week of his surgery, Hans was home. Although the first few days were slightly uncomfortable, on the whole he was surprised and delighted with how good he actually felt. Nervous about venturing too far from the house, he began his walking regime in his own yard and slowly increased his speed. He and Susan made further dietary changes and got used to counting fat grams.

In addition to changing their daily lives, they also began reevaluating their long-term goals. They decided to gradually sell off their factory holdings with the aim of moving to Switzerland, but also decided to keep the pace of the change very slow, in order to be sure of Hans's health before changing health-care systems.

However, when I saw Hans eight weeks after his operation, his weight was essentially unchanged and his cholesterol values were alarming:

	Hans's Level	Desirable Level
Total cholesterol	251 mg/dl	Less than 200 mg/dl
Triglycerides	191 mg/dl	Less than 150 mg/dl
HDL cholesterol	41 mg/dl	Greater than 45 mg/dl
LDL cholesterol	172 mg/dl	Less than 100 mg/dl
Lipoprotein (a)	95 mg/dl	Less than 20 mg/dl

These numbers helped me understand why Hans's cardiac disease had progressed so rapidly in just three years, despite quitting smoking and exercising regularly. With numbers like these, he would need not only an aggressive dietary program, but also medication. My choice for him was niacin, a B vitamin with cholesterol-lowering properties.

Hans and Susan were a bit surprised by my stress on the need for a more radical approach to diet. Over the past few years, they had made many dietary changes, and since his bypass, they had restricted their fat intake still further. They said they were honestly at a loss as to what more they could do. "You haven't met Mary Card," I told them, smiling. Most of my patients agree that Mary (our team's registered dietitian) is a minor miracle worker when it comes to food and nutrition. Not only is she able to detect hidden fats in even the most streamlined diets, but, more important, she creates new diets to take their place that are low in fat, delicious, and easy to live with. She had already designed a plan for Hans and Susan and would meet them later the morning of their appointment with me, to go over the fine points with them. I assured them that if they followed their new dietary program faithfully, they could expect to see an improvement of at least 20 percent in Hans's cholesterol numbers.

Before introducing Hans and Susan to Mary Card, I reviewed the other components of his treatment plan with them. Diet alone would not be sufficient to normalize his cholesterol levels. In order to improve his lipid profile, he would require a vigorous exercise program. If he chose to continue with walking, he would need to increase both his speed and distance. We discussed how to exercise to achieve maximum benefit, and I gave him a heart rate to strive for (see Chapter 3 to determine your own training heart rate).

Both Hans and Susan were eager to put Mary's and my suggestions into practice. But they were still concerned about his laboratory report. In addition to wondering how they would ever lower his LDL (the bad cholesterol) level to below 100 mg/dl, they were particularly worried about his lipoprotein (a)—or Lp(a)—result. This blood fat had not been measured in his earlier tests and they wondered what it was and why it was so high.

I explained that a person's level of the blood fat Lp(a) (which is examined in detail in Chapter 1) is entirely genetically predetermined, and unfortunately, neither diet nor exercise seems to help in lowering it. The only way to bring Hans's level down would be with the use of medications. My earlier suggestion of niacin was specifically linked to his high Lp(a): in addition to lowering LDL and triglycerides and raising HDL, niacin also works to lower Lp(a). While conclusive evidence does not yet exist as to the importance of lowering Lp(a) for the purpose of avoiding future cardiac disease, common sense would seem to indicate a strong connection. All other things being equal, I preferred to do whatever I could to bring Hans's level down (especially since the treatment would also improve his other lipid profiles—that is, the LDL, HDL, and triglycerides).

Hans and Susan met Mary Card after seeing me and returned home armed with a stricter diet, an exercise prescription, instructions on how to begin taking niacin, and the determination to start fresh. When I saw them six weeks later, it was clear that they had been determined indeed. Hans's weight was down by five pounds and his commitment to cardiac health was reflected in his blood report:

	Hans's Level	Desirable Level
Total cholesterol	166 mg/dl	Less than 200 mg/dl
Triglycerides	168 mg/dl	Less than 150 mg/dl
HDL-cholesterol	43 mg/dl	Greater than 45 mg/dl
LDL cholesterol	89 mg/dl	Less than 100 mg/dl

LP(a) was not measured at this follow-up visit because it takes about three months to see the full effect of niacin.

Eight weeks later, after more fine tuning of his diet, a 10-pound additional weight loss, a small increase in his niacin dose, and an even greater investment in exercise, no one would have ever believed Hans had a cholesterol problem:

	Hans's Level	Desirable Level
Total cholesterol	155 mg/dl	Less than 200 mg/dl
Triglycerides	116 mg/dl	Less than 150 mg/dl
HDL-cholesterol	48 mg/dl	Greater than 45 mg/dl
LDL cholesterol	84 mg/dl	Less than 100 mg/dl
Lipoprotein (a)	32 mg/dl	Less than 20 mg/dl

I told him that his was one of the most profound improvements I had ever seen.

It has been over two years since Hans's bypass. He remains firmly committed to maintaining his now excellent health, his cholesterol levels have been consistently excellent—and his Lp(a) is now 16 mg/dl. He and Susan have sold off most of their business equipment and plan to move to Switzerland in the near future. The "good life" that they dreamed of a few years ago is now within their reach. And best of all, the chances are very promising that Hans will be around to enjoy it.

Recipes

A Note About Ingredients

When you first start cutting back on the fat in your diet, you will miss it. Fat has a wonderful "mouth-feel." Eventually, you won't miss the fat at all—for example, if you drink a glass of whole milk after a month of drinking skim, it will seem unpleasant, as if you were drinking a glass of heavy cream. So when you begin your new diet, you need to give your mouth something else besides fat to wake it up.

Use the freshest, most seasonal products you can find. Don't try to make a fresh tomato sauce in December, for instance. The sauce will not be flavorful and you will blame it on the missing fat; but the truth is that December tomatoes are as tasteless as balls of wax.

Most of the recipes here call for fresh herbs. Fresh herbs really add a lot of flavor. They can be very expensive in the supermarket, but it is easy to start a small window garden of fresh herbs, including for example, basil, parsley, chives, oregano, rosemary, thyme, and tarragon. You should be able to do this for under $20. Fresh herbs will give your dishes much more flavor than dried herbs, particularly if you are like me and tend to buy a jar of dried herbs and keep it around for years. My mother uses allspice in her pumpkin pies every Thanksgiving—she bought the can in 1959 when she got married. How much flavor can it still have 37 years later?

What's in a Serving?

At the bottom of each recipe you will notice that I have listed the fat, cholesterol, sodium, fiber, and protein of each dish. You will also notice how many servings of vegetable, fruit, protein, bread, or meat the protein provides. This will help to balance your food intake. Remember, try to aim for at least 5 servings of vegetables, 4 servings of fruit.

Generally a serving of fruit or vegetable is ½ cup or 1 fresh fruit.

Recipe Substitution

Don't throw out your favorite family recipes now that you're changing your diet. The substitutions listed here will help you create low-fat versions of your beloved high-fat casseroles and desserts. You may be surprised at how great the low-fat versions taste. Please feel free to send me any of your masterpieces—I'm always on the lookout for a new low-fat dish.

WHEN A RECIPE CALLS FOR	SUBSTITUTE WITH
All white flour	¼ whole wheat flour, ¾ white flour
Butter, lard, margarine	Lower fat margarine or vegetable oil (use slightly less oil)
Salt	Very often salt is unnecessary and can be omitted entirely.
Eggs	2 egg whites for each whole egg or ¼ cup egg substitute for each whole egg
Whole milk or 2% milk	Use skim or 1% low-fat milk
Sour cream	Nonfat sour cream, reduced-fat sour cream, low-fat or nonfat plain yogurt
Cheddar, Swiss, American, or cream cheese	Cheese with 5 grams of fat or less per ounce; nonfat or lite cream cheese
Ricotta or cottage cheese	Nonfat or lite varieties
Whipping cream	Chilled evaporated skim milk, whipped
Nuts	Reduce amount: use ¼ to ½ cup per recipe
Mayonnaise	Nonfat or reduced-calorie mayonnaise; half the amount, plus nonfat yogurt
Bouillon or broth	½ broth and ½ water, low-sodium bouillon, nonfat chicken broth in can
Baking chocolate	3 tablespoons baking cocoa and 1 tablespoon oil or margarine = 1 ounce baking chocolate

Sugar	Reduce amount called for by ⅓ initially, then work up to a ½ reduction
Oil	It is often possible to cut the amount of oil in baking by half and in place substitute applesauce

THINGS TO CONSIDER IN MAKING SUBSTITUTIONS

Before you change a recipe, consider the function of each ingredient. Can the recipe be altered without changing the appearance, taste, or texture of the dish?

For example: Yogurt used in place of sour cream will not change the taste or consistency of a sauce; skim milk in place of sour cream will make a significant difference.

ecipe Contents

Soups

♥ VEGETABLE SOUP WITH TORTELLINI

14 ounces canned reduced-fat beef broth

1 pound canned diced, peeled tomatoes, with juice

6 ounces canned tomato paste

2 cups water

2 stalks celery, chopped

2 small onions, chopped

1 carrot, sliced

2 cloves garlic, minced

¼ teaspoon salt

1 cup cooked meat-filled or cheese-filled tortellini

1 small zucchini, sliced

½ cup sliced mushrooms

½ cup chopped fresh spinach leaves

½ cup chopped parsley

¼ cup chopped basil leaves

½ teaspoon pepper

Grated Parmesan cheese

Spray nonstick saucepan with vegetable oil spray. Saute celery, onion, and garlic for about 5 minutes. Add carrot, cook one minute more. Add beef broth, tomatoes with juice, tomato paste, water, salt, and pepper. Bring to a boil, reduce heat, and simmer over low heat for 20 minutes. Add tortellini, zucchini, and mushrooms, simmer 5 minutes longer or until zucchini is tender. Add spinach, parsley, and basil, cook one minute more.

Ladle soup into bowls and top with a sprinkling of Parmesan cheese. Serves 8.

Per serving: 125 calories; 3.3 grams fat, 1 gram saturated fat; 10 mg cholesterol; 575 mg sodium; 2 grams fiber; 7 grams protein. 1 serving = 2 vegetables + 1 bread.

♥ APPLE-SQUASH SOUP

4 medium onions, diced

2 medium butternut squash, about 3 pounds total

2 14½ ounces cans nonfat chicken broth

1¼ cups apple juice

1 unpeeled Granny Smith apple, for garnish

Juice of ½ lemon (2 tablespoons)

Pepper to taste

4 teaspoons curry powder

4 apples, peeled, cored, and diced

Water as needed

½ teaspoon salt

Spray saucepan with vegetable oil spray. Saute onions with curry powder until onions are translucent.

Peel the squash, scrape out seeds, and chop coarsely. When onions are tender, pour in the stock and water, add squash and apples, and bring to a boil. (Make sure squash and apples are covered by liquid. If not, add more water.) Reduce heat and simmer, partially covered, until squash and apples are very tender, about 25 minutes. Drain liquid, but save it. Process vegetables and fruit in a blender until smooth. Return pureed soup to the pot and add apple juice and additional cooking liquid, about 2 cups, until soup is of the desired consistency. Add lemon juice and season to taste with salt, pepper, and additional curry powder. Simmer to heat through and serve immediately, garnished with grated apple.

Serves 6.

Per serving: 234 calories; 1 gram fat, 0 grams saturated fat;
0 mg cholesterol; 529 mg sodium; 8 grams fiber; 5 grams protein.
1 serving = 1 vegetable + 2 fruits + 1 bread.

♥ **CHUNKY MINESTRONE**

2 medium onions, chopped	2 6 ounce cans vegetable juice
1 medium carrot, sliced	1 medium zucchini, halved
2 stalks celery, chopped	lengthwise and sliced
1 clove garlic, minced	15½ ounces canned cannellini
½ cup long grain rice, uncooked	beans, rinsed and drained
1 teaspoon dried Italian seasoning	1 10 ounce package frozen
2½ cups water	chopped spinach, thawed and
2 16 ounce cans diced, peeled	drained
tomatoes with juice	Salt and pepper to taste
14½ ounces canned nonfat	6 tablespoons Parmesan cheese
chicken broth	

Spray saucepan with vegetable oil spray. Add onion, carrot, and celery and saute until onions are translucent. Add garlic, saute 1 minute more. Stir in rice, Italian seasoning, water, diced tomatoes, chicken broth, and vegetable juice. Bring to a boil. Cover, reduce heat, and simmer 20 minutes. Add zucchini, beans, and spinach; bring to a boil. Remove from heat, add salt and pepper as needed, and ladle into individual bowls. Top with Parmesan cheese.

Serves 7 (each serving 1½ cups).

Per serving: 217 calories;   2.5 grams fat, 1 gram saturated fat;
   4.2 mg cholesterol;   994 mg sodium;   7 grams fiber;   10 grams protein.
   1 serving = 2 breads + 2 vegetables

TIP: To decrease sodium, eliminate ½ teaspoon salt and use low-sodium
V-8 juice.

♥ NEW ENGLAND CLAM CHOWDER

2 ounces Canadian bacon, diced
½ tablespoon olive oil
1 medium onion, chopped
2 tablespoons flour
2 sprigs fresh thyme, picked
¼ teaspoon ground black pepper

3 cups skim milk
6½ ounces canned minced clams,
   drained, liquid reserved*
1 8 ounce bottle clam juice
3 large potatoes, peeled and diced
   into ½ inch cubes

Heat oil in saucepan. Add onion and Canadian bacon. Cook over medium heat, stirring frequently, until onion is soft. Stir in flour, thyme,
and pepper. Stir in milk slowly, stirring to remove lumps. Add reserved
clam liquid, clam juice, and potatoes. Bring to a boil, stirring constantly.
Lower heat and simmer until potatoes are tender. Add clams. Heat completely.
   *Try using fresh clams if available.
   Serves 4.

Per serving: 316 calories;   4 grams fat, 1 gram saturated fat;
   36 mg cholesterol;   591 mg sodium;   4 grams fiber;   17 grams protein.
   1 serving = 1 milk + 2 breads + 1 meat + ½ fat.

♥ VEGETABLE SOUP

2 quarts boiling water
1 cup orzo pasta
1 medium onion, diced
3 stalks celery, diced
3 ounces canned tomato paste

1 can stewed tomatoes (chopped)
4 to 5 beef bouillon cubes
1 10 ounce package frozen mixed
   vegetables

Spray saucepan with vegetable oil spray. Saute onion and celery until
onion is translucent. Add pasta, boiling water, and bouillon cubes. Cook
about 8 minutes. Add tomato paste and mixed vegetables, bring to a
boil, remove from heat, and serve.
   Serves 8 (each serving 1 cup).

Per serving: 139 calories;   0.7 grams fat, 0 grams saturated fat;
0 mg cholesterol;   627 mg sodium;   2 grams fiber;   3 grams protein.
1 serving = 1 bread + 2 vegetables.

♥ GAZPACHO

2 large cucumbers, peeled, halved
  lengthwise, and seeded
2 large tomatoes, peeled and
  seeded
1 green pepper, halved and
  seeded
1 medium onion, peeled
4 cloves garlic, minced
3 cups tomato juice or vegetable
  juice

⅓ cup red wine vinegar
2 teaspoons olive oil
¼ teaspoon Tabasco
2 teaspoons Worcestershire sauce
½ teaspoon salt
Ground pepper to taste
½ cup chopped parsley
¼ cup chopped basil

In a blender or food processor, combine one of the cucumbers, one of the tomatoes, ½ of the green pepper, ½ of the onion, and the garlic. Puree with the tomato juice.

Chop the remaining vegetables. Add the pureed mixture, vinegar, oil, Tabasco, Worcestershire sauce, and the chopped vegetables. Chill mixture for at least 2 hours. Remove from refrigerator, mix thoroughly, and season to taste with salt and pepper.

Serves 6.

Per serving: 81 calories;   2 grams fat, 0 grams saturated fat;
0 mg cholesterol;   971 mg sodium;   6.5 grams fiber;   4 grams protein.
1 serving = 2 vegetables + ½ fat.

♥ BROCCOLI SOUP WITH RED PEPPER AND MUSHROOMS

1 small onion, peeled and
  chopped
1 stalk celery, chopped
½ cup rice, uncooked
3½ cups chicken stock (nonfat)
1 medium stalk broccoli, chopped
1 red pepper, seeded and
  chopped

5 mushrooms, sliced
1 teaspoon curry powder
3 sprigs fresh tarragon
1 cup skim milk
⅛ teaspoon salt
Ground pepper to taste

Spray nonstick saucepan with vegetable oil spray. Saute onions and celery about 10 minutes, or until onions are translucent. Stir in rice. Add chicken stock, bring to a boil, reduce to a simmer, and cook 15 minutes. Add broccoli, red pepper, mushrooms, curry powder, tarragon, and skim milk. Bring to a boil, then simmer about 5 minutes until broccoli is tender. Puree in several batches in a blender or food processor. Pour back into saucepan and heat through. Season to taste with salt and pepper.

Serves 6.

Per serving: 100 calories; 0.4 grams fat, 0 grams saturated fat; 1 mg cholesterol; 404 mg sodium; 1.5 grams fiber; 5 grams protein. 1 serving = 1 vegetable + 1 bread.

Breads and Muffins

♥ BUTTERNUT-OATMEAL BREAD

2 packages dry yeast
1¼ cups warm water
5 cups all-purpose flour, divided
1¼ cups mashed cooked fresh
   butternut squash
¼ cup molasses

1 cup whole-wheat flour
2 tablespoons vegetable oil
1½ teaspoons salt
1 cup + 1 tablespoon quick
   cooking oats, uncooked and
   divided

Dissolve yeast in warm water. Let stand 5 minutes. Combine yeast mixture, 3 cups flour, squash, molasses, vegetable oil, and salt in large mixing bowl. Beat at medium speed on an electric mixer for 2 minutes or until smooth. Stir in oats and 2 cups flour to form a moderately stiff dough. Turn dough out onto a lightly floured surface. Knead until smooth and elastic, about 15 minutes. Add enough of remaining flour, ¼ cup at a time, to prevent dough from sticking to hands. Place in a large bowl coated with cooking spray. Coat all sides of dough ball with spray. Cover and let rise in a warm place—about 85 degrees—free from drafts, for 45 minutes or until the dough doubles in bulk.

Coat two 8½ × 4½ × 3 inch loaf pans with vegetable oil spray. Punch dough down and knead 5 times. Divide dough in half, shaping each portion in a 14 × 7 inch rectangle. Roll up dough, starting at short edge, pressing firmly to eliminate air pockets. Pinch edges and ends to seal. Place seam side down in loaf pan. Repeat with remaining dough. Brush loaves with 1 tablespoon water and sprinkle with a few oats. Cover and let rise in a warm place, free from drafts, 35 minutes or until the dough doubles in bulk. Bake at 350 degrees for 45 minutes or until loaves sound hollow when tapped. Remove from pans immediately and cool on wire racks.

Per ½ inch slice: 98 calories;   1 gram fat, 0 grams saturated fat;
   0 mg cholesterol;   101 mg sodium;   1.2 grams fiber;   3 grams protein;
   2 grams sugar.
   ½ inch slice = 1 bread + 1 vegetable.

♥ NO-KNEAD BREAD

1 teaspoon salt	3½ cups whole wheat or white
1 package dried yeast	flour, or a mixture of both
1¼ cups warm water	3 tablespoons sugar

Dissolve yeast in warm water. Add sugar, salt, and flour. Mix, let rise in a covered bowl in a warm place one hour. Shape into loaf, place into loaf pan coated with vegetable spray. Bake about 50 minutes at 350 degrees. Loaf is done when it sounds hollow when tapped on bottom.

To make 5 loaves, use:

1 tablespoon salt, 5 pounds flour, 5 packages yeast in 5 cups warm water, ⅞ cup sugar.

10 slices per loaf.

Per slice: 169 calories;   0.5 grams of fat, 0.1 gram saturated fat;
   0 mg cholesterol;   214 mg sodium;   2 grams fiber;   5 grams protein;
   4.2 grams sugar.
   1 slice= 2 bread.

Variation: Cinnamon Raisin Swirl Bread

Make dough as above. After rising for ½ hour, roll out to about 10 × 17 × 1 inch thick. Sprinkle with a mixture of ½ cup sugar, 2 teaspoons cinnamon, ½ cup raisins plumped in ¼ water and drained. Roll up mixture. Tuck seams underneath. Put in loaf pan or on cookie sheet sprayed with vegetable spray. Let rise ½ hour more. Bake as above.

Per slice: 59 calories;   0.05 grams fat, 0 grams saturated fat;
   0 mg cholesterol;   1 mg sodium;   1 gram fiber   0.4 grams protein;
   14 grams sugar.
   Per cinnamon raisin bread slice: 2 breads + 1 fruit.

ZUCCHINI-PINEAPPLE BREAD

¾ cup egg substitute
½ cup applesauce
2 cups sugar
1 teaspoon salt
1 teaspoon baking soda
1 teaspoon baking powder
3 cups flour

8 ounces canned crushed
   pineapple
2 cups zucchini, grated
2 tablespoons vanilla
½ cup raisins, plumped in ¼ cup
   water

Combine egg substitute, applesauce, and sugar. Add salt, baking soda, baking powder, and flour. Mix until well blended. Stir in pineapple, zucchini, raisins, and vanilla. Pour mixture into 2 loaf pans which have been sprayed with vegetable oil spray. Bake at 350 degrees for about 40 minutes or until toothpick inserted in center of loaf comes out clean.

   12 slices per loaf.

Per Slice: 139 calories;   0 grams fat, 0 grams saturated fat;
   0 mg cholesterol;   153 mg sodium;   1 gram fiber;   3.0 grams protein;
   18 grams sugar.
   1 slice = 1 bread + 1 fruit.

Tip: To plump raisins, put the raisins in a saucepan, cover them halfway with water, bring water to a boil, turn off heat, and cover pan. Let raisins stand for about 5 minutes, then drain and use. This makes the raisins plumper and juicier. It's a step that can be skipped if you're in a real rush, but the extra 5 minutes is well spent.

▸ LEMON TEA BREAD

Bread:
½ cup skim milk
¼ cup egg substitute
1 cup sugar
⅓ cup applesauce
1¼ cups flour
1 teaspoon baking powder

1 teaspoon salt
1½ teaspoons grated lemon peel

Glaze:
¼ cup sugar
3 tablespoons fresh lemon juice

Combine all ingredients for bread. Pour into loaf pan which has been sprayed with vegetable oil spray. Bake at 350 degrees for about 45 minutes, or until toothpick inserted in center of loaf comes out clean. While bread is baking, combine ingredients for glaze. Pour glaze on while bread is still hot from oven. Allow to cool before serving.

   10 slices per loaf.

Per slice: 157 calories;   0.1 grams fat; 0 grams saturated fat;
  0 mg cholesterol;   265 mg sodium;   0.6 grams fiber;   2 grams protein;
  24 grams sugar.
  1 slice = 2 breads.

Tip: This bread is great at brunch, as dessert after a light luncheon, or
for a bridal shower.

♥ BLUEBERRY MUFFINS

2 tablespoons light margarine
¾ cup sugar
½ cup egg substitute
½ cup skim milk
1 pint fresh blueberries, rinsed
    well, or 1 can of blueberries,
    drained

2 tablespoons applesauce
2 cups flour
2 teaspoons baking powder
½ teaspoon salt

On low speed of electric mixer, cream margarine and sugar until fluffy.
Add applesauce and egg substitute. Add dry ingredients, alternating
with milk. Fold in blueberries with a spatula. Spray muffin tin with vegetable oil spray. Fill each cup ¾ full with mixture. Bake at 375 degrees
for 30 minutes. Makes 12 muffins.

One muffin: 157 calories;   1.5 grams fat, 0.3 grams saturated fat;
  0 mg cholesterol;   193 mg sodium;   1.3 grams fiber;   4 grams protein;
  14 grams sugar.
  One muffin = 1½ breads + ½ fruit.

♥ PUMPKIN MUFFINS

1 cup flour
⅔ cup brown sugar
1 teaspoon baking powder
¼ teaspoon nutmeg
¼ teaspoon cloves
¼ teaspoon ginger
¼ cup pureed plums or
    applesauce
1 pound canned pumpkin

1⅓ cups nonfat milk powder
1 teaspoon baking soda
1 teaspoon vanilla
1 teaspoon cinnamon
¼ teaspoon salt
1 8-ounce box egg substitute
½ cup raisins, plumped in ¼ cup
    water (see p. 245)

Mix all ingredients in a bowl. Spray muffin tin with vegetable oil spray.
Fill each cup ¾ full with mixture. Bake at 350 degrees for 20 to 25
minutes. Makes 12 muffins.

One muffin: 151 calories; 0.5 grams fat, 0 grams saturated fat;
  1.3 mg cholesterol; 200 mg sodium; 1 gram fiber; 6.5 grams protein;
  18.5 grams sugar.
  One muffin = ½ fruit + 1 bread + ½ milk.

♥ ORANGE-CORNBREAD MUFFINS

1½ cups flour	½ cup egg substitute
1½ cups cornmeal	1⅓ cups orange juice
4 teaspoons baking powder	4 teaspoons grated orange rind
⅔ cup sugar	

Combine all ingredients. Pour mixture into muffin tins which have been sprayed with vegetable oil spray. Bake at 350 degrees for 25 minutes. Makes 20 muffins.

One muffin: 105 calories; 0.2 grams fat, 0 grams saturated fat;
  0 mg cholesterol; 68 mg sodium; 0.3 grams fiber; 2 grams protein;
  8 grams sugar.
  One muffin = 1 bread + ½ fruit.

Tip: Instead of baking this in muffin tins, try baking it in an 8-inch round cake pan. After cooking, cut into wedges. Place the wedges on the grill and cook until toasted on each side. This is a great accompaniment to grilled chicken.

Salads

♥ HAWAIIAN SPINACH SALAD

1 bag spinach, washed and drained	1 can grapefruit sections, drained
1 head Boston or iceberg lettuce, washed and drained	*8 ounces mixed dried fruit (no nuts or coconut)
2 small cans mandarin oranges, drained	Oregano Salad Dressing, see p. 251.

Tear spinach and lettuce into small pieces. Toss with fruit. Serve with Oregano Salad Dressing.

Suggestion: Papaya, pineapple, apricots, bananas, or raisins may be substituted.

Serves 6.

Per serving: 151 calories; 0.5 grams fat, 0 grams saturated fat;
 0 mg cholesterol; 50 mg sodium; 2 grams fiber 3 grams protein.
1 serving = 1 fruit + 2 vegetables.

♥ **CAESAR SALAD**

Dressing:

⅔ cup nonfat mayonnaise
2 teaspoons Worcestershire sauce
1 teaspoon Dijon mustard
3 cloves garlic, minced
Ground black pepper, to taste
½ cup grated Parmesan cheese,
    divided

Salad:

2 cups low-fat croutons (recipe
    follows)
2 heads romaine lettuce

Wash romaine, pat dry, and tear leaves into bite-size pieces. Combine dressing ingredients, using half (¼ cup) of the Parmesan. Toss with romaine and croutons. Place on 6 plates, and sprinkle with additional cheese before serving.
    Serves 6.

Per serving: 69 calories; 2.6 grams fat, 1.6 grams saturated fat;
 6.6 mg cholesterol; 383 mg sodium; 1 gram fiber; 4.5 grams protein.
    You may want to top this delicious salad with homemade low-fat croutons.

Low-fat Croutons

Slice French bread across in very thin slices. Place on a baking sheet that has been sprayed with vegetable cooking spray. Sprinkle bread rounds with a little salt and lots of freshly ground pepper. Bake in a 350-degree oven until golden brown. Note: Watch them carefully! One minute they will be white, the next minute they will have just a touch of golden brown, then before you know it they are burned.

TIP 1: Serve these croutons with whole roasted garlic (see p. 275)

TIP 2: The calorie and fat breakdown for the above Caesar Salad assumes that you are using dry grated Parmesan cheese (the kind you buy in the pasta aisle in your supermarket). The real Parmesan has 6 more grams of fat per ounce than the dry grated Parmesan. This probably explains why the freshly grated Parmesan tastes so much better. If you occasionally want to indulge in the full flavor of real Parmesan cheese, then plan to cut one fat serving out of your diet earlier in the day.

♥ SPINACH MOLD

1 3 ounce package lemon gelatin
1 cup boiling water
2 tablespoons white vinegar
¾ cup nonfat mayonnaise
¾ cup nonfat cottage cheese

1 cup raw spinach, chopped
½ cup cucumber, chopped very
  small
½ cup onion, grated or chopped
  very small

Puree cottage cheese in blender or food processor for a few seconds to get rid of the lumps. Dissolve gelatin in boiling water. Add vinegar and mayonnaise to gelatin and beat with rotary beater. Chill until partially set. Beat again until frothy. Add cottage cheese, spinach, cucumber, and onion. Combine well. Pour into mold and chill until set.
Serves 8.

Per serving: 75 calories;   0.3 grams fat, 0 grams saturated fat;
  1 mg cholesterol;   250 mg sodium;   1 gram fiber;   4 grams protein.
  1 serving = 1 vegetable + ½ bread.

♥ STRAWBERRY GELATIN SALAD

2 3 ounce packages strawberry
  gelatin
2 cups boiling water
1 pound frozen strawberries

16 ounces nonfat yogurt
16 ounces canned crushed
  pineapple, not drained
2 mashed bananas

Dissolve gelatin in boiling water. Add all remaining ingredients except yogurt. Pour ½ of the mixture into gelatin mold, and refrigerate this until set. Leave the other half of the mixture out of the refrigerator. When set, put the yogurt on top of the gelatin, then pour the other half of the mixture over this. Refrigerate until set.
Serves 8.

Per serving: 205 calories;   0.5 grams fat, 0.13 grams saturated fat;
  1 mg cholesterol;   45 mg sodium;   2 grams fiber;   6 grams protein.
  1 serving = 3 fruits + ½ milk.

TIP: This makes a yogurt "sandwich" with the gelatin as the bread. The recipe also works if you mix the yogurt into the second half of the gelatin mixture and pour this over the jelled first half. This makes a pretty, two-layer salad or dessert.

♥ DAZZLING RASPBERRY SALAD

1 3 ounce package raspberry
  gelatin
1 10 ounce package frozen
  raspberries, thawed

1 cup nonfat yogurt
¾ cup water

Combine all ingredients in a saucepan, using a wire whisk to remove lumps of yogurt. Bring to a boil over medium heat, stirring frequently. Remove from heat. Pour into mold. Chill several hours before serving.
  Serves 6.

Per serving: 116 calories;   0.14 grams fat, 0 grams saturated fat;
  0 mg cholesterol;   29 mg sodium;   2 grams fiber;   4 grams protein.
  1 serving = 1 fruit + ½ milk

♥ COLESLAW

1 head finely chopped cabbage
1 carrot, shredded
1 green pepper, finely chopped

Dressing:
⅓ cup sugar
½ teaspoon salt

¼ teaspoon ground pepper
1 teaspoon celery seed
¼ cup skim milk
½ cup nonfat mayonnaise
⅓ cup nonfat yogurt
1½ tablespoons white vinegar
Juice of 1 lemon

Combine dressing ingredients. Pour over vegetables and mix well. Best if made and chilled at least 1 hour before serving.
  Serves 6.

Per serving: 98 calories;   0.3 grams fat, 0 grams saturated fat;
  0.4 mg cholesterol;   350 mg sodium;   2 grams fiber;   2.5 grams protein.
  1 serving = 1 vegetable + 1 fruit.

♥ EGGPLANT SALAD

1 large eggplant, sliced in half
2 tomatoes, seeded and diced
1 green pepper, diced
1 red onion, thinly sliced
2 cloves garlic, crushed
½ teaspoon salt
¼ teaspoon ground pepper

¼ cup red wine vinegar
1 tablespoon olive oil
1 tablespoon sugar
2 tablespoons chopped fresh
  parsley
2 tablespoons chopped fresh basil

Place eggplant halves cut side down on baking sheet and put under broiler. Broil for a few minutes until the skin peels off easily. Dice the eggplant. Combine with all other ingredients, toss and serve.

Serves 6.

Per serving: 85 calories;   2.5 grams fat, 0.6 grams saturated fat;
0 mg cholesterol;   1.3 grams protein;   2.7 grams fiber.
1 serving = 1½ vegetables + ½ fat.

♥ **MARK'S SUMMER SLAW**

Serve this slaw with grilled fish or crabcakes. It's a real winner.

½ cup champagne vinegar
3½ tablespoons sugar
1 tablespoon water

1 teaspoon olive oil
½ teaspoon salt
¼ teaspoon pepper

5 cups of vegetables, such as finely shredded cabbage, grated carrots, corn kernels which have been blanched and cut off the ears, thinly sliced red and green peppers, thinly sliced red onion, grated summer squash, grated zucchini, snow peas which have been blanched and thinly sliced—the bigger the variety of vegetables, the better.

Combine the 5 cups of vegetables in a large bowl. In a separate bowl mix vinegar, sugar, water, oil, salt, and pepper briskly with a wire whisk. Pour over vegetables and toss well.

Serves 5 (each serving 1 cup).

Per serving: 75 calories;   1.2 grams fat, 0.2 grams saturated fat;
0 mg cholesterol;   2 grams fiber;   1.3 grams protein.
1 serving = 3 vegetables.

Dressings

♥ **OREGANO SALAD DRESSING**

4 teaspoons sugar
¼ cup white vinegar
½ cup nonfat mayonnaise

1 teaspoon oregano
Ground pepper, to taste

Whisk all ingredients together. Store in refrigerator.

Entire recipe: 155 calories;   0 grams fat, 0 grams saturated fat;
0 mg cholesterol;   841 mg sodium   0 grams fiber;   0 grams protein.
2 tablespoons = 26 calories.

♥ NO-OIL DRESSING

1 cup ice water
1 tablespoon honey
½ teaspoon salt
½ teaspoon thyme
½ teaspoon chives
½ teaspoon oregano
Juice of ½ lemon

½ cup cider vinegar
1 garlic clove, minced
2 tablespoons chopped fresh
    parsley
½ teaspoon basil leaves
1 teaspoon pepper

Place all ingredients in a blender. Whirl and store in the refrigerator.

Entire recipe: 87 calories;   0.3 grams fat, 0 grams saturated fat;
    0 mg cholesterol;   1074 mg sodium;   1 gram fiber;   1 gram protein.
    2 tablespoons = 14 calories.

♥ ITALIAN DRESSING

¼ cup lemon juice
¼ cup cider vinegar
¼ cup apple juice
½ teaspoon oregano
½ teaspoon dry mustard
½ teaspoon onion powder

1 garlic clove, minced
½ teaspoon paprika
½ teaspoon basil
⅛ teaspoon thyme
⅛ teaspoon rosemary

Whisk all ingredients together. Store in refrigerator.

Entire Recipe: 60 calories;   0.3 grams fat, 0 grams saturated fat;
    0 mg cholesterol;   5 grams sodium;   0.3 grams fiber;   1 gram protein.
    2 tablespoons = 10 calories.

♥ TARRAGON-DIJON DRESSING

1 tablespoon olive oil
5 tablespoons red wine vinegar
2 tablespoons lemon juice
6 tablespoons water
1 teaspoon Dijon mustard
1¼ teaspoons tarragon

1 garlic clove, minced
2 tablespoons shallots, minced
1 tablespoon honey
¼ teaspoon paprika
Pepper to taste

Whisk all ingredients together. Store in refrigerator. Makes 1 cup.

Per 2 tablespoons: 29 calories;   1.75 grams fat, 0.25 grams saturated fat;
    0 mg cholesterol;   24 mg sodium;   0 grams fiber;   1 gram protein.
    2 tablespoons = ½ fat.

♥ CUCUMBER-DILL DRESSING

1 cup nonfat yogurt
1 tablespoon white vinegar
2 cucumbers, peeled and seeded

¼ cup fresh dill, snipped
½ teaspoon salt
½ teaspoon pepper

Combine all ingredients in blender or food processor. Process until smooth. This dressing tastes best if chilled for 24 hours before using.

Entire recipe: 236 calories;   1.6 grams fat, 0 grams saturated fat;
   4 mg cholesterol;   1271 mg sodium;   8.6 grams fiber;   19 grams protein.
   2 tablespoons = 20 calories.

♥ PARMESAN PEPPERCORN SALAD DRESSING

½ cup plain yogurt
½ cup nonfat mayonnaise
¼ cup dry grated Parmesan
   cheese

2 teaspoons cracked black pepper
¼ teaspoon salt
2 tablespoons lemon juice

Combine all ingredients. Chill overnight or for several hours before serv-ing—the flavor takes several hours to develop.
   Makes 1¼ cups.

Per 2 tablespoons: 26 calories;   0.7 grams fat, 0.5 grams saturated fat;   2 mg
   cholesterol;   192 mg sodium;   0 grams fiber;   1.5 grams protein.

TIP ON VINEGAR: Vinegar is a great way to spice up foods without adding fat. There are so many tasty vinegars on the market now, including:

Balsamic vinegar
Fruited vinegars (i.e., raspberry or apple cider)
Red or white wine vinegar
Champagne vinegar
Rice wine vinegar
Herbed vinegar (i.e., basil or tarragon)
Malt vinegar

When you see a recipe that calls for a certain type of vinegar, experiment a little and try some of the other vinegars too. Rice wine and champagne vinegars can be great on their own as a salad dressing. Vinegars may also be substituted for wine—the recipe won't taste the same but it will taste just as good, just a bit different.

Beans

♥ BAKED BEANS

1 cup small white navy beans
4 cups water
2 medium onions, chopped
2 slices Canadian bacon, diced
1 bay leaf
¼ teaspoon salt
¼ teaspoon pepper

1 cup ketchup
1 cup brown sugar
2 tablespoons vinegar
1½ tablespoons Worcestershire
   sauce
½ tablespoon dry mustard

Soak beans in water overnight or during the day while you are at work. There should be enough water in the container to cover beans by 2 inches. Dried beans will generally expand to 3 times their size when soaked, so 1 cup of dried beans will become 3 cups of soaked beans.

After soaking for at least 8 hours, drain beans and rinse with cold water. Put into a saucepan. Add 3 cups of water and remaining ingredients. Bring to a boil, reduce heat, and simmer one hour or until beans are tender. Add more water if needed.

Serves 6.

Per serving: 320 calories;   1.25 grams fat, 0.2 grams saturated fat;
    4.5 mg cholesterol;   680 mg sodium;   5.3 grams fiber;   10 grams protein.
    1 serving = 2 breads + 1½ meats + 2 vegetables.

♥ QUICK BAKED BEANS

3 cups canned red beans or pinto
   beans
2 medium onions, chopped
2 slices Canadian bacon, diced
1 cup ketchup

⅓ cup molasses
1 teaspoon prepared mustard
½ teaspoon chili powder
¼ cup cider vinegar
¼ cup brown sugar

Combine all ingredients, and pour into a bean pot or casserole dish. Bake at 350 degrees uncovered for 1 hour. Cover and continue baking for 30 minutes.

Serves 6.

Per serving: 295 calories;   1.3 grams fat, 0.3 grams saturated fat;
    4.5 mg cholesterol;   165 mg sodium;   6 grams fiber;   13 grams protein.
    1 serving = 2 breads + 1 meat + 2 vegetables.

♥ **MEATLESS CHILI**

2 medium onions, chopped	15 ounces canned kidney beans
3 cloves garlic, minced	2 bay leaves
1 green pepper, chopped	½ teaspoon pepper
1½ cups water	¼ teaspoon crushed red pepper
16 ounces canned diced tomatoes in juice	1 teaspoon oregano
	2 tablespoons chili powder
28 ounces canned crushed tomatoes	1 tablespoon cumin

Spray a large saucepan with vegetable oil spray. Saute onion for about 10 minutes, until it is lightly browned. Add garlic and pepper, saute 2 minutes more. Add remaining ingredients. Bring to a boil, then reduce to a simmer for 30 minutes. Season to taste with additional chili powder. Serves 6.

Per serving: 152 calories; 1.67 grams fat, 0.1 grams saturated fat; 0 mg cholesterol; 665 mg sodium; 7 grams fiber; 8 grams protein. 1 serving = 2½ vegetables + 1 bread.

TIP: If served over rice, count ⅓ cup cooked rice as 1 additional bread serving.

♥ **MEXICAN CASSEROLE**

3 medium onions, chopped	16 ounces canned nonfat refried beans
3 stalks celery, chopped	
2 cloves garlic, minced	1 cup frozen corn
1 teaspoon cumin	1 16 ounce jar taco sauce, divided
1 teaspoon chili powder	12 corn tortillas
4 cups Meatless Chili, see recipe on this page	1 cup grated low-fat cheese.
	Nonfat sour cream (optional)

Spray frying pan with vegetable oil spray. Saute onions for 5 minutes, add celery, saute 5 minutes more, add garlic and saute 1 more minute. Stir in cumin, chili powder, chili, refried beans, corn, and 1 cup taco sauce. Remove from heat.

Spray 9 × 13 baking dish with vegetable oil spray. Cut tortillas into small wedges. Put ½ of the wedges on the bottom of the baking dish. Top with ½ of the chili mixture. Put the other half of the wedges on this and top with the remainder of the chili mixture. Bake in a 350 degree oven for 45 minutes. Sprinkle cheese on top, and bake for an additional

5 minutes, until cheese has melted. Serve with additional taco sauce and nonfat sour cream.

Serves 8.

Per serving: 280 calories; 6.5 grams fat, 1.83 grams saturated fat;
12 mg cholesterol; 985 mg sodium; 4.5 grams fiber; 15 grams protein.
1 serving = 2 breads + 1 meat + 2 vegetables.

TIP: When shopping for cheese, choose brands with 3 grams of fat per ounce or less. There are many fat-free cheeses available, but these often fail to provide the same flavor as the reduced-fat cheeses. In large part this is due to the high moisture content of the fat-free cheeses. It should be noted that reduced-fat cheese tends to be higher in sodium than full-fat cheese. If sodium is a concern, make sure to read the labels.

♥ ENCHILADAS

16 ounces canned nonfat refried
    beans
1 can black, kidney, or pinto
    beans, rinsed and drained
1 medium onion, chopped
1 medium green pepper, chopped
2 cloves garlic, minced
1 teaspoon chili powder
1 teaspoon ground cumin
2 cups picante sauce or salsa,
    divided

1 cup frozen corn
8 flour tortillas
1 small tomato, chopped
¼ cup shredded part-skim
    mozzarella
¼ cup nonfat cheddar
½ cup shredded lettuce (optional)
Nonfat sour cream (optional)

Spray nonstick skillet with vegetable oil spray and saute onion about 5 minutes. Add green pepper and garlic, saute 1 minute more. Add 1 cup of the picante sauce, the chili powder, cumin, the refried beans, kidney beans, and corn, and heat through.

Spoon ½ cup of the mixture down center of each tortilla, fold up like an envelope. Place seam side down on baking dish which has been sprayed with vegetable oil spray. Combine ½ cup picante sauce and tomato, spoon over enchiladas. Cover with foil and bake at 350 degrees until heated through, about 15 minutes. Uncover and sprinkle with cheese. Return to oven until cheese melts, about 5 minutes. Serve with shredded lettuce, a dollop more of picante sauce, and nonfat sour cream.

Serves 8.

Per serving (excluding optional sour cream): 230 calories;
   5 grams fat, 0 grams saturated fat; 6 mg cholesterol; 487 mg sodium;
   3.8 grams fiber; 10 grams protein.
2 tablespoons of nonfat sour cream will add: 20 calories;
   0 grams fat, 0 grams saturated fat; 0 mg cholesterol; 50 mg sodium;
   0 mg protein.
   1 serving = 1 vegetable + 2 bread + 1 meat

TIP: Watch fat content of tortillas as it varies from brand to brand.

♥ STUFFED MUSHROOMS

1½ pounds large mushrooms (about 24)	½ teaspoon cumin
1 can nonfat refried beans	½ teaspoon chili powder
⅔ cup picante sauce	½ teaspoon pepper
2 tablespoons thinly sliced onions	¼ cup fresh cilantro, chopped
	½ cup grated nonfat cheese

Clean and remove the stems from mushrooms. Place the caps in a baking dish sprayed with vegetable oil spray. In a small bowl mix the refried beans, picante sauce, onions, cumin, chili powder, pepper, and cilantro. Fill mushroom caps with bean mixture. Bake in a 325 degree oven for 20 minutes until hot and cooked through. Top with nonfat cheese and return to oven for 5 more minutes.

   Makes 24 mushrooms.

Per mushroom: 30 calories; 0.4 grams fat, 0 grams saturated fat;
   0 mg cholesterol; 121 mg sodium; 0.5 grams fiber; 2.7 grams protein.
   1 mushroom = 1 vegetable.

Vegetable Entrees

♥ STUFFED SHELLS

1 12-ounce package shells	½ cup egg substitute
1½ pounds nonfat cottage cheese	¼ cup chopped parsley
½ cup grated part-skim mozzarella cheese	¼ cup bread crumbs
¼ cup grated Parmesan cheese	4 cups tomato sauce

Boil 4 quarts water. Add shells and cook until done, 12 to 15 minutes. Drain water from shells.

   Combine cheeses, egg substitute, parsley, and bread crumbs. Stuff shells with cheese mixture. Pour 2 cups of tomato sauce into a large shallow casserole that has been sprayed with vegetable spray. Arrange shells in sauce. Top with additional tomato sauce. Cover dish and bake at 350 degrees for 30 minutes.

Serves 8.

Per serving: 338 calories;   5 grams fat, 2.6 grams saturated fat;   14 mg cholesterol;   557 mg sodium;   1.5 grams fiber;   25 grams protein.   1 serving = 3 breads + 1 vegetable + 2 meats

TIP: For a comparison of fresh versus dry grated Parmesan cheese, see Caesar Salad recipe page 248.

♥ TOMATO SAUCE

32 ounces canned tomato sauce (no salt added)
2 tablespoons brown sugar
2 teaspoons oregano
2 teaspoons rosemary

1 teaspoon garlic powder
½ cup fresh parsley, chopped
½ cup fresh basil, chopped
1 teaspoon crushed red pepper flakes

Combine all ingredients in medium saucepan. Cook for at least 20 minutes.

Serves 8 (each serving ½ cup).

Per serving: 63 calories;   0 grams fat, 0 grams saturated fat;   0 mg cholesterol;   35 mg sodium;   0 grams fiber;   2.2 grams protein;   3 grams sugar.   1 serving = 2 vegetables.

♥ EASY LASAGNA

9 lasagna noodles, uncooked
24 ounces canned tomato sauce
16 ounces nonfat ricotta cheese
2 tablespoons grated Parmesan cheese
2 egg whites, beaten

2 teaspoons Italian seasoning
1 10 ounce package frozen chopped spinach, thawed, drained, squeezed dry as possible

Spray 9 inch square pan with vegetable spray. Spread ½ cup tomato sauce over bottom of pan. Place 3 lasagna noodles, broken off at 9" length, in tomato sauce. Combine cheeses, egg whites, Italian seasoning, and spinach. Put half the cheese mixture over the lasagna noodles. Top with 1 cup sauce, and 3 more noodles. Top this with remaining cheese mixture and more sauce. Layer 3 noodles on top. Spread remaining sauce over noodles. Bake, covered, in 350 degree oven, for 45 minutes. Remove from oven and let rest 15 minutes before cutting.

Serves 6.

Per serving: 318 calories; 1.56 grams fat, 0.4 grams saturated fat;
8 mg cholesterol; 220 mg sodium; 1.5 grams fiber; 24 grams protein.
1 serving = 2 vegetables + 2 breads + 2 meats

TIP: This recipe tastes great with added mushrooms. Saute mushrooms in 1 to 2 tablespoons of nonfat chicken broth or wine before adding to tomato sauce.

♥ POTATO PESTO

1 medium potato, peeled and
thinly sliced
½ cup nonfat chicken broth
4 cloves roasted garlic, see recipe
p. 275, or 4 cloves fresh garlic,
minced

Juice of 1 lemon
2 cups firmly packed fresh basil
1 cup fresh Italian parsley
¼ cup grated Parmesan cheese
Ground black pepper to taste

In small saucepan over medium heat, simmer the potato, garlic, and broth, covered, for 10 minutes. Remove the cover, increase the heat to medium-high, and continue to cook until any remaining broth evaporates, about 1 minute. Place the potato mixture in a blender or food processor and blend until smooth. Let the mixture cool slightly. Add lemon juice, herbs, and Parmesan. Blend.

Makes 2 cups.

Entire recipe: 325 calories; 8 grams fat, 5 grams saturated fat;
20 mg cholesterol; 834 mg sodium; 9 grams fiber; 18 grams protein.
1 serving = 2 tablespoons.

Per 2 tablespoons: 40 calories; 1 gram fat, 0.67 grams saturated fat;
2.5 mg cholesterol; 104 mg sodium; 1.1 grams fiber; 2.25 grams protein.

♥ BROCCOLI PESTO

4 cups broccoli florets, chopped
14½ ounces canned chicken broth
4 cloves roasted garlic, see recipe,
p. 276, or 4 cloves fresh garlic,
minced

1 cup tightly packed basil leaves
¼ cup grated Parmesan cheese
Ground black pepper to taste

Steam broccoli over the broth for about 5 minutes, until tender. Process garlic in blender or food processor until smooth. Add the broccoli, Parmesan, and chicken broth. Add basil leaves. Process until very smooth. If you would like a creamy sauce, add 2 to 3 tablespoons of skim buttermilk.

Makes 3 cups.

Entire recipe: 278 calories; 9 grams fat, 5 grams saturated fat; 20 mg cholesterol; 1711 mg sodium; 15 grams fiber; 23 grams protein. 1 serving = 2 tablespoons.

Per 2 tablespoons: 11 calories; 0 grams fat, 0 grams saturated fat; 1 mg cholesterol; 71 mg sodium; 1 gram fiber; 1 gram protein.

♥ BASIL PESTO

6 cloves roasted garlic, see recipe p. 275, or 6 cloves fresh garlic, minced

2 cups tightly packed basil leaves
¼ cup grated Parmesan cheese
1 tablespoon extra-virgin olive oil

Turn blender or food processor on. Drop in garlic. Add the basil and process until smooth. Add the oil and cheese and blend until smooth. Cover and refrigerate or freeze until needed.

Makes 2 cups.

Entire recipe: 296 calories; 21 grams fat, 7 grams saturated fat; 20 mg cholesterol; 523 mg sodium; 5 grams fiber; 14 grams protein. 1 serving = 2 tablespoons.

Per 2 tablespoons: 19 calories; 1.3 grams fat, 0.4 grams saturated fat; 1 mg cholesterol; 33 mg sodium; 0 grams fiber; 1 gram protein.

♥ PASTA WITH SWEET PEPPER AND BEAN SAUCE

1 pound pasta, cooked according to package directions
2 red peppers, seeded and diced
1 medium onion, chopped
2 cloves garlic, minced
28 ounces canned Italian tomatoes, chopped, with juice
½ cup tomato paste
1 teaspoon fresh thyme leaves
¼ cup fresh basil leaves, chopped

¼ cup fresh parsley, chopped
16 ounces canned Great Northern white beans, rinsed and drained
1¼ cup nonfat chicken broth or white wine
¼ teaspoon crushed red pepper
Salt and ground black pepper to taste

Spray large saute pan with vegetable oil spray. Saute onions for about 10 minutes, until very tender. Add peppers and garlic, saute 1 minute more. Add chicken broth or wine, tomatoes, tomato paste, and thyme. Stir in the beans and crushed red pepper. Cover and simmer 30 minutes or until thickened. Stir in basil leaves and parsley. Top pasta with sauce.
  Serves 6.

Per serving: 423 calories;   2.6 grams fat, 0 grams saturated fat;
    0 mg cholesterol;   363 mg sodium;   6 grams fiber;   18 grams protein.
    1 serving = 3 breads + 2 meats + 2 vegetables

♥ FETTUCCINE ALFREDO

½ tablespoon olive oil
2 cloves garlic, minced
1 tablespoon flour
1¼ cups skim milk
¼ cup nonfat plain yogurt

½ cup Parmesan cheese
2 tablespoons chopped parsley
Ground black pepper to taste
4 cups hot cooked fettuccine

Spray nonstick saucepan with vegetable oil spray. Heat olive oil over medium heat. Add garlic, saute 1 minute. Add flour. Gradually add milk, stirring with a wire whisk to eliminate lumps of flour. Cook 8 minutes or until thickened and bubbly, stirring occasionally. Add yogurt and ½ cup Parmesan, stirring until cheese melts. Add pepper, and toss with hot fettuccine. Sprinkle serving with chopped parsley.
  Serves 4.

Per serving: 306 calories;   6.6 grams fat, 2.7 grams saturated fat;
    11 mg cholesterol;   285 mg sodium;   1 gram fiber;   16 grams protein.
    1 serving = ½ milk + 2 breads + 2 meats

♥ SUMMER VEGETABLE CASSEROLE

2 cups cubed, unpeeled potatoes
2 medium carrots, sliced
1 medium onion, chopped
1 clove garlic, minced
2 tablespoons margarine (lower
    fat)
¼ cup flour
2½ cups skim milk
1¼ cups shredded, reduced-fat
    cheddar cheese, divided

⅛ cup fresh basil, chopped
¼ teaspoon dry mustard
1 cup sliced zucchini
½ cup frozen green beans
½ cup frozen corn
⅔ cup bread crumbs

Place potatoes in large pot, cover with cold water and bring to a boil. Boil for 8 minutes. Drain and set aside.

Melt margarine in medium saucepan. Add onion, saute 3 minutes. Add carrots, saute 3 minutes, add garlic and saute 1 minute more. Add flour. Gradually add milk, mixing with a wire whisk to eliminate lumps of flour. Add basil and dry mustard. Cook an additional 10 minutes or so, until thickened and bubbling, stirring constantly. Stir in ¾ cup of cheese. Remove from heat.

Mix in potatoes, zucchini, corn, and beans. Put into a 9 x 13 inch baking dish which has been sprayed with vegetable spray. Bake, uncovered at 350 degrees for 20 minutes. Top with bread crumbs and remaining cheese, bake 10 minutes more.

Serves 8.

Per serving: 224 calories; 5.6 grams fat, 2.7 grams saturated fat;
    12.5 mg cholesterol; 273 mg sodium; 2 grams of fiber; 6.3 grams protein.
    1 serving = 1 vegetable + 2 breads + 1 fat

♥ CORN CASSEROLE

1 tablespoon margarine (lower fat)	½ teaspoon salt
	3 dashes Tabasco
½ cup sliced green onions	⅓ cup flour
1 red pepper, diced	¾ cup egg substitute
1 green pepper, diced	3½ cups fresh corn cut from cob
2¼ cups skim milk	
3 teaspoons sugar	

Melt margarine in a medium saucepan. Add green onions and red and green peppers, saute 2 minutes. Add milk, sugar, salt, and Tabasco, heat through, then remove from heat.

Combine flour and egg substitute in a bowl. Add hot milk mixture in gradually, scraping down sides of bowl. Add corn. Bake in 9 x 13 inch pan which has been sprayed with vegetable spray. Bake at 350 degrees for about 1 hour, check for doneness. It is done when a toothpick inserted near center comes out clean.

Serves 6.

Per serving: 156 calories; 2 grams fat, 0.4 grams saturated fat;
    1.5 mg cholesterol; 317 mg sodium; 5 grams fiber; 9 grams protein.
    1 serving = ½ milk + 1 bread + 1 vegetable

♥ GRILLED PIZZAS

The inspiration for these pizzas comes from Al Forno, a restaurant in Providence, Rhode Island. Its pizzas are wonderful—thin crusts, topped with very fresh ingredients. The grilled flavor and the fresh ingredients more than make up for the flavor of the fat you are leaving out.

Crust:

1 cup warm water

1 packet active dry yeast

1 teaspoon sugar

3 cups flour, divided

1 tablespoon olive oil

In a large bowl, dissolve the sugar and yeast in warm water. Let sit 5 minutes. Add olive oil and 2½ cups flour. Knead the dough in the bowl for about 5 minutes, adding flour by tablespoons as needed so that the dough will not stick to your fingers. Spray the doughball on all sides with vegetable spray, and let bowl of dough sit in a warm place, covered, for about 1 hour, until doubled in bulk.

At this point, you can use the dough immediately, or you can refrigerate it until needed. It will keep for 2 days tightly wrapped in plastic film in the refrigerator.

Take ⅙ of the dough, and roll it out into a large free-form plate-size pizza crust. Spray with vegetable spray, then put on a very hot grill for 1 to 2 minutes per side, until it is cooked and grill marks appear. (If weather is inclement, you can cook indoors on a cookie sheet in a 500 degree oven.) You can also grill the pizzas ahead, then finish them later if you are doing a bunch. Top with toppings and finish on grill covered with a bowl to make toppings heat through, or pop in hot oven for a minute.

Makes 6 pizza crusts.

Per crust: 253 calories; 2.7 grams fat, 0.4 grams saturated fat;
  0 mg cholesterol; 1 mg sodium; 2 grams fiber; 7 grams protein.
  1 crust = 3 breads

Suggested toppings for pizza:

¼ cup pesto (see pp. 260), 1 thinly sliced tomato, and 1 teaspoon Parmesan cheese per pizza

¼ cup Grilled Ratatouille (see p. 277) and 1 teaspoon Parmesan cheese per pizza

Assorted sliced mushrooms sauteed with garlic (use vegetable oil spray to saute)

Shrimp scampi pizza—4 shrimp per pizza, cut in half the long way, marinated in lemon juice and garlic, sauteed in vegetable oil spray

Spinach, garlic, and white beans sauteed together, with 1 teaspoon Parmesan cheese

Canadian bacon and pineapple

Tomato sauce and part-skim mozzarella

♥ SWEET AND SOUR BROCCOLI

1 pound broccoli pieces

1 medium onion

2 green peppers, seeded and sliced into 8 pieces

2 cloves garlic, minced

20 ounces canned pineapple chunks, drained

8 ounces canned water chestnuts, drained

⅓ cup sugar

¼ cup ketchup

3 tablespoons white vinegar

¼ cup soy sauce

1 tablespoon cornstarch mixed with ⅓ cup water

Boil a large pot of salted water. Add broccoli, cook until bright green and tender. Drain broccoli and rinse with cold water. Set aside.

Combine sugar, ketchup, vinegar, and soy sauce. Set aside.

Spray a large frying pan or wok with vegetable cooking spray. Over high heat, saute garlic, onions, and peppers for 2 minutes. Add soy sauce mixture, bring to a boil. Add cornstarch mixture, bring to a boil again. Add broccoli, pineapple chunks, and water chestnuts, cook only until heated through. Serve over rice.

Serves 4.

Per serving: (without shrimp or chicken);   231 calories
0.7 grams fat, 0 grams saturated fat;   0 mg cholesterol;   0 mg sodium;
8 grams fiber;   6 grams protein.
1 serving = 1 fruit + 3 vegetables + 1 bread

TIP: To reduce sodium in this recipe use reduced-sodium soy sauce. This recipe is also great with cooked shrimp or chicken added at the last minute.

♥ CAJUN VEGETABLE STEW

2 medium onions, chopped
1 tablespoon olive oil
1 green pepper, chopped
1 red pepper, chopped
2 stalks celery, chopped
3 cloves garlic, minced
4 cups nonfat chicken broth
14 ounces canned tomatoes, chopped, with juice
½ cup rice, uncooked
2 bay leaves
½ teaspoon dried rosemary

½ teaspoon dried oregano
½ teaspoon dried basil
1 10 ounce package frozen corn kernels
1 cup shredded Swiss chard or spinach
16 ounces canned black-eyed peas
¾ teaspoon paprika
¼ teaspoon crushed red pepper
½ cup chopped parsley
Ground black pepper to taste

In a large saucepan, heat olive oil and saute onions for 7 to 8 minutes, until tender. Add green pepper, red pepper, celery, and garlic. Cook 5 minutes more. Stir in rice.

Add the chicken broth, tomatoes, bay leaves, rosemary, oregano, and basil. Bring to a boil. Cover and simmer 20 minutes. Add corn, Swiss chard or spinach, black-eyed peas, paprika, and crushed red pepper. Heat through, stir in parsley, then season to taste with black pepper.

Serves 4.

Per serving: 345 calories;   5.25 grams fat, 1 gram saturated fat;
0 mg cholesterol;   215 mg sodium;   12 grams fiber;   15 grams protein.
1 serving = 2½ vegetables + 3 breads + 1 fat

Chicken

♥ CHICKEN-MUSHROOM TOSTADAS

1 medium onion, sliced
1 garlic clove, minced
½ red pepper, cut in thin strips, divided
½ green pepper, cut in thin strips, divided
2 cups thinly sliced mushrooms
2 cups chopped, cooked chicken breast

1 cup picante sauce
1 teaspoon cumin
1 tablespoon fresh chopped cilantro
Juice of ½ lime
6 flour tortillas
¾ cup shredded nonfat cheese

Spray nonstick skillet with vegetable spray, saute onion for about 5 minutes. Add garlic and most of pepper strips, reserving just a few for garnish. Cook 1 minute more. Add mushrooms and cook, stirring occasionally, until liquid from mushrooms is evaporated, about 4 minutes. Add chicken, picante sauce, and cumin, heat through. Take off heat, stir in cilantro and lime juice.

While chicken mixture simmers, broil tortillas 8 inches from heat source until golden brown and crisp, about 1 minute per side. Top with chicken mixture and cheese, broil for 1 minute until cheese has melted. Garnish with pepper strips. Serve with additional picante sauce and a dollop of nonfat sour cream, if desired.

Serves 6.

Per serving: 235 calories;   4 grams fat, 0.5 grams saturated fat;
32 mg cholesterol;   600 mg sodium;   1 gram fiber;   24 grams protein.
1 serving = 1 bread + 1 vegetable + 2 meats

♥ SPICY GRILLED CHICKEN

4 boneless, skinless split chicken breasts (16 ounces)

4 lemon wedges

2 teaspoons dry mustard

1½ teaspoons ground turmeric

½ teaspoon ground coriander

½ teaspoon ground allspice

½ teaspoon ground cloves

½ teaspoon cayenne pepper

½ teaspoon ground black pepper

4 teaspoons paprika

Grated zest of one orange

½ cup orange juice

½ cup white wine

½ cup water

Rinse the chicken and pat it dry. Rub the chicken with lemon wedges and place in a shallow dish.

Using a wire whisk, combine all remaining ingredients in a bowl. Pour marinade over the chicken. Cover and refrigerate for at least 8 hours. Grill the chicken over hot coals for 4 to 6 minutes on each side, basting with marinade.

Serves 4.

Per serving: 188 calories;   3.5 grams fat, 1 gram saturated fat;
73 mg cholesterol;   84 mg sodium;   0 grams fiber;   27 grams protein.
1 serving = 3 meats + ½ fruit.

♥ GRILLED BALSAMIC CHICKEN

4 boneless, skinless split chicken
  breasts (16 ounces)
¼ cup nonfat chicken broth
½ cup balsamic vinegar
2 scallions, chopped

2 tablespoons Dijon mustard
2 cloves garlic, minced
1 tablespoon sugar
2 teaspoons Worcestershire sauce
½ teaspoon ground black pepper

Rinse the chicken and pat dry. Arrange pieces in a shallow dish. In a small bowl, combine the remaining ingredients and whisk to blend well. Pour the marinade over the chicken. Cover and refrigerate for at least 6 to 8 hours, turning occasionally.

Grill the chicken over hot coals for 4 to 6 minutes on each side, basting occasionally with some of the marinade.

To make a dipping sauce, take the remaining marinade, strain to remove scallions and garlic pieces, and bring to a boil. Serve with chicken.

Serves 8.

Per serving: 210 calories;   4 grams fat, 1.1 grams saturated fat;
  96 mg cholesterol;   205 mg sodium;   0 grams fiber;   35 grams protein.
  1 serving = 4 meats.

♥ OVEN-BAKED DIJON CHICKEN

4 boneless, skinless split chicken
  breasts (16 ounces)
8 teaspoons Dijon mustard
½ cup bread crumbs

1 teaspoon dried basil leaves
2 tablespoons Parmesan cheese
½ cup dry white wine

Rinse the chicken and pat dry. Spread 1 teaspoon mustard on the top of each chicken breast. Combine the bread crumbs, basil, and Parmesan and dip the mustard-coated side of the chicken into the crumb mixture.

Place the chicken breasts, crumb side up, in a shallow baking dish which has been sprayed with vegetable spray. Pour in white wine. Bake, uncovered, at 350 degrees 25 to 30 minutes, until crumbs have browned and chicken is cooked through.

Serves 8.

Per serving: 237 calories;   4.8 grams fat, 1.5 grams saturated fat;
  97 mg cholesterol;   287 mg sodium;   0 grams fiber;   37 grams protein.
  1 serving = 5 meats.

♥ OLD-FASHIONED CHICKEN AND BISCUITS

Chicken mixture:

1 medium onion, chopped

2 10½ ounce cans low-fat chicken broth

2 cups diced potatoes

3 carrots, thinly sliced

2 stalks celery, chopped

½ cup frozen green peas

½ teaspoon poultry seasoning

1 cup sliced mushrooms

½ teaspoon pepper

½ cup skim milk

¼ cup flour

½ teaspoon salt

2 cups chopped, cooked chicken breast

Biscuits:

1¾ cup flour

1 teaspoon baking powder

½ teaspoon salt

1 teaspoon sugar

⅔ cup nonfat plain yogurt

¼ cup egg substitute

2 tablespoons skim milk

3 scallions, thinly sliced

Spray medium saucepan with vegetable oil spray and saute onion for about 5 minutes. Add carrots and celery and saute 2 minutes more. Add chicken broth and potatoes, bring to a boil, cover, and cook about 6 minutes, until potatoes are tender.

Combine flour, salt, pepper, poultry seasoning, and skim milk in a bowl, stirring well. Add to the vegetable mixture, mixing with a wire whisk to eliminate lumps of flour. Bring to a boil and cook over medium heat until thickened and bubbling, about 3 minutes. Stir in peas, mushrooms, and chicken. Pour into 9 × 13 inch baking dish which has been sprayed with vegetable oil spray.

Make biscuit dough by combining flour, baking powder, salt, and sugar. In a separate bowl, combine yogurt, egg substitute, and skim milk. Stir in flour, mixing only enough to combine. Add in scallions, again mixing as little as possible.

Drop pieces of biscuit dough on top of chicken mixture. Bake in a 350 degree oven for about 35 minutes at 350 degrees, until biscuits are golden brown.

Serves 8.

Per serving: 321 calories;   2.6 grams fat, 0.7 grams saturated fat;
   49 mg cholesterol;   605 mg sodium;   2.6 grams fiber;   24 grams protein.
   1 serving = 2 meats + 2½ breads + 1 vegetable.

♥ BAKED CHICKEN NUGGETS

1 pound boneless, skinless
chicken breast
⅓ cup nonfat ranch or Italian
salad dressing, plus additional
for dipping

1 cup seasoned bread crumbs

Rinse the chicken and pat dry. Put in a bowl and add salad dressing, turning to coat all sides of chicken. Shake chicken in a plastic bag with bread crumbs. Place chicken pieces on baking sheet which has been sprayed with vegetable spray. Bake at 350 degrees for 25 to 30 minutes. Serve with additional salad dressing as dipping sauce.
Serves 4.

Per serving: 325 calories;   5 grams fat, 0 grams saturated fat;
96 mg cholesterol;   707 mg sodium;   0 grams fiber;   39 grams protein.
1 serving = 4 meats + ½ bread.

Fish

A word on cooking fish: Many people shy away from cooking and serving fish because they are not sure about its preparation. Seafood is really very easy to bake, broil, or grill. It readily picks up the flavor of whatever spices, seasonings, or sauces you add to it. In general, seafood is very low in fat, especially saturated fat. Crab, shrimp, and lobster are excellent replacements for red meat even though they are higher in cholesterol. The fat content of these shellfish is about one gram per 3 ounces. When choosing seafood at the market make sure it is fresh—fresh fish should never smell fishy.

♥ BIRTHDAY PASTA

½ pound small, fresh unpeeled
shrimp
½ pound scallops
1 small onion, sliced
2 cloves garlic, minced
¼ cup sliced sun-dried tomatoes
½ cup water
1 green pepper, chopped

½ cup dry white wine
1 tablespoon fresh basil leaves,
chopped
1 bay leaf
1 tablespoon fresh parsley,
chopped
1 pound fresh linguine pasta,
cooked

Place sun-dried tomatoes in ½ cup water, heat to boiling, and simmer for 5 minutes. Drain and reserve liquid. Peel and devein shrimp, set aside.

Coat a medium nonstick skillet with vegetable oil spray, place over medium heat. Add onion, saute about 5 minutes. Add garlic and pepper, saute 1 minute more. Add reserved tomato liquid, white wine, basil and bay leaf. Bring to a boil. Reduce heat. Simmer, uncovered, 10 minutes. Add shrimp, scallops, and sun-dried tomatoes, cover and simmer 4 minutes or until seafood is cooked. Discard bay leaf. Serve over linguine, sprinkle with parsley.

Serves 4.

Per serving: 312 calories;   2.1 grams fat, 0.24 grams saturated fat;
129 mg cholesterol;   241 mg sodium;   2 grams fiber;   28 grams protein.
1 serving = 2½ meats + 2 breads + 1 vegetable.

TIP: In the summer, use 2 to 3 tomatoes, peeled, seeded, and diced. When you can't get good fresh tomatoes or sun-dried tomatoes, use 14 ounces canned diced tomatoes with juice.

♥ SEAFOOD SHISH KEBABS

Marinade:
¼ cup olive or canola oil
Juice of 1 lemon
¼ cup white wine
2 tablespoons red or white wine
    vinegar
½ cup chopped fresh herbs—
    either one of or a combination
    of the following: basil, parsley,
    thyme, or oregano

Kebabs:
½ pound medium shrimp, peeled
½ pound scallops
1 pound swordfish cut into
    scallop-sized cubes
1 red pepper, cut in squares
1 green pepper, cut in squares
1 zucchini, sliced in ¼ inch thick
    slices
4 scallions, cut in 1 inch pieces
Fresh basil leaves

Place the shrimp, scallops, and swordfish in a flat 9 × 12 inch glass baking dish. Mix the marinade and pour over the seafood, turning gently. Let marinate in refrigerator for at least one hour, turning occasionally.

Divide the seafood and vegetables among six large skewers, placing a leaf of fresh basil next to each piece of seafood. Grill over red-hot coals for about 3 to 5 minutes on each side, depending on the thickness of the fish. Test with a fork; the seafood and vegetables should be tender and the shrimp should be pink.

Serves 6.

Per serving: 288 calories;   14 grams fat (9 grams due to the oil in the
marinade);
2.5 grams saturated fat;   124 mg cholesterol;   242 mg sodium;
1 gram fiber; 34 grams protein.
1 serving = 4 meats + 1 vegetable + 1 fat.

TIP: Even though oil is used in most marinades, not much oil is actually
absorbed into the poultry, fish, or meat. Oil is used in this situation to
seal out air, thereby allowing the poultry, fish or meat to absorb the full
flavor of the marinade.

♥ TUNA PASTA SALAD

¼ cup plain nonfat yogurt
2 tablespoons nonfat mayonnaise
1 tablespoon vinegar or 1
   tablespoon balsamic vinegar
1 teaspoon honey
2 teaspoons snipped fresh dill
¼ teaspoon celery seed
¼ teaspoon paprika
½ teaspoon pepper
1½ cups cooked pasta

6½ ounces canned light tuna,
   packed in water, drained, and
   flaked
⅓ cup frozen peas, thawed
⅓ cup frozen corn, thawed
⅓ cup chopped celery
¼ cup chopped green pepper
¼ cup chopped red pepper
1 carrot, thinly sliced
2 scallions, thinly sliced

In large bowl, combine yogurt, mayonnaise, vinegar, honey, dill, celery
seed, paprika, and pepper. Stir in remaining ingredients. Store in refrigerator until serving time.
    Serves 4.

Per serving: 151 calories;   0.5 grams fat, 0.12 grams saturated fat;
0.25 mg cholesterol;   192 mg sodium;   2 grams fiber; 16 grams protein.
1 serving = 1 bread + 1 meat + 1 vegetable.

♥ GRILLED SALMON STEAKS

2 tablespoons Dijon mustard
¼ teaspoon pepper
2 tablespoons frozen orange juice
   concentrate, thawed

2 minced scallions
4 salmon steaks

In shallow glass dish, stir together mustard, pepper, orange juice concentrate, and scallions. Add salmon steaks and turn to coat both sides.

Cover with plastic wrap and marinate in refrigerator at least 15 minutes.
Grill over hot coals 3 to 5 minutes per side, or until cooked through.
Serves 4.

Per serving: 229 calories; 8.5 grams fat, 1.6 grams saturated fat;
56 mg cholesterol; 247 mg sodium; 0 grams fiber; 31 grams protein.
1 serving = 4 meats.

♥ TERIYAKI SWORDFISH

⅔ cup soy sauce
½ cup dry sherry
¼ cup rice vinegar
1 tablespoon sugar

1 garlic clove, minced
2 teaspoons peeled, grated ginger
  root
2 pounds swordfish steaks

Combine soy sauce, sherry, vinegar, sugar, garlic, and ginger in a small
saucepan. Bring to a boil over moderate heat, then pour into a glass
baking dish. Let cool, then put fish in marinade, turning to coat both
sides. Marinate fish for 30 minutes in refrigerator, turning occasionally.
Drain and reserve marinade. Grill or broil fish until cooked. Bring marinade to a boil, strain, and use as a dipping sauce.
Serves 6.

Per serving: 188 calories; 4.3 grams fat, 1.2 grams saturated fat;
43 mg cholesterol; 1937 mg sodium (1838 mg due to the sodium in
regular soy sauce); 0 grams fiber; 24.5 grams protein.
1 serving = 4 meats.

TIP: Use low-sodium soy sauce and recipe will have 1072 mg sodium per
serving)

♥ LINGUINE WITH CLAM SAUCE

½ pound linguine, cooked
  according to package
  directions, then rinsed,
  drained, and set aside
1 tablespoon olive oil
2 medium onions, chopped
3 cloves garlic, minced

2 8 ounce cans minced clams,
  drained, with juice reserved
½ cup white wine
½ teaspoon ground pepper
Juice of 1 lemon
¼ cup chopped parsley

Heat oil in medium skillet. Saute onion in oil for about 5 minutes. Add
garlic, saute 1 minute more. Add juice from clams and wine. Cook over

medium heat until total volume of liquid is reduced by half, about 10 to 12 minutes. Add pepper, lemon juice, and clams. Cover. Reduce heat and simmer 5 minutes. Add pasta, heat through. Serve topped with chopped parsley.

Serves 4.

Per serving: 215 calories;   5.2 grams fat, 0.8 grams saturated fat;
70 mg cholesterol;   80 mg sodium; 1 gram fiber;   13 grams protein.
1 serving = 1½ meats + 1½ breads.

♥ CRABCAKES WITH REMOULADE SAUCE

12 ounces canned pasteurized
crabmeat (available in the
fresh seafood department of
your supermarket)
1¼ cups bread crumbs, divided
1 medium onion, minced
2 ribs celery, minced

¼ cup nonfat mayonnaise
1 egg white, lightly beaten
2 teaspoons Dijon mustard
2 teaspoons Worcestershire sauce
3 to 4 dashes Tabasco
1 tablespoon lemon juice
1 teaspoon Old Bay seasoning

Drain crabmeat. Pick through for pieces of shell. Combine crabmeat, 1 cup bread crumbs, and remainder of ingredients. Shape into 10 patties. Coat outsides with additional bread crumbs. Refrigerate for 30 minutes.

Spray a large nonstick skillet with vegetable oil spray, place over medium heat. Cook crabcakes 4 to 5 minutes on each side or until golden. Serve with remoulade sauce.

Serves 5.

Remoulade Sauce

1 cup nonfat mayonnaise
2 tablespoons drained, finely
chopped cornichons or sweet
pickles
1 tablespoon drained, chopped
capers

1 tablespoon chopped pimento
2 teaspoons Dijon mustard
1 tablespoon chopped fresh
parsley
1 teaspoon chopped fresh
tarragon

Combine all ingredients. Refrigerate until serving. Serves 5

Per serving: 223 calories;   3 grams fat, 0.5 grams saturated fat;
68 mg cholesterol;   1085 mg sodium;   0.5 grams fiber;   16 grams protein.
1 serving = 1½ meats + 2 breads.

♥ FLAVORFUL FISH

1 pound haddock or cod
1 tablespoon lemon juice (more if
   you wish)
⅓ cup dry bread crumbs
1 tablespoon fresh basil or ½
   teaspoon dry basil

½ tablespoon canola oil
2 tablespoons dry sherry
Freshly ground black pepper
   (optional)

Place fish in a baking dish which has been coated with vegetable oil spray. Season fish with lemon juice and black pepper if desired. Combine bread crumbs, basil, canola oil, and sherry. Spread bread crumb mixture evenly over the fish.* Bake fish uncovered in a preheated 350 degree oven for 20 to 25 minutes.
   Serves 4.

Per serving: 180 calories; 3.1 grams fat, 0.4 grams saturated fat;
   84 mg cholesterol; 201 mg sodium; 0.5 grams fiber; 27 grams protein.
   1 serving = 3 ounces fish.

*Colorful variation: Slice 1 tomato into thin slices and layer over fish, top with 2 to 3 tablespoons chopped onion and ½ cup chopped green and red peppers before adding bread crumb mixture.

TIP: Do not use cooking sherry or cooking wines. When compared with regular sherry or white wine, the cooking varieties are much higher in sodium.

Potatoes and Other Side Dishes

♥ OVEN-FRIED POTATOES

2 medium-size baking potatoes,
   washed and sliced into ¼ inch
   slices
½ tablespoon olive oil or canola
   oil

1 teaspoon garlic powder
½ teaspoon paprika

Spray cookie sheet with vegetable spray. Place potato slices on cookie sheet and brush with oil. Sprinkle with garlic powder and paprika. Bake in 400 degree oven for 20 to 30 minutes.
   Serves 4.

Per serving: 130 calories;   2 grams fat, 0.3 grams saturated fat;
 0 mg cholesterol;   8 mg sodium;   2 grams fiber;   2.5 grams protein.
 1 serving = 2 breads.

♥ TWICE-BAKED POTATOES

4 baking potatoes, scrubbed
1 cup nonfat cottage cheese
4 teaspoons grated Parmesan
  cheese

1 tablespoon/chives, chopped
Ground pepper, to taste
3 egg whites

Bake potatoes until tender. (Microwave potatoes or bake the day ahead of serving to save time.) Cut in half and scoop out insides. Combine with cheeses, chives, and pepper. In a separate bowl, whip egg whites until stiff peaks form. Fold into cheese mixture. Stuff back into potatoes and bake in a 350 degree oven for 30 to 35 minutes.
 Serves 4.

Per serving: 284 calories;   1.4 grams fat, 0.8 grams saturated fat;
 4 mg cholesterol;   322 mg sodium;   5 grams fiber;   15 grams protein.
 1 serving = 2 breads + 1 meat.

♥ LEO'S ACORN SQUASH

2 acorn squash
Boiling water

2 cups applesauce
Cinnamon

Cut squash in half, scoop out seeds, place open side down in a baking pan, and then pour ½ inch of boiling water in pan. Place pan in 400 degree oven. Bake until squash is tender, about 30 minutes. Remove from oven, place cut side up in a baking pan without water. Fill cavities with applesauce, sprinkle with cinnamon, and return to oven until heated through, about 10 minutes.
 Serves 4.

Per serving: 113 calories;   0.2 grams fat, 0 grams saturated fat;
 0 mg cholesterol;   7.5 mg sodium;   4 grams fiber;   1.4 grams protein.
 1 serving = 1 bread + 1 fruit.

♥ ROASTED GARLIC

Wrap whole, unpeeled heads of garlic in aluminum foil. Bake at 350 degrees for 1 hour and 15 minutes. Cut heads in half and serve. The garlic comes out buttery and spreadable, very mildly flavored. This tastes great spread on bread or crackers, or as the basis for other recipes. For example, you can use this garlic in the pestos on pages 259–260; they still have the garlic flavor but not the bite. The roasted garlic keeps for several days, and can be reheated for serving.

1 clove: 4 calories;   0 grams fat, 0 grams saturated fat;
     0 mg cholesterol;   1 mg sodium;   0 grams fiber;   0 grams protein.

♥ GARLIC MASHED POTATOES

3 pounds potatoes, peeled and
    cubed
2 heads roasted garlic, (see recipe
    on p. 276)

½ cup skim milk
¼ cup nonfat yogurt
½ teaspoon salt
1 teaspoon pepper to taste

Boil the potatoes until tender. While potatoes are cooking, combine skim milk and yogurt. Cut garlic heads in half, and squeeze out roasted garlic into milk mixture. Drain potatoes, mash, and mix in milk mixture.
    Serves 8.

Per serving: 157 calories;   0.2 grams fat, 0 grams saturated fat;
     0.4 mg cholesterol;   156 mg sodium;   2 grams fiber;   4 grams protein.
     1 serving = 2 breads.

♥ RICE PILAF

2 cups nonfat chicken broth
1 medium onion, chopped small
1 cup rice
1 bay leaf

½ cup sliced fresh mushrooms
¼ cup frozen green peas, thawed
2 tablespoons chopped pimento

Spray ovenproof saucepan with vegetable oil spray. Saute onion for about 5 minutes, until just tender. Add rice, bay leaf, and mushrooms. Saute 1 minute more. Add broth, bring to a boil. Cover and put into 350 degree oven for 20 minutes. Remove from oven, stir in peas and pimento, remove bay leaf, and serve.
    Serves 4.

Per serving: 218 calories;   0.7 grams fat, 0 grams saturated fat;
     0 mg cholesterol;   309 mg sodium;   1.5 grams fiber;   6.6 grams protein.
     1 serving = 2½ breads + 1 vegetable.

♥ SPANISH RICE

1 cup chicken stock or water
1 cup tomato juice
1 rib celery, sliced
3 scallions, white and green parts,
    sliced thin
1 green pepper, diced small
2 tomatoes, peeled, seeded, and
    chopped

1 cup rice
1 clove garlic, minced
1 teaspoon paprika
2 to 3 drops Tabasco
1 small pinch crumbled saffron
    threads (optional)

Spray ovenproof saucepan with vegetable oil spray. Saute celery, scallions, and green pepper for about 3 minutes. Add garlic and rice, saute 1 minute more. Add remaining ingredients, bring to a boil, then cover and place in 350 degree oven for 20 minutes.
    Serves 6.

Per serving: 136 calories;   0.4 grams fat, 0 grams saturated fat;
    0 mg cholesterol;   167 mg sodium;   2 grams fiber;   3.3 grams protein.
    1 serving = 1½ breads + 1 vegetable.

TIP: At first glance saffron seems very expensive-about $13.00 for a normal size spice bottle at a local supermarket. When you open the bottle and find there are really only about 2 teaspoons of saffron in it, you are surprised. However, when the recipe calls for a few threads, it means a few threads. ⅟₃₂nd of a teaspoon should be enough for the above recipe.

♥ GRILLED RATATOUILLE

1 pound eggplant, peeled and cut
    into ½ inch slices
1 teaspoon salt
1 medium zucchini, thinly sliced
1 large onion, thinly sliced
1 red pepper, seeded and cut into
    1 inch squares
1 green pepper, seeded and cut
    into 1 inch squares

2 large, ripe tomatoes, cut into
    cubes
½ cup chopped basil (optional)
½ cup chopped parsley
2 cloves garlic, minced
½ teaspoon olive oil
1 tablespoon oregano leaves
Salt and pepper to taste

Place eggplant in a colander and sprinkle with salt. Let rest for 30 minutes, then rinse with cold water and pat dry.
    Spray the eggplant, zucchini, onion, and peppers with vegetable oil spray. Place over red-hot coals, and cook for 3 minutes on each side, or

until just tender. Remove from the grill and place on a large piece of heavy-duty aluminum foil. Add remaining ingredients and seal the foil tightly. Place the wrapped packet back on the grill and cook another 10 minutes, until the vegetables are tender.

Rainy weather version, for when you can't cook out:

Cut the peeled eggplant in 1 inch cubes, sprinkle with salt, and leave in colander for ½ hour. Rinse and pat dry.

Put olive oil into a nonstick skillet, heat, and saute onions for about 5 minutes. Add garlic, peppers, and zucchini, saute about 2 minutes more. Put this mixture and all remaining ingredients into a 9 × 13 inch baking dish, cover and bake in 350 degree oven for about 30 minutes or until vegetables are tender.

Serves 6.

Per serving: 67 calories;   1.7 grams fat, 0.3 gram saturated fat;
   0 mg cholesterol;   543 mg sodium;   4.5 grams fiber;   2.3 grams protein.
   1 serving = 2 vegetables.

♥ BAKED TOMATOES

4 medium tomatoes
1 small onion, minced
½ red bell pepper, minced
1 clove garlic, minced
¼ cup chopped parsley
2 tablespoons chopped basil

¼ cup nonfat mayonnaise
2 tablespoons grated Parmesan
   cheese
1 cup bread crumbs
Pepper to taste

Cut tomatoes in half and squeeze out seeds. Place upside down on paper towels to drain while you make stuffing.

Saute onion, pepper, and garlic for 1 minute. Remove from heat and add parsley, basil, tomatoes, mayonnaise, Parmesan, and bread crumbs. Top tomatoes with this mixture, and bake in a 400 degree oven for 25 minutes. If not browned in this much time, broil for a minute more to brown tops.

Serves 8.

Per serving: 45 calories;   1 gram fat, 0 grams saturated fat;
   1.2 mg cholesterol;   100 mg sodium;   1.5 grams fiber;   2 grams protein.
   1 serving = 1 vegetable + ½ bread.

TIP: This is a fun recipe to change and experiment with herbs. If you don't have basil or parsley, try substituting dill, mint, or other herbs.

♥ BRAISED BUTTERNUT SQUASH

1½ pounds butternut squash,
    peeled, seeded, and cut into
    cubes
1 medium onion, thinly sliced

14½ ounces canned nonfat
    chicken broth
Pepper to taste

Preheat oven to 350 degrees. Spray a baking dish with vegetable spray. Put onion and squash into baking dish. Sprinkle with pepper. Bring broth to a boil, pour over squash. Cover the baking dish with foil. Bake for 30 minutes. Remove foil and bake 15 minutes more.
    Serves 4.

Per serving: 90 calories;   0.2 grams fat, 0 grams saturated fat;
    0 mg cholesterol;   420 mg sodium;   3.6 grams fiber;   2 grams protein.
    1 serving = 1 bread.

Desserts for Special Occasions

By including recipes for desserts in this book we do not want to imply that you should have dessert every day. We view the following as recipes for special occasions. We suggest fresh fruit, fruit salad, or nonfat yogurt for daily desserts.
Some desserts do not require recipes, these include:
    Angel food cake with strawberries
    Low-fat cookies
    Popsicles
    Fruit bars

♥ OATMEAL RAISIN COOKIES*

3 egg whites
1 cup brown sugar
¼ cup granulated sugar
½ cup flour
2 tablespoons lower fat
    margarine, melted

1 teaspoon vanilla
1 cup old-fashioned rolled oats
½ cup raisins, plumped in 1 cup
    water and drained

Preheat oven to 350 degrees. Spray at least two large baking sheets with vegetable cooking spray.
    With a rotary mixer, beat the egg whites until soft peaks form. Beat in brown sugar, then granulated sugar. Stir in the flour, oats, margarine, and vanilla, then fold in the raisins.

Drop the batter from a teaspoon onto the prepared cookie sheets, leaving about 2 inches of space between them—these cookies spread. Bake 8 to 10 minutes until very lightly browned. Remove cookie sheet from oven and allow cookies to cool on the sheet for 10 minutes before removing with a spatula.

Makes about 30 cookies.

Per cookie: 67 calories;   1 gram of fat, 0.1 gram saturated fat;
   0 mg cholesterol;   18 mg sodium;   0.4 grams fiber;   1 gram protein;
   9.7 grams sugar (58% of calories).

*This is *not* an appropriate recipe if you are limiting sugar due to high triglycerides.

♥ **STRAWBERRY-RHUBARB CRISP**

Filling:

1 pound fresh or frozen and
   partially thawed strawberries,
   hulled and cut in half (about
   2½ cups)
¾ pound fresh or frozen and
   partially thawed rhubarb
   stalks, cut into 1 inch pieces
   (about 2 cups)
1¼ cups sugar
¼ cup all-purpose white flour
½ teaspoon nutmeg
Pinch salt

Topping:

½ cup flour
¾ cup rolled oats
½ cup brown sugar
4 tablespoons diet margarine

Combine strawberries, rhubarb, sugar, flour, nutmeg, and salt. Put into 9 × 13 inch pan that has been coated with vegetable oil spray. Mix topping ingredients together, sprinkle over filling. Bake at 350 degrees for about 45 minutes.

Serves 10.

Per serving: 270 calories;   3 grams fat, 0.5 grams saturated fat;
   0 mg cholesterol;   57 mg sodium;   2 grams fiber;   2.4 grams protein;
   36 grams sugar (9 teaspoons)*.
   1 piece = 2 fruits + 2 breads.

*If you have diabetes or an elevated triglyceride level, you should replace the sugar in this recipe with a sugar substitute (Equal, Sweet and Low).

♥ ZUCCHINI-STREUSEL BUNDT CAKE

Cake:
2 cups shredded zucchini
3 cups flour
1¼ cups sugar
1½ teaspoon baking powder
1 teaspoon baking soda
½ teaspoon salt
1⅓ cups plain nonfat yogurt
⅓ cup applesauce
1 tablespoon vanilla extract
¼ cup egg substitute

Streusel:
⅓ cup firmly packed brown sugar
⅓ cup raisins, plumped in ¼ cup
    water (see recipe p. 245)
1 tablespoon cinnamon

Topping:
¾ cup sifted powdered sugar
3 teaspoons lemon juice

Combine streusel ingredients, set aside. Combine flour, sugar, baking powder, baking soda, and salt. Add yogurt, applesauce, vanilla, and egg substitute. Mix well. Add zucchini, stir until just combined.

Spray a 12 cup Bundt pan with vegetable spray. Pour in ½ of cake mixture. Sprinkle streusel over cake mixture. Spoon remaining batter into pan. Bake at 350 degrees for one hour or until a toothpick inserted in center comes out clean. Cool 10 minutes, remove from pan onto wire rack. When cake has cooled, combine topping ingredients and drizzle over cake.

Serves 18.

Per slice: 183 calories;   0.2 grams fat, 0 grams saturated fat;
    0.3 mg cholesterol;   155 mg sodium;   1 gram fiber;   3.4 grams protein;
    24 grams sugar (6 teaspoons).
    1 slice = 2 breads + ½ fruit.

♥ CHOCOLATE CAKE

1¼ cups flour
⅔ cup baking cocoa
1 teaspoon baking soda
3 tablespoons light margarine
3 tablespoons applesauce

½ cup no-sugar raspberry
    preserves
1 cup sugar
1 cup skim milk
1 tablespoon white vinegar

Melt margarine in saucepan. Remove from heat. Stir in sugar, set aside. In large bowl, combine flour, cocoa, baking soda. Add applesauce, skim milk, and vinegar. Whisk in sugar and margarine. Pour into 9 × 13 inch pan that has been sprayed with vegetable oil spray. Bake 20 minutes or until a toothpick inserted in center comes out clean. Cool cake. Top with raspberry preserves and frosting, refrigerate until serving time.

Chocolate frosting: In small bowl, stir together 1 envelope dry whipped topping mix, ½ cup skim milk, 1 tablespoon baking cocoa, and ½ teaspoon vanilla. Beat with electric mixer for about 2 minutes or until soft peaks form. Spread on cake.

Serves 12.

Per slice with frosting: 158 calories; 3 grams fat, 1 gram saturated fat; 0.5 mg cholesterol; 113 mg sodium; 0.5 grams fiber; 3 grams protein; 24 grams sugar (6 teaspoons).
1 piece = 2 breads.

♥ YOGURT POUND CAKE

1½ cups sugar	¾ cup applesauce
⅔ cup egg substitute	¾ cup nonfat yogurt
½ teaspoon baking soda	2¼ cups flour
Pinch salt	1 teaspoon vanilla extract

Mix sugar, egg substitute, and applesauce. Add yogurt. Add remaining ingredients, stir until well combined. Pour into 9 inch round cake pan which has been sprayed with vegetable spray. Bake at 350 degrees for 45 minutes or until a toothpick inserted in center comes out clean.

Serves 12.

Per slice: 199 calories; 0.2 grams fat, 0 grams saturated fat; 0.25 mg cholesterol; 95 mg sodium; 1 gram fiber; 5 grams protein; 24 grams sugar (6 teaspoons).
1 slice = 3 breads.

♥ GRAHAM CRACKER CRUST

1½ cups graham cracker crumbs (10 crackers)	2 tablespoons honey
	¼ cup applesauce

Combine all ingredients. Press into bottom and sides of pie plate or onto bottom of springform pan which has been coated with vegetable oil spray. Bake at 350 degrees for 10 minutes. Cool to room temperature before filling.

Per crust: 706 calories; 10 grams fat, 2 grams saturated fat; 0 mg cholesterol; 663 mg sodium; 5 grams fiber; 10 grams protein; 40 grams sugar (10 teaspoons).

♥ STRAWBERRY CHEESECAKE

Graham cracker crust prebaked in
 10 inch springform pan
1 15-ounce package nonfat ricotta
 cheese
¾ cup sugar
⅔ cup flour
½ cup egg substitute
2 tablespoons grated lemon peel
2 teaspoons vanilla
1 cup nonfat plain yogurt

Topping:
2 pints strawberries, washed and
 hulled
¼ cup sugar
2 tablespoons lemon juice

Using an electric mixer, beat the ricotta until smooth. Add the sugar.
Beat for 5 minutes—you cannot overbeat, you are trying to incorporate
some air into the mixture and make it lighter. Add the flour, egg substitute, lemon peel, and vanilla. Mix well. Blend in yogurt. Pour the
cheese mixture into the crust and smooth the top. Bake at 350 degrees
for 45 minutes. To prevent cake from drying out and cracking, place a
baking dish full of boiling water in the oven at the same time you put
the cheesecake in.

   After baking, allow cake to cool and then refrigerate until serving
time. Slice strawberries. Puree about ½ the strawberries in a blender or
food processor. Add the sugar and lemon juice, combine well, and serve
over cheesecake.

   Serves 14.

Per serving (includes crust):   169 calories;   1 gram fat, 0.1 grams saturated fat;
   1.7 mg cholesterol;   78 mg sodium;   1 gram fiber;   6.4 grams protein;
   17 grams sugar (4¼ teaspoons).
   1 piece = 1 fruit + ½ meat + 1 bread.

♥ CARROT CAKE

2 cups flour
2 cups sugar
1 teaspoon salt
2 teaspoons baking soda
2 teaspoons cinnamon
2 tablespoons canola oil

½ cup applesauce
1 cup egg substitute
3 cups shredded carrots
8 ounces canned crushed
 pineapple, drained (reserve
 juice for icing)

Sift all dry ingredients together. Add oil, applesauce, egg substitute, carrots, and pineapple. Pour into a 9 × 13 inch pan that has been sprayed
with vegetable oil spray. Bake at 350 degrees for 40 to 45 minutes until

toothpick inserted in center comes out clean. Let cool to room temperature before frosting.

Nonfat Cream Cheese Icing
1 cup confectioner's sugar
8 ounces nonfat cream cheese, softened
2 teaspoons vanilla

Beat well until smooth. Serves 12.

Per slice with frosting: 305 calories;   2.5 grams fat, 0.33 grams saturated fat;
3.3 mg cholesterol;   472 mg sodium;   1.7 grams fiber;   5 grams protein;
42 grams sugar (11 teaspoons).
1 slice = 2 breads + 2 fruits + ½ fat.

♥ APPLE PIE

6 cups fresh, peeled, sliced
   Granny Smith or other firm
   apples
1 tablespoon lemon juice
½ cup sugar
¼ cup brown sugar
3 tablespoons flour
¼ teaspoon salt
½ teaspoon cinnamon
½ teaspoon nutmeg
Graham cracker crust, prebaked
   in 9 inch pan

Topping:
¾ cup flour,
¼ cup sugar,
¼ cup brown sugar
¼ cup applesauce

Combine sliced apples, lemon juice, sugars, flour, salt, cinnamon, and nutmeg. Mix well and spoon into crust. In another bowl, combine topping ingredients with a fork or pastry blender until crumbly. Sprinkle topping over apples. Bake at 350 degrees until topping is golden and filling is bubbling, about 45 minutes.

This is also wonderful as an apple crisp, without the bottom crust. Serves 8.

Per slice: 337 calories;   1.8 grams fat, 0.4 grams saturated fat;
0 mg cholesterol;   154 mg sodium;   3 grams fiber;   3 grams protein;
51 grams sugar (13 teaspoons).
1 slice = 3 fruits + 2 breads.

♥ MRS. DUNLOP'S FRUIT PIE

20 ounces canned crushed
pineapple, with juice
20 ounces canned red sour
cherries, drained
1 cup sugar

⅓ cup flour
3 ounce box orange gelatin
5 or 6 bananas, sliced
2 graham cracker crusts, prebaked

Mix pineapple, cherries, sugar, and flour together and cook over medium heat until thick. Add orange gelatin, stir until gelatin is dissolved. Cool 15 minutes. Add sliced bananas. Pour into pie shells. Refrigerate. Will keep several days.

Makes 2 pies. Each pie serves 8.

Per slice: 254 calories;   1.5 grams fat, 0.33 grams saturated fat;
0 mg cholesterol;   86 mg sodium;   2 grams fiber;   3.9 grams protein;
40 grams sugar (10 teaspoons).
1 slice = 1½ fruits + 2 breads.

♥ WHIPPED CREAM SUBSTITUTE

⅓ cup evaporated skim milk
½ teaspoon unflavored gelatin
1 tablespoon cold water

1 teaspoon sugar
½ teaspoon vanilla
1 to 2 teaspoons lemon juice

Chill evaporated skim milk in a small bowl along with beaters. Sprinkle gelatin over cold water in a small saucepan. Stir over low heat until gelatin dissolves, then add to milk. Beat mixture until stiff. Add sugar, vanilla, and lemon juice. Use immediately or chill and rewhip before serving.

Entire recipe: 84 calories;   0 grams fat, 0 grams saturated fat;
3 mg cholesterol;   100 mg sodium;   0 grams fiber;   6.5 grams protein;
4 grams sugar (1 teaspoon).

Appendix

FAMILIAL HYPERCHOLESTEROLEMIA

If, based on the discussion in Chapter 1 titled "Am I at Risk for Developing Heart Disease," you think you may have familial hypercholesterolemia (FH), it will be important for you to try to make contact with one of the MED-PED (Make Early Diagnosis—Prevent Early Death) FH centers listed here.

Physicians all over the world are asking FH patients to fill out a family questionnaire, which will be used to track down and identify other persons at risk for FH. And remember, if you have FH, roughly half of your first-degree relatives will also have it.

Dr. Roger Williams, the director of MED-PED, Dr Susan Stephenson, the coordinator of MED-PED, and their staff are seeking family members of FH patients no matter where they live, because cholesterol-lowering medications can save lives in persons with FH. In the United States, there are five centers that are collaborating with Dr. Williams. I am assisting Dr. Robert Lees, the Northeast Regional Collaborator, so if you think you might have FH or would like more information about the project, please feel free to contact me or the center closest to you. Here is a list of Dr. Williams's collaborators:

Dr. Roger Illingsworth
University of Oregon Health Science Center. 3181 S. W. Sam Jackson Park Road, L465. Portland Oregon 97201-3098.

Dr. John Kane
University of California San Francisco. 505 Parnassus Avenue. San Francisco, California 94143.

Dr. Peter Kwiterovich
Johns Hopkins University Hospital. 550 Building, Suite #308. 550 North Broadway. Baltimore, Maryland 21205.

Dr. Robert Lees
The Boston Heart Foundation. 139 Main Street. Cambridge, Massachusetts 02142.

Dr. Mary P. McGowan
The New England Heart Institute. 100 McGregor Street. Manchester, New Hampshire 03102.

Dr. Evan Stein
The Christ Hospital. 2139 Auburn Avenue. Cincinnati, Ohio 45219.

Dr. Roger Williams
Director MED-PED. 410 Chipeta Way #161. Salt Lake City, Utah 84108.

In addition to the MED-PED project, individuals who suspect they may have FH can contact The Inherited High Cholesterol Foundation (David Hardy, president) at their toll free #: 1-888-2 HI-Chol, for information on support services available to them. The Inherited High Cholesterol Foundation was started in 1995 by a dear friend of mine, Laura Therrien. Laura, who has FH and has now entered Dartmouth Medical School, plans someday to develop a cure for FH. I am sure you will be hearing from Dr. Laura Therrien in the future.

Glossary

Aerobic exercise Exercise in which the muscles utilize oxygen (aerobic means "with oxygen") to burn both sugar and body fat. Examples include walking, running, swimming, skiing, and cycling.

Anaerobic exercise Exercise which is performed in short intense bursts and does not utilize oxygen. Examples include weight lifting and sprinting.

Angina pectoris Chest pain or pressure resulting from insufficient blood flow (and oxygen delivery) to the heart muscle—typically, the result of blockages within the coronary arteries. In some people angina is felt as arm, jaw, or neck pain.

Angioplasty See **Coronary artery balloon angioplasty**.

Antioxidant A dietary supplement or medication which prevents LDL cholesterol (the bad cholesterol) from becoming oxidized. Studies indicate that oxidized LDL cholesterol is a major component of the cholesterol plaque within diseased arteries. Examples of antioxidants include estrogen, probucol, and vitamins E, C, and beta-carotene.

Arrhythmia An electrical disturbance in the heart rhythm that is often the result of underlying coronary artery disease.

Atherosclerosis A disease process that begins in childhood, characterized by the gradual buildup of plaque within the artery wall. Cholesterol is a major constituent of the plaque. When a plaque becomes large, it can block the artery and lead to angina or a heart attack.

Atromid-S See Chapter 8.

Beta-blocker A medication used for the treatment of high blood pressure or angina (chest pain or pressure). Beta-blockers reduce the work of the heart by slowing heart rate. Side effects can include nausea, fatigue, and diarrhea. Beta-blockers can also result in an increase in triglycerides and a reduction in HDL cholesterol (the protective cholesterol).

Bypass See **Coronary artery bypass grafting**

Carbohydrate A sugar or starch. One gram of carbohydrate contains four calories.

Cardiac Pertaining to the heart.

Cardiac catheterization See **Coronary angiography**.

Cardiac rehabilitation program A thrice weekly, medically supervised exercise program attended by people with cardiac disease. Such programs also generally include advice on diet, smoking cessation, and stress reduction.

Cardiac risk factors Aspects of one's life which predispose to the development of cardiac disease. These include: elevated LDL cholesterol (bad cholesterol), depressed HDL cholesterol (the good cholesterol), elevated triglycerides, smoking, diabetes, a family history of heart disease, obesity, a sed-

289

entary lifestyle, high blood pressure, stress, an elevated lipoprotein(a), an elevated homocysteine level and being a male over the age of 45 or being a postmenopausal female.

Catheterization   See **Coronary angiography**.

Cholesterol   A white waxy chemical found only in products of animal origin, including egg yolks, meat, cheese, milk, and ice cream. Cholesterol is also produced by the human liver; small amounts are necessary to make cell membranes and hormones.

Clofibrate   See Chapter 8.

Colestid   See Chapter 8.

Colestipol   See Chapter 8.

Coronary angiography   A procedure in which dye is injected into the coronary arteries via a flexible catheter (a thin, hollow plastic tube) to determine if these arteries have significant blockages.

Coronary artery   An artery that supplies blood and oxygen to the heart muscle. Coronary arteries arise from the aorta. The major arteries include the right coronary artery and the left main artery which quickly divides into the circumflex and left anterior descending arteries.

Coronary artery balloon angioplasty   A procedure in which a thin catheter containing an inflatable balloon is used to open a blocked coronary artery.

Coronary artery bypass grafting   Open heart surgery in which a leg vein (saphenous vein) or breast artery (mammary artery) is used to connect the aorta with a coronary artery just beyond a cholesterol blockage.

Coronary artery disease (CAD)   A progressive disorder caused by blockages within the coronary arteries. Aftereffects of this disease include angina pectoris, heart attack, and sudden cardiac death. Individuals with coronary artery disease may require coronary artery bypass grafting or angioplasty.

Coronary care unit (CCU)   An intensive care unit within a hospital in which cardiac patients receive specialized monitoring and care. Such units are equipped with defibrillators, respirators, and other life-sustaining equipment.

Diabetes   Fasting blood sugar levels greater than 140 mg/dl when measured on three separate occasions.

Directional coronary atherectomy (DCA)   A procedure in which a cholesterol deposit (plaque) is actually shaved off the wall of the diseased artery and removed from the body by an X-ray guided catheter.

Electrocardiogram   Often referred to as an EKG or ECG, an electrocardiogram is a painless procedure in which electrodes are placed on the chest wall, arms, and legs and used to monitor electrical impulses as they pass through the heart muscle, controlling its activity. In some situations the EKG is combined with exercise (a stress test). This is done to detect electrical disturbances that might not be evident at rest.

Endothelium   The inner lining of an artery.

Estrogen   A female sex hormone produced by the ovaries. After menopause the production of estrogen is drastically reduced. Estrogen deficiency is believed to be one of the major causes for the increase in cardiac events in postmenopausal women.

Familial combined hyperlipidemia (FCH)   A genetic cholesterol disorder. Afflicted persons may have an elevated LDL cholesterol (bad cholesterol), an elevated triglyceride level, or elevations of both these lipoproteins. Regardless of the specific cholesterol abnormality, people with FCH are at high risk for the development of premature cardiac disease. FCH is the most common inherited cholesterol abnormality, affecting roughly one person in every 100 in the United States.

Familial hypercholesterolemia (FH)   A genetic cholesterol disorder that prevents affected individuals from processing LDL cholesterol (the bad cholesterol) properly. Persons who have inherited two genes for this disorder may have a total cholesterol level of up to 1000 mg/dl and will often have their first heart attack in the first decade of life.

Those who have inherited only one gene for this disorder typically have a cholesterol level of 300 to 500 mg/dl. If left untreated, a heart attack can be expected in middle age.

Highly effective therapies are available for people who have inherited a single gene for this disorder. Therapy for the rare person who has inherited two genes for familial hypercholesterolemia is not as effective but has greatly improved in the last few years.

Fiber   Roughage: material found in plants and vegetables that is resistant to digestion. Fiber may be either water soluble or water insoluble. Water soluble fiber is found in fruits, beans, oatmeal, and legumes. This type of fiber helps to reduce cholesterol levels. Water insoluble fiber, found mostly in grains and vegetables, reduces constipation and has been linked with a reduction in colon cancer.

Folic acid   A dietary constituent found in foods such as lima beans, broccoli, spinach, asparagus, potatoes, whole wheat bread, and dried beans. Folic acid is necessary for homocysteine metabolism. Elevated homocysteine levels are a risk factor for the development of cardiac disease.

Gemfibrozil   See Chapter 8.

Heart attack   See **Myocardial infarction**.

Heparin   A medication which prevents the blood from clotting.

High blood pressure   See **Hypertension**.

High-density lipoprotein cholesterol (HDL-C)   Often referred to as the good cholesterol, high levels of this lipoprotein protect against the development of cardiac disease through a process called reverse cholesterol transport.

HMG CoA reductase inhibitor   A class of cholesterol-lowering drugs including lovastatin (Mevacor), simvastatin (Zocor), pravastatin (Pravachol), and fluvastatin (Lescol). See Chapter 8.

Hypercholesterolemia   An elevated blood cholesterol level.

Hypertension   A condition characterized by sustained high blood pressure and an increased risk for heart disease and stroke. While salt and alcohol restriction, exercise and weight reduction may normalize blood pressure, there are cases when medications are necessary.

Hypothyroidism   A condition in which the thyroid gland is underactive. This condition may lead to marked triglyceride elevations. Therapy involves daily thyroid hormone replacement in the form of a pill.

Hysterectomy   Surgery to remove the uterus.

Insulin   A hormone produced by the pancreas which promotes the entry of sugar into the cells.

Legume   Edible seeds enclosed in pods. Examples include soy beans, lima beans, peas, lentils, black beans, kidney beans, black-eyed peas, chickpeas, and cannellini beans.

Linoleic acid   An essential fatty acid which is not produced by the body and must be consumed through the diet.

Lipid profile   A blood test which reports total cholesterol, triglycerides, HDL cholesterol, and LDL cholesterol.

Lipitor   See Chapter 8.

Lipoprotein (a)   An LDL-like particle with an attached protein called apolipoprotein (a) found in the bloodstream. Elevated levels of this blood lipid increase a person's risk of developing early heart disease.

Lipoprotein lipase   An enzyme necessary for the breakdown of triglyceride-rich particles. This enzyme promotes the transfer of fat from the bloodstream into fat cells.

Lopid   See Chapter 8.

Low-density lipoprotein cholesterol (LDL-C)   Often referred to as the bad cholesterol, elevated levels of this blood fat increase the risk of developing premature heart disease.

Mediterranean diet   A diet in which up to 40 percent of calories are obtained from fat. The major fat source in this diet is olive oil.

Menopause   The time in a woman's life when the ovaries cease to produce the female sex hormones estrogen and progesterone. In the United States the average woman enters menopause at about age 51. Heavy smokers enter menopause at an earlier age.

Mevacor   See Chapter 8.

Monounsaturated fat   The type of fat found in olive oil, canola oil, and peanut oil. When this type of fat is substituted for saturated fat, total cholesterol level will fall and HDL cholesterol level may rise.

Myocardial infarction   A heart attack. This condition develops when an area of heart muscle is deprived of oxygen. The result is cellular death and eventual scar formation.

Nephrology   The study of the kidney in health and disease.

Niacin   See Chapter 8.

Oat bran   A water soluble fiber known to lower cholesterol and relieve constipation.

Pectin   The cholesterol-lowering, water soluble fiber found in fruit.

Plaque   A blockage within an artery composed of cholesterol, cellular debris, and fibrous material.

Platelet   Blood-clotting cell.

Polyunsaturated fat   The type of fat found in corn, sunflower, and safflower oils. When this type of fat is substituted for saturated fat, both total and HDL cholesterol levels may fall. In some studies polyunsaturated fats have been linked to the development of colon cancer.

Progesterone   A female sex hormone produced by the ovaries. Like estrogen, progesterone ceases to be produced at menopause.

Protein   An essential element of the diet which contains amino acids, carbon, hydrogen, oxygen, and nitrogen. Protein is plentiful in grains, poultry, and dairy products and can be obtained in sufficient amount without consuming meat. Each gram of protein contains four calories.

Psyllium   A cholesterol-lowering, water-soluble fiber found in products like Metamucil and Citrucel.

Questran   See Chapter 8.

Regression   In the context of cardiac disease, regression refers to the shrinkage of plaques within diseased arteries. Regression tends to occur when the LDL cholesterol falls below 100 mg/dl.

Saturated fat   The type of fat found in butter, cheese, whole milk, ice cream, white marbling in meat, palm oil, and coconut oils. This type of fat is known to increase cholesterol levels dramatically.

Step One diet   An American Heart Association diet which calls for the restriction of fat to 30 percent (or less) of total calories, saturated fat to no more than 10 percent of total daily calories, and cholesterol to less than 300 mg per day.

Step Two diet   An American Heart Association diet which calls for the restriction of fat to 30 percent (or less) of total calories, saturated fat to no more than 7 percent of total daily calories, and cholesterol to less than 200 mg per day.

Stress test   See **Electrocardiogram**.

Tissue plasminogen activator (TPA)   A clot dissolving agent.

Trans fat   The type of fat created when liquid oils (such as canola, olive, corn, or sunflower) undergo the hydrogenation process. The resulting fat behaves much the way saturated fat does, leading to an increase in cholesterol levels. Trans fats are found in fast foods and commercially prepared baked goods.

Triglyceride   One of the blood fats. Triglycerides may be made by the liver or ingested through the diet. An elevated triglyceride level appears to be a strong predictor of cardiac disease, especially in women.

Wheat bran   A water insoluble fiber which has been linked to a reduction in colon cancer risk. This type of fiber does not reduce cholesterol levels.

Xanthelasma   A yellowish deposit of cholesterol on the eyelid or under the eye which suggests that the cholesterol level is likely to be elevated.

Xanthoma   A cholesterol deposit typically found in the tendons of the hand or ankle. Xanthomas are found in approximately 75 percent of adults with familial hypercholesterolemia.

Suggested Reading

Introduction

The Scandinavian Simvastatin Survival Study Group. Randomized trial of cholesterol lowering in 4444 patients with coronary artery disease: the Scandinavian Simvastatin Survival Study (4S). *Lancet*. 1994; 344:1383–1389.

J. Sheperd, S. M. Cobbe, I. Ford, et al. Prevention of coronary heart disease with pravastatin in men with hypercholesterolemia. *New England Journal of Medicine*. 1995; 333:1301–1307.

F. M. Sacks, M. A. Pfeffef, L. A. Moye, et al. The effect of pravastatin on coronary events after myocardial infarction in patients with average cholesterol levels. *New England Journal of Medicine*. 1996; 335:1001–1009.

Chapter 1. Am I At Risk for Developing Heart Disease?

Heart and Stroke Facts—1994 Statistical Supplement. Dallas, TX: American Heart Association, 1994.

Summary of the second report of the National Cholesterol Education Program (NCEP) Expert Panel on detection, evaluation, and treatment of high blood cholesterol in adults (Adult Treatment Panel II). *Journal of the American Medical Association*. 1993; 269:3015–3023.

K. Berg. A new serum type system in man: the Lp system. *Acta Pathologia Microbiologia et Immunologica Scandinavica*. 1963; 59:369–382.

A. M. Scanu, R. M. Lawn, K. Berg. Lipoprotein (a) and Atherosclerosis. *Annals of Internal Medicine*. 1991; 115:209–218.

R. L. Desmarais, I. J. Sarembock, C. R. Ayers, et al. Elevated serum Lipoprotein (a) is a risk factor for clinical recurrence after coronary balloon angioplasty. *Circulation*. 1995; 91:1403–1409.

V. M. Maher, G. B. Brown, S. M. Marcovina, et al. Effects of lowering elevated LDL cholesterol on the cardiovascular risk of lipoprotein (a). *Journal of the American Medical Association*. 1995; 274:1771–1774.

H. F. Hoff, G. J. Beck, M. S. Skibinski, et al. Serum Lp (a) level as a predictor of vein graft stenosis after coronary artery bypass surgery in patients. *Circulation*. 1988; 77:1238–1244.

J. K. Williams, J. A. Vita, S. B. Manuck, A. P. Selwyn, J. R. Kaplan. Psychosocial factors impair vascular responses of coronary arteries. *Circulation*. 1991; 84:2146–2153.

A. S. Krolewski, J. H. Warram, P. Valsania, et al. Evolving natural history of coronary artery disease in diabetes mellitus. *American Journal of Medicine.* 1991; 90 (suppl 2A): 56S–61S.

C. E. Walden, R. H. Knopp, P. W. Wahl, K. W. Beach, E. Strandness, Jr. Sex differences in the effect of diabetes mellitus on lipoprotein triglyceride and cholesterol concentrations. *New England Journal of Medicine.* 1984; 311:953–959.

J. K. Ockene. Smoking intervention: a behavioral, educational, and pharmacological perspective. In I. S. Ockene, J. K. Ockene, eds. *Prevention of Coronary Heart Disease.* Boston: Little, Brown, 1992.

R. J. Kuczmarski, K. M. Flegal, S. M. Campbell, C. L. Johnson. Increasing prevalence of overweight among U.S. adults: The National Health and Nutrition Examination Survey, 1960 to 1991. *Journal of the American Medical Association.* 1994; 272:205–211.

R. C. Klesges, M. L. Shelton, L. M. Klesges. Effects of television on metabolic rate: potential implications for childhood obesity. *Pediatrics.* 1993; 91:281–286.

N. D. Wong, T. K. Hei, P. Y. Qaqundah, et al. Television viewing and pediatric hypercholesterolemia. *Pediatrics.* 1992; 90:75–79.

M. A. Austin, J. L. Breslow, C. H. Hennekens, J. E. Buring, W. C. Willett, R. M. Krauss. Low-density lipoprotein subclass patterns and risk of myocardial infarction. *Journal of the American Medical Association.* 1988; 260:1917–1921.

A. H. Slyper. Low-density lipoprotein density and atherosclerosis. *Journal of the American Medical Association.* 1994; 272:305–308.

A. M. Dattilo, P. M. Kris-Etherton. Effects of weight reduction on blood lipids and lipoproteins: a meta-analysis. *American Journal of Clinical Nutrition.* 1992; 56:320–328.

J. G. Warner, P. H. Brubaker, Y. Zhu, et al. Long-term (5-year) changes in HDL cholesterol in cardiac rehabilitation patients: Do sex differences exist? *Circulation.* 1995; 92:773–777.

D. E. Bild, R. R. Williams, H. B. Brewer, J. A. Herd, T. A. Pearson, E. Stein. Identification and management of heterozygous familial hypercholesterolemia: Summary and recommendations from an NHLBI workshop. *American Journal of Cardiology.* 1993; 72:1D–5D.

P. O. Kwiterovich. *Beyond Cholesterol: The Johns Hopkins Complete Guide for Avoiding Heart Disease.* Baltimore: The Johns Hopkins University Press, 1989.

R. R. Williams, M. C. Schumacher, G. K. Barlow, et al. Documented need for more effective diagnosis and treatment of familial hypercholesterolemia according to data from 502 heterozygotes in Utah. *American Journal of Cardiology.* 1993; 72:18D–24D.

D. G. Franken, G. H. J. Boers, H. J. Blom, F. J. M. Trijbels, P. W. C. Kloppenborg. Treatment of mild hyperhomocysteinemia in vascular disease patients. *Arteriosclerosis and Thrombosis.* 1994; 14:465–470.

S. Torri. Homocysteine: a potentially independent, modifiable cardiovascular disease risk factor. *Pulse.* 1996; 15:2–4.

J. Selhub, P. F. Jacques, P. W. F. Wilson, D. Rush, I. H. Rosenberg. Vitamin status and intake as primary determinants of homocysteinemia in an elderly population. *Journal of the American Medical Association.* 1993; 270:2693–2698.

High Cholesterol and Early Heart Disease—It May Be Your Genes: The Cases of Susan and Lorraine

1. Since this chapter was written, Lorraine was diagnosed with laryngeal cancer (cancer of the voicebox). She fought valiantly, but after many surgical procedures and extensive radiation therapy she died at home with her entire family around her.

Moved and inspired by her struggle to overcome her cancer, her son Ron and his family have created a lasting memorial to Lorraine: an aggressive lifestyle modification program of diet, exercise, and weight loss. Ron has already lost 20 pounds and reduced his cholesterol level by nearly 100 mg/dl. I'm sure Lorraine's spirit is cheering him and his family on.

P. O. Kwiterovich. *Beyond Cholesterol: The Johns Hopkins Complete Guide for Avoiding Heart Disease.* Baltimore: The Johns Hopkins University Press, 1989.

D. E. Bild, R. R. Williams, H. B. Brewer, J. A. Herd, T. A. Pearson, E. Stein. Identification and management of heterozygous familial hypercholesterolemia: Summary and recommendations from an NHLBI workshop. *American Journal of Cardiology.* 1993; 72:1D–5D.

W. E. Connor, S. L. Connor. Importance of diet in the treatment of familial hypercholesterolemia. *American Journal of Cardiology.* 1993; 72:42D–53D.

V. M. G. Maher, B. G. Brown, S. M. Marcovina, L. A. Hillger, X. Q. Zhao, J. J. Albers. Effects of lowering elevated LDL cholesterol on the cardiovascular risk of lipoprotein (a). *Journal of the American Medical Association.* 1995; 274: 1771–1774.

R. P. Mensink, M. B. Katan. Effect of a diet enriched with monounsaturated or polyunsaturated fatty acids on levels of low-density and high-density lipoprotein cholesterol in healthy women and men. *New England Journal of Medicine.* 1989; 321:436–441.

D. M. Dreon, K. M. Vranizan, R. M. Krauss, M. A. Austin, P. D. Wood. The effects of polyunsaturated fat vs. monounsaturated fat on plasma lipoproteins. *Journal of the American Medical Association.* 1990; 263:2462–2466.

M. A. Denke, J. L. Breslow. Effects of a low-fat diet with and without intermittent saturated fat and cholesterol ingestion on plasma lipid, lipoprotein, and apolipoprotein levels in normal volunteers. *Journal of Lipid Research.* 1988; 29:963–969.

J. M. Sullivan, R. Vander Zwang, J. P. Hughes, et al. Estrogen replacement and coronary artery disease: Effect on survival in postmenopausal women. *Archives of Internal Medicine.* 1990; 150:2557–2562.

Chapter 2. A Heart-Healthy Diet: Planning the Diet You Can Live With

W. P. Newman III, W. Wattigney, G. S. Berenson. Autopsy studies in U.S. children and adolescents. Relationship of risk factors to atherosclerotic lesions. *Annals of the New York Academy of Sciences.* 1991;623:16–25.

R. P. Mensink, M. B. Katan. Effect of a diet enriched with monounsaturated or polyunsaturated fatty acids on levels of low-density and high-density lipoprotein cholesterol in healthy women and men. *New England Journal of Medicine.* 1989;321:436–441.

D. M. Dreon, K. M. Vranizan, R. M. Krauss, M. A. Austin, P. D. Wood. The effects of polyunsaturated fat vs. monounsaturated fat on plasma lipoproteins. *Journal of the American Medical Association*. 1990;263:2462–2466.

D. Schardt, B. Liebman, S. Schmidt. Going Mediterranean. *Nutrition Action*. 1994; 21:1–8.

S. M. Bailey, J. B. Blumberg, et al., eds. On the margarine-butter controversy. *Tufts University Diet and Nutrition Letter*. 1994;12:1–2.

A. H. Lichtenstein, L. M. Ausman, W. Carrasco, J. L. Jenner, J. M. Ordovas, E. J. Schaefer. Hydrogenation impairs the hypolipidemia effect of corn oil in humans. *Arteriosclerosis and Thrombosis*. 1993;13:154–161.

M. Wootan, B. Liebman. The great trans wreck. *Nutrition Action*. 1993;20:10–12.

Hypertriglyceridaemia and vascular risk: Report of a meeting of physicians and scientists, University College London Medical School. *Lancet*. 1993;342: 781–787.

J. H. Rapp, A. Lespine, R. L. Hamilton, et al. Triglyceride-rich lipoproteins isolated by selected-affinity anti-apolipoprotein B immunosorption from human atherosclerotic plaque. *Arteriosclerosis and Thrombosis*. 1994;14:1767–1774.

W. C. Willett, J. E. Manson, M. J. Stampfer, et al. Weight, weight change and coronary heart disease in women: Risk within the "normal" range. *Journal of the American Medical Association*. 1995;273:461–465.

T. J. Orchard. Intervention for the prevention of coronary heart disease in diabetes. In I. S. Ockene, J. K. Ockene, eds. *Prevention of Coronary Heart Disease*. Boston: Little, Brown, 1992.

P. W. F. Wilson, W. B. Kannel, K. M. Anderson. Lipids, glucose intolerance and vascular disease: the Framingham study monograph. *Atherosclerosis*. 1985; 13:1–11.

G. M. Reaven. Role of insulin resistance in human disease. *Diabetes*. 1988;37:1595–1607.

B. Liebman. Fiber: Separating fact from fiction. *Nutrition Action*. 1994;21:1–11.

S. Renaud, M. DeLorgeril. Wine, alcohol, platelets, and the French paradox for coronary heart disease. *Lancet*. 1992;339:1523–1525.

J. M. Gaziano, J. E. Buring, J. L. Breslow, et al. Moderate alcohol intake, increased levels of high-density lipoprotein and its subfractions, and decreased risk of myocardial infarction. *New England Journal of Medicine*. 1993;329:1829–1834.

D. Steinberg. Antioxidants, vitamins and coronary heart disease. *New England Journal of Medicine*. 1993;328:1487–1489.

D. Steinberg, J. L. Witzum. Lipoproteins and atherogenesis: current concepts. *Journal of the American Medical Association*. 1990;264:3047–3052.

M. J. Stampfer, C. H. Hennekens, J. E. Manson, G. A. Colditz, B. Rosner, W. C. Willett. Vitamin E consumption and the risk of coronary heart disease in women. *New England Journal of Medicine*. 1993;328:1444–1449.

J. M. Gaziano, J. E. Manson, L. G. Branch, G. A. Colditz, J. E. Buring, C. H. Hennekens. Dietary beta-carotene and decreased cardiovascular mortality in an elderly cohort (abstract). *Journal of the American College of Cardiology*. 1992;19:377.

J. M. Gaziano, J. E. Manson, P. M. Ridker, J. E. Buring, C. H. Hennekens. Beta-carotene therapy for chronic stable angina (abstract). *Circulation*. 1990;82 (suppl. 3):202.

E. B. Rimm, M. J. Stampfer, A. Ascherio, E. Giovannucci, G. A. Colditz, W. C. Willett. Vitamin E consumption and the risk of coronary heart disease in men. *New England Journal of Medicine*. 1993;328:1450–1456.

J. Selhub, P. F. Jacques, A. G. Bostom, et al. Association between plasma homocysteine concentrations and extracranial carotid-artery stenosis. *New England Journal of Medicine*. 1995;332:286–291.

M. J. Stampfer, M. R. Malinow. Can lowering homocysteine levels reduce cardiovascular risk? *New England Journal of Medicine*. 1995;332:328–329.

B. Liebman Folic Acid: for the young and heart. *Nutrition Action*. 1995;22:1–7.

Using Diet To Increase Your Odds: The Case of Jack

A. I. MacIsaac, J. D. Thomas, E. J. Topol. Toward the quiescent coronary plaque. *Journal of the American College of Cardiology*. 1993;22:1228–1241.

E. Falk, P. K. Shah, V. Fuster. Coronary plaque disruption. *Circulation*. 1995;92: 657–671.

V. Fuster, L. Badimon, J. J. Badimon, J. H. Chesebro. The pathogenesis of coronary artery disease and acute coronary syndromes. *New England Journal of Medicine*. 1992;326:242–250.

Summary of the second report of the National Cholesterol Education Program (NCEP) Expert Panel on detection, evaluation, and treatment of high blood cholesterol in adults (Adult Treatment Panel II). *Journal of the American Medical Association*. 1993;269:3015–3023.

H. R. Superko, R. M. Krauss. Coronary Artery Disease Regression: Convincing evidence for the benefit of aggressive lipoprotein management. *Circulation*. 1994;90:1056–1069.

Chapter 3. Making Exercise a Lifetime Commitment

C. Bailey. *The New Fit or Fat*. Boston: Houghton Mifflin, 1991.

A. Ward, P. A. Taylor, L. Ahlquist, D. R. Brown, D. C. Carlucci, J. M. Rippe. Exercise and exercise intervention. In I. S. Ockene, J. K. Ockene, eds. *Prevention of Coronary Heart Disease*. Boston: Little, Brown, 1992.

G. A. V. Borg. Psychophysical basis of perceived exertion. *Medicine and Science in Sports and Exercise*. 1982;14: 377–381.

G. F. Fletcher, G. Balandy, V. F. Froelicher, L. H. Hartley, W. L. Haskell, M. L. Pollack, Exercise standards: a statement for health-care professionals from the American Heart Association. *Circulation*. 1995;86: 340–344.

R. M. Lampman, J. T. Santinga, M. F. Hodge, W. D. Block, J. D. Flora, D. R. Bassett. Comparative effects of physical training and diet in normalizing serum lipids in men with type IV hyperlipoproteinemia. *Circulation*. 1977; 55:652–659.

P. D. Wood, W. L. Haskell, S. N. Blair, et al. Increased exercise level and plasma lipoprotein concentrations: A one-year randomized controlled study in sedentary middle-aged men. *Metabolism*. 1983;32:31–39.

J. O. Holloszy, J. S. Skinner, G. Toro, T. K. Cureton. Effects of a six-month program of endurance exercise on the serum lipids of middle-aged men. *American Journal of Cardiology.* 1964;14:753–760.

High Triglycerides and Low HDL Cholesterol—The Impact of Exercise and Other Lifestyle Changes on Cardiac Risk: The Case of Wayne

G. Franceschini, A. Bondioli, D. Granata, et al. Reduced HDL$_2$ levels in myocardial infarction patients without risk factors for atherosclerosis. *Atherosclerosis.* 1987;68:213–219.

M. Miller, A. Seidler, P. O. Kwiterovich, T. A. Pearson. Long-term predictors of subsequent cardiovascular events with coronary artery disease and "desirable" levels of plasma total cholesterol. *Circulation.* 1992;86:1165–1170.

F. M. Sacks. Desirable serum total cholesterol with low HDL cholesterol levels: An undesirable situation in coronary artery disease. *Circulation.* 1992;86: 1341–1343.

J. E. Buring, G. T. O'Connor, S. Z. Goldhaber, et al. Decreased HDL$_2$ and HDL$_3$ cholesterol, apo A-I and apo A-II, and increased risk of myocardial infarction. *Circulation.* 1992;85:22–29.

M. J. Stampfer, F. M. Sacks, S. Salvini, W. C. Willett, C. H. Hennekens. A prospective study on cholesterol, apolipoproteins, and the risk of myocardial infarction. *New England Journal of Medicine.* 1991;325:373–381.

R. A. Kreisberg. Low high-density lipoprotein cholesterol: What does it mean, what can we do about it, and what should we do about it? *American Journal of Medicine.* 1993;94:1–5.

G. Assmann, H. Schulte, A. von Eckardstein. Hypertriglyceridemia and elevated lipoprotein (a) are risk factors for major coronary events in middle-aged men. *American Journal of Cardiology.* 1996;77:1179–1184.

M. J. Stampfer, R. M. Krauss, J. Ma, et al. A prospective study of triglyceride level, low-density lipoprotein particle diameter, and risk of myocardial infarction. *Journal of the American Medical Association.* 1996; 276:882–888.

M. A. Austin, M. C. King, K. M. Vranizan, R. M. Krauss. Atherogenic lipoprotein phenotype: A proposed genetic marker for coronary heart disease risk. *Circulation.* 1990;82:495–506.

M. A. Austin, J. L. Breslow, C. H. Hennekens, J. E. Buring, W. C. Willett, R. M. Krauss. Low-density lipoprotein subclass patterns and risk of myocardial infarction. *Journal of the American Medical Association.* 1988;260:1917–1921.

M. Miller, P. S. Bachorik, B. W. McCrindle, P. O. Kwiterovich. Effect of gemfibrozil in men with primary isolated low high-density lipoprotein cholesterol: A randomized, double-blind, placebo-controlled, crossover study. *American Journal of Medicine.* 1993;94:7–12.

P. D. Wood, W. L. Haskell, S. N. Blair, et al. Increased exercise level and plasma lipoprotein concentrations: A one-year randomized controlled study in sedentary middle-aged men. *Metabolism.* 1983;32:31–39.

P. D. Wood, M. L. Stefanick, D. M. Dreon, et al. Changes in plasma lipids and lipoproteins during weight loss by dieting vs. exercise in overweight men. *New England Journal of Medicine.* 1988;319:1173–1179.

J. G. Warner, P. H. Brubaker, Y. Zhu, et al. Long-term (5-year) changes in HDL cholesterol in cardiac rehabilitation patients: Do sex differences exist? *Circulation*. 1995;92:773–777.

R. D. Hawkins, H. Kalant. The metabolism of ethanol and its metabolic effects. *Pharmacology Review*. 1972;24:67–157.

J. H. Mendelson, N. K. Mello. Alcohol-induced hyperlipidemia and beta lipoproteins. *Science*. 1973;180:1372–1374.

J. Kabat-Zinn. *Full Catastrophe Living: Using the Wisdom of Your Body and Mind to Face Stress, Pain and Illness*. New York: Delacorte/Dell, 1990.

C. Dodds, G. L. Mills. Influence of myocardial infarction on plasma-lipoprotein concentration. *Lancet*. 1959; June:1160–1163.

H. B. Rubins, S. J. Robins, M. K. Iwane, et al. Rationale and design of the Department of Veterans Affairs high-density lipoprotein cholesterol intervention trial (HIT) for secondary prevention of coronary artery disease in men with low high-density lipoprotein cholesterol and desirable low-density lipoprotein. *American Journal of Cardiology*. 1993;71:45–52.

Chapter 4. Quitting: A Tough Task With Great Rewards

K. O. Fagerstrom. Measuring degree of physical dependence to tobacco smoking with reference to individualization of treatment. *Addictive Behaviors*. 1978; 3:235–241.

K. O. Fagerström. Reducing the weight gain after stopping smoking. *Addictive Behaviors*. 1987;12:91–93.

J. K. Ockene, R. C. Benfari, R. L. Nuttall, I. Hurwitz, I. S. Ockene. Relationship of psychosocial factors to smoking behavior change in an intervention program. *Preventive Medicine*. 1982;11:13–28.

J. K. Ockene. Physician-delivered interventions for smoking cessation: Strategies for increasing effectiveness. *Preventive Medicine*. 1987;16:723–737.

J. K. Ockene. Smoking intervention: a behavioral, educational, and pharmacological perspective. In I. S. Ockene, J. K. Ockene, eds. *Prevention of Coronary Heart Disease*. Boston: Little, Brown, 1992.

M. C. Fiore, S. S. Smith, D. E. Jorenby, T. B. Baker. The effectiveness of the nicotine patch for smoking cessation. *Journal of the American Medical Association*. 1994; 271:1940–1947.

J. Hung, J. Y. T. Lam, L. Lacoste, G. Letchacovski. Cigarette smoking acutely increases platelet thrombus formation in patients with coronary artery disease taking aspirin. *Circulation*. 1995;92:2432–2436.

When Smoking and Genes Don't Mix: The Case of George

J. L. Goldstein, H. G. Schrott, W. R. Hazzard, E. L. Bierman, A. G. Motulsky. Hyperlipidemia in coronary heart disease, II: genetic analysis of lipid levels in 176 families and delineation of a new, inherited disorder, combined hyperlipidemia. *Journal of Clinical Investigation*. 1973;52:1544–1568.

J. D. Brunzell, M. A. Austin, S. S. Deeb, et al. Familial combined hyperlipidemia and genetic risk of atherosclerosis. In F. P. Woodford, J. Davignon, A. Sniderman, eds. *Atherosclerosis X*. Proceedings of the 10th International Symposium on Atherosclerosis, Montréal, October 9–14, 1994. Amsterdam: Elsevier, 1995.

M. Austin. State of the art symposium: Triglycerides, small dense LDL, and coronary heart disease. At the 10th International Symposium on Atherosclerosis in Montreal, Canada. October 1994 (unpublished remarks).

P. O. Kwiterovich. *Beyond Cholesterol: The Johns Hopkins Complete Guide for Avoiding Heart Disease*. Baltimore: The Johns Hopkins University Press, 1989.

J. H. Rapp, A. Lespine, R. L. Hamilton, et al. Triglyceride-rich lipoproteins isolated by selected-affinity anti-apolipoprotein B immunosorption from human atherosclerotic plaque. *Arteriosclerosis and Thrombosis.* 1994;14:1767–1774.

Hypertriglyceridaemia and vascular risk: report of a meeting of physicians and scientists, University College London Medical School. *Lancet.* 1993;342: 781–787.

H. R. Superko, R. M. Krauss. Coronary Artery Disease Regression: Convincing evidence for the benefit of aggressive lipoprotein management. *Circulation.* 1994;90:1056–1069.

Chapter 5. Estrogen Replacement Therapy and Your Heart: Sorting Out the Risks and Benefits

P. H. Wolf, J. H. Madans, F. F. Finucane, M. Higgins, J. C. Kleinman. Reduction in cardiovascular disease-related mortality among postmenopausal women who use hormones: Evidence from a national cohort. *American Journal of Obstetrics and Gynecology.* 1991;164:489–494.

M. J. Stampfer, G. A. Colditz, W. C. Willett, et al. Postmenopausal estrogen therapy and cardiovascular disease: Ten-year follow-up from the Nurses' Health Study. *New England Journal of Medicine.* 1991;325:756–762.

J. M. Sullivan, R. Vander Zwang, J. P. Hughes, et al. Estrogen replacement and coronary artery disease: Effect on survival in postmenopausal women. *Archives of Internal Medicine.* 1990;150:2557–2562.

V. T. Miller, R. A. Muesing, J. C. LaRosa, et al. Effects of conjugated equine estrogen with and without three different progestogens on lipoproteins, high-density lipoprotein subfractions and apolipoprotein A-1. *American Journal of Obstetrics and Gynecology.* 1991;77:235–240.

B. G. Wren. HRT and the cardiovascular system. *Australian Family Physician.* 1992; 21:226–229.

A. A. Nabulsi, A. R. Folsom, A. White, et al. Association of hormone replacement therapy with various cardiovascular risk factors in postmenopausal women. *New England Journal of Medicine.* 1993;328:1069–1075.

C. J. Kim, H. C. Jang, D. H. Cho, Y. K. Min. Effects of hormone replacement therapy on lipoprotein (a) and lipids in postmenopausal women. *Arteriosclerosis and Thrombosis.* 1994;14:275–281.

A. Gurakar, J. M. Hoeg, G. Kostner, N. M. Papadopoulos, H. B. Brewer, Jr. Levels of lipoprotein Lp (a) decline with neomycin and niacin treatment. *Atherosclerosis.* 1985;57:293–301.

F. Lepre, B. Campbell, S. Crane, P. Hickman. Low-dose sustained release nicotinic acid (Tri-B3) and lipoprotein (a). *American Journal of Cardiology.* 1992;70: 133.

Writing Group for the PEPI Trial. Effects of estrogen or estrogen/progestin regimens on heart disease risk factors in postmenopausal women. *Journal of the American Medical Association.* 1995;273:199–208.

G. A. Colditz, S. I. Hankinson, D. J. Hunter, et al. The use of estrogens and progestins and the risk of breast cancer in postmenopausal women. *New England Journal of Medicine.* 1995;332:1589–1593.

J. L. Stanford, N. S. Weiss, L. F. Voigt, et al. Combined estrogen and progestin hormone replacement therapy in relation to risk of breast cancer in middle-aged women. *Journal of the American Medical Association.* 1995;274:137–142.

P. E. Belchetz. Hormonal treatment of postmenopausal women. *New England Journal of Medicine.* 1994;330:1062–1071.

American College of Obstetrics and Gynecology (ACOG) Technical Bulletin. Hormone replacement therapy. 1992;166:1–8.

F. Grodstein, M. J. Stampfer, J. E. Manson, et al. Postmenopausal estrogen and progestin use and the risk of cardiovascular disease. *New England Journal of Medicine.* 1996;335:453–461.

M. A. Cobleigh, R. F. Berris, T. Bush, et al. Estrogen replacement therapy in breast cancer survivors. A time for change. *Journal of the American Medical Association.* 1994;272:540–544.

Too Little Estrogen: The Case of Patricia

V. T. Miller, R. A. Muesing, J. C. LaRosa, et al. Effects of conjugated equine estrogen with and without three different progestogens on lipoproteins, high-density lipoprotein subfractions and apolipoprotein A-1. *American Journal of Obstetrics and Gynecology.* 1991;77:235–240.

A. A. Nabulsi, A. R. Folsom, A. White, et al. Association of hormone-replacement therapy with various cardiovascular risk factors in postmenopausal women. *New England Journal of Medicine.* 1993;328:1069–1075.

P. E. Belchetz. Hormonal treatment of postmenopausal women. *New England Journal of Medicine.* 1994;330:1062–1071.

American College of Obstetrics and Gynecology (ACOG) Technical Bulletin. Hormone replacement therapy. 1992;166:1–8.

Chapter 6. Reducing Stress in Your Life

B. S. Dohrenwend, B. P. Dohrenwend, eds. *Stressful Life Events: Their Nature and Effects.* New York: Wiley, 1974.

R. S. Eliot. *Stress and the Heart: Mechanisms, Measurements, and Management.* Mount Kisco, N.Y.: Futura, 1988.

J. Kabat-Zinn. *Full Catastrophe Living: Using the Wisdom of Your Body and Mind to Face Stress, Pain and Illness.* New York: Delacorte/Dell, 1990.

J. Kabat-Zinn. *Wherever You Go, There You Are.* New York: Hyperion, 1994.

J. K. Williams, J. A. Vita, S. B. Manuck, A. P. Selwyn, J. R. Kaplan. Psychosocial factors impair vascular responses of coronary arteries. *Circulation.* 1991;84: 2146–2153.

J. Goldstein, and J. Kornfield. *Seeking the Heart of Wisdom: The Path of Insight Meditation.* Boston: Shambhala, 1987.

T. Dixon. *Zen Mind, Beginner's Mind.* Edited by S. Suzuki. New York: Weatherhill, 1970.

D. T. Jaffe. *Healing from Within: Psychological Techniques to Help the Mind Heal the Body.* New York: Simon & Schuster, 1986.

D. Ornish. *Dr. Dean Ornish's Program for Reversing Heart Disease.* New York: Random House, 1990.

Diabetes, Stress, and the Heart: The Case of Bill

National Diabetes Data Group. Classification and diagnosis of diabetes mellitus and other categories of glucose intolerance. *Diabetes.* 1979;28:1039–1057.

American Diabetes Association. Nutritional recommendations and principles for individuals with diabetes mellitus: 1986. *Diabetes Care.* 1987;10:126–32.

P. K. Shah, J. Amin. Low high-density lipoprotein level is associated with increased restenosis rate after coronary angioplasty. *Circulation.* 1992;85: 1279–1285.

B. S. Dohrenwend, B. P. Dohrenwend, eds. *Stressful Life Events: Their Nature and Effects.* New York: Wiley, 1974.

R. S. Eliot. *Stress and the Heart: Mechanisms, Measurements, and Management.* Mount Kisco, N.Y.: Futura, 1988.

J. Kabat-Zinn. *Full Catastrophe Living: Using the Wisdom of Your Body and Mind to Face Stress, Pain and Illness.* New York: Delacorte/Dell, 1990.

J. Kabat-Zinn. *Wherever You Go, There You Are.* New York: Hyperion, 1994.

D. Ornish. *Dr. Dean Ornish's Program for Reversing Heart Disease.* New York: Random House, 1990.

Chapter 7. Elevated Blood Pressure: What Can You Do to Lower Your Level?

Joint National Committee on Detection, Evaluation, and Treatment of High Blood Pressure. The fifth report of the Joint National Committee on detection, evaluation, and treatment of high blood pressure (JNC V). *Archives of Internal Medicine.* 1993;153:154–183.

J. Stamler. Dietary salt and blood pressure. *Annals of the New York Academy of Science.* 1993;676:122–156.

C. Lenfant. High blood pressure: Some answers, new questions, continuing challenges. *Journal of the American Medical Association.* 1996; 275:1604–1606.

K. L. Nelson, G. L. Jennings, M. D. Elser, et al. Effect of changing levels of physical activity on blood pressure and haemodynamics in essential hypertension. *Lancet.* 1986;2:473–476.

S. MacMahon. Alcohol consumption and hypertension. *Hypertension.* 1987;9:111–121.

J. J. Rohlfing, J. D. Brunzell. The effect of diuretics and adrenegic-blocking agents on plasma lipids. *Western Journal of Medicine.* 1986;145:210–218.

Sometimes Diet and Exercise Can Do It All: The Case of Jim

Joint National Committee on Detection, Evaluation, and Treatment of High Blood Pressure. The fifth report of the Joint National Committee on detection, evaluation, and treatment of high blood pressure (JNC V). *Archives of Internal Medicine.* 1993;153:154–183.

C. Dodds, G. L. Mills. Influence of myocardial infarction on plasma-lipoprotein concentration. *Lancet.* 1959;1160–1163.

J. J. Rohlfing, J. D. Brunzell. The effect of diuretics and adrenegic-blocking agents on plasma lipids. *Western Journal of Medicine.* 1986;145:210–218.

Chapter 8. The Crucial Role of Medications in Lowering Cholesterol and Blood Pressure

G. Schonfeld. HMG CoA Reductase Inhibitors. In J. C. La Rosa, ed. *Practical Management of Lipid Disorders.* Fort Lee, N.J.: Health Care Communications; 1992:75–90.

H. R. Superko, P. Greenland, R. A. Manchester, et al. Effectiveness of low-dose colestipol therapy in patients with moderate hypercholesterolemia. *American Journal of Cardiology.* 1992; 70:135–140.

H. N. Ginsberg. Nicotinic acid. In J. C. La Rosa, ed. *Practical Management of Lipid Disorders.* Fort Lee, N.J.: Health Care Communications; 1992:49–59.

S. M. Grundy, G. L. Vega. Fibric acids: Effects on lipids and lipoprotein metabolism. *American Journal of Medicine.* 1987; 83 (suppl. 5B): 9–20.

M. A. Pfeffer, F. M. Sacks, L. A. Moyé, et al. Cholesterol and recurrent events: A secondary prevention trial for normolipidemic patients. *American Journal of Cardiology.* 1995; 76:98C–106C.

The Scandinavian Simvastatin Survival Study Group. Randomized trial of cholesterol lowering in 4444 patients with coronary heart disease: the Scandinavian simvastatin survival study (4S). *Lancet.* 1994; 344:1383–1389.

J. Shepherd, S. M. Cobbe, I. Ford et al. Prevention of coronary heart disease with pravastatin in men with hypercholesterolemia. *New England Journal of Medicine.* 1995;333:1301–1307.

The Post Coronary Artery Bypass Graft Trial Investigators. The effect of aggressive lowering of low-density lipoprotein cholesterol levels and low-dose anticoagulation on obstructive changes in saphenous-vein coronary-artery bypass grafts. *New England Journal of Medicine.* 1997; 336:153–162.

Joint National Committee on Detection, Evaluation, and Treatment of High Blood Pressure. The fifth report of the Joint National Committee on detection, evaluation, and treatment of high blood pressure (JNC V). *Archives of Internal Medicine.* 1993; 153:154–183.

M. A. Weber, J. H. Laragh. Hypertension: Steps forward and steps backward. The Joint National Committee fifth report. *Archives of Internal Medicine.* 1993; 153:149–152.

M. Pahor, J. M. J. M. Guralnik, M. E. Salive, et al. Do calcium channel blockers increase the risk of cancer? *American Journal of Hypertension.* 1996;9:695–699.

J. R. Daling. Calcium channel blockers and cancer: Is an association biologically plausible? *American Journal of Hypertension*. 1996; 9:713–714.

C. D. Furberg, B. M. Psaty, J. V. Meyer. Nifedipine: dose related increase in mortality in patients with coronary heart disease. *Circulation*. 1995; 92:1326–1331.

H. J. Dargie. Calcium Channel blockers and the clinician. *Lancet*. 1996; 348:488.

A. M. Walker, M. J. Stampfer. Observational studies of drug safety. *Lancet*. 1996; 348:489.

The Importance of Knowing All Your Risk Factors: The Case of Hans

K. Berg. A new serum type system in man: the Lp System. *Acta Pathologia Microbiologia et Immunologica Scandinavica*. 1963;59:369–382.

A. M. Scanu, R. M. Lawn, K. Berg. Lipoprotein (a) and atherosclerosis. *Annals of Internal medicine*. 1991; 115:209–218.

R. L. Desmarais, I. J Sarembock, C. R. Ayers, et al. Elevated serum lipoprotein (a) is a risk factor for clinical recurrence after coronary balloon angioplasty. *Circulation*. 1995; 91:1403–1409.

Index

ACAT inhibitors. *See* acyl coenzyme A (ACAT) inhibitors

Accupril. *See* quinapril

ACE inhibitors, as antihypertensives, 222–224

acetylcholine, nicotine activation of, 120

Achilles tendons, cholesterol deposits in familial hypercholesterolemia, 28, 32, 34

acorn squash [recipe], 275

acyl coenzyme A (ACAT) inhibitors, as cholesterol-lowering drugs, 216–217

addiction, smoking as, 121–124

adrenal gland, role in stress, 163

adrenaline. *See* epinephrine

adrenergic inhibitors, as antihypertensive drugs, 218, 220–222

aerobic dancing
  caloric expenditure in, 94
  program for, 99

aerobic exercise
  benefits, 89–90, 101
  definition, 289
  three stages of, 96–101

African Americans, response to salt restriction, 187

Afrikaaners, familial hypercholesterolemia in, 20, 27

alcohol
  avoidance by diabetics, 13
  effects on blood pressure, 14
  perceived need for smoking with, 123, 124
  possible beneficial effects of, 62–63

alcoholic beverages, calories in, 63

alcoholism
  adverse effects of, 63

in America, 62
  triglyceride overproduction in, 18

alcohol restriction, 5, 15
  for blood-pressure control, 7
  desirable effect on triglyceride levels, 21, 45

Alexander, Franz, M.D., 163

All-Bran (Kellogg), fiber in, 53

Alpert, Joseph, M.D., 5–6

alpha-beta-blockers, as antihypertensive drugs, 220, 222

alpha-blockers, as antihypertensive drugs, 220, 221–222

Altace. *See* ramipril

Alzheimer's disease, 150

American Heart Association Doctors' Road Race, 6

American Heart Association Scientific Statement on Exercise, 92

amlodipine, as antihypertensive, 225

anaerobic exercise, definition, 289

angina pectoris. *See also* chest pain
  definition, 289

angiography. *See* coronary angiography

angioplasty. *See* balloon angioplasty

angiotensin-converting enzyme (ACE) inhibitors, as antihypertensives, 222–224

Antihypertensive and Lipid-Lowering Treatment to Prevent Heart Attack (ALLHAT), 224–226

anti-inflammatories
  effect on diuretic therapy, 219
  interactions with other drugs, 221

antioxidant(s)
  definition and examples, 289
  as dietary supplements, 64
  estrogen as, 145

apple pie [recipe], 284

307